WORLD HEALTH ORGANIZATION

INTERNATIONAL AGENCY FOR
RESEARCH ON CANCER

ENVIRONMENTAL CARCINOGENS METHODS OF ANALYSIS AND EXPOSURE MEASUREMENT

VOLUME 10 – Benzene and Alkylated Benzenes

EDITORS
L. FISHBEIN & I.K. O'NEILL

IARC Scientific Publications No. 85

INTERNATIONAL AGENCY FOR RESEARCH ON CANCER
LYON
1988

The International Agency for Research on Cancer (IARC) was established in 1965 by the World Health Assembly, as an independently financed organization within the framework of the World Health Organization. The headquarters of the Agency are at Lyon, France.

The Agency conducts a programme of research concentrating particularly on the epidemiology of cancer and the study of potential carcinogens in the human environment. Its field studies are supplemented by biological and chemical research carried out in the Agency's laboratories in Lyon and, through collaborative research agreements, in national research institutions in many countries. The Agency also conducts a programme for the education and training of personnel for cancer research.

The publications of the Agency are intended to contribute to the dissemination of authoritative information on different aspects of cancer research.

Distributed for the International Agency for Research on Cancer by
Oxford University Press, Walton Street, Oxford OX2 6DP, UK

London   New York   Toronto
Delhi   Bombay   Calcutta   Madras   Karachi
Kuala Lumpur   Singapore   Hong Kong   Tokyo
Nairobi   Dar es Salaam   Cape Town
Melbourne   Auckland

Oxford is a trade mark of Oxford University Press

Distributed in the USA
by Oxford University Press, New York

ISBN 92 832 1185 5
ISSN 0300-5085

© International Agency for Research on Cancer 1988
150 cours Albert Thomas, 69372 Lyon Cedex 08, France

PRINTED IN SWITZERLAND

IARC MANUAL SERIES:

ENVIRONMENTAL CARCINOGENS – METHODS OF ANALYSIS AND EXPOSURE MEASUREMENT[1]

Volume 1 (1978)   *Analysis of Volatile Nitrosamines in Food (IARC Scientific Publications No. 18)*

Volume 2 (1978)   *Methods for the Measurement of Vinyl Chloride in Poly(Vinyl Chloride), Air, Water and Foodstuffs (IARC Scientific Publications No. 22)*

Volume 3 (1979)   *Analysis of Polycyclic Aromatic Hydrocarbons in Environmental Samples (IARC Scientific Publications No. 29)*

Volume 4 (1982)   *Some Aromatic Amines and Azo Dyes in the General and Industrial Environments (IARC Scientific Publications No. 40)*

Volume 5 (1982)   *Some Mycotoxins (IARC Scientific Publications No. 44)*

Volume 6 (1982)   N-*Nitroso Compounds (IARC Scientific Publications No. 45)*

Volume 7 (1985)   *Some Volatile Halogenated Hydrocarbons (IARC Scientific Publications No. 68)*

Volume 8 (1986)   *Some Metals: As, Be, Cd, Cr, Ni, Pb, Se, Zn (IARC Scientific Publications No. 71)*

Volume 9 (1987)   *Passive Smoking (IARC Scientific Publications No. 81)*

Volume 10 (1988)   *Benzene and Alkylated Benzenes (IARC Scientific Publications No. 85)*

Volume 11 (in preparation)   *Polychlorinated Dioxins, Dibenzofurans and Biphenyls*

Volume 12 (in preparation)   *Indoor Air Contaminants*

---

[1] For volumes 1 through 8, the title of the series was 'Environmental Carcinogens – Selected Methods of Analysis'.

ENVIRONMENTAL CARCINOGENS – METHODS OF ANALYSIS
AND EXPOSURE MEASUREMENT
VOLUME 10 – BENZENE AND ALKYLATED BENZENES

In order to ensure that future volumes in this series meet the needs of workers in this field, we would be pleased if you could return this questionnaire.

1) How did you get to know of this publication?

....

2) Why did you decide to obtain it?

....

3) What is your main interest in this book?

Methods .... Chapters ....

4) Does this book meet your needs?

....

5) Do you have any suggestions to improve content, format or presentation?

....

6) Do you know of or use other volumes in this Manual series?

Volume ....

7) Do you have suggestions for further volumes?

....

8) Other comments ....

....

Name ....

Address ....

Thank you for returning this page to

Dr I.K. O'Neill
International Agency for Research on Cancer
150 cours Albert Thomas
69372 Lyon Cedex 08
France

CONTENTS

METHODS FOR INDUSTRIAL AND AMBIENT AIR

METHODS FOR BIOLOGICAL MONITORING

FOREWORD

The widespread, large-scale use of benzene and alkylated benzenes as solvents and chemical intermediates, as well as their ubiquitous presence in the general environment arising from combustion and household products and vehicle fuels, emphasize the need for standard detection techniques both in exposure control and in epidemiological studies. Provision of clear information on efficient and reliable techniques and on the practicability of an overall approach are the aims of this series. Benzene is a human carcinogen, and there are conflicting reports from experimental studies on the carcinogenicity of xylene which have been widely introduced as replacement for benzene. Air, food and water exposure routes are covered in this volume, with emphasis on appropriate sampling techniques that render possible exposure assessment. Included also are very recent advances in biological monitoring *via* breath analysis, as well as established blood and urine measurements.

Thanks are due to the many workers in government and research laboratories who freely contributed chapters or re-wrote and clarified their techniques for inclusion in these pages.

L. Tomatis, M.D.
Director, IARC

INTRODUCTION

The volumes in the series *Environmental Carcinogens: Methods of Analysis and Exposure Measurement* are designed to meet the need for methods of sampling and analysis of environmental carcinogens, both known and suspected, in the context of epidemiological and analytical studies. A major objective of this series in relation to the IARC is to provide a focus of past and present sampling and analytical procedures. This is necessary for a more reliable assessment of exposure.

The present volume deals with benzene, toluene and the xylenes. Benzene has been assessed in two IARC Monographs (Volumes 7 and 29), as well as in IARC Monographs Supplement 7. Benzene, toluene and the xylenes are produced on a massive scale (in the millions of tonnes annually in many industrialized countries) and are employed in a great variety of applications as chemical intermediates, solvents and components in gasoline. They have often been employed together and it should be noted that commercial toluene can contain varying amounts of benzene. Toluene and xylenes are increasingly employed as 'safe' replacements for benzene in solvent applications. Major sources of these aromatic hydrocarbons in the environment are losses during production, transportation and processing of petroleum, refueling and operation of motor vehicles, and their use (particularly toluene and xylene) as solvents.

There is a broad potential for the exposure of industrial workers engaged in production and use of these agents as solvents and chemical intermediates (particularly in the rubber and plastics industry), and of the general public through dissipation into the environment, vehicle exhausts, consumer products, etc. Toluene and the xylenes are present in a wide range of commonly available household products, such as paint and varnish removers, rust removers, adhesives and glues. Toluene, moreover, has been widely abused by 'glue sniffers'.

Indoor concentrations of aromatic hydrocarbons, such as benzene, toluene and xylene, have often been found at levels which exceed those outdoors. The presence of benzene and toluene indoors arises primarily from tobacco smoke.

In order to furnish as comprehensive a treatment as possible, reviews concerning the epidemiology, use and occurrence, carcinogenicity, genetic toxicity, metabolism and pharmacokinetics of the title compounds are included in this volume. The importance of sampling and analytical techniques is stressed in six review chapters dealing with industrial, ambient and indoor air, chemical waste disposal sites, water and food and biological monitoring. Three analytical methods written in the ISO format cover the determination of the designated aromatic hydrocarbons in industrial and ambient air, while seven procedures described for the determination of benzene, toluene and xylene in breath, and their metabolites in blood and urine, reflect the increasing recognition of the utility of biological monitoring in providing data related to recent or accumulated exposures.

The Editorial Board continues to be aware of the need to recognize advances in the state-of-the-art and to incorporate procedures reflecting enhanced sampling proficiency, accuracy, sensitivity, specificity, reproducibility, ease of manipulation and, as far as possible, economy, particularly since analytical chemists and other scientists in developing countries may often find the facilities at their disposal to be less advanced than those available in more affluent societies.

Volumes in preparation include *Polychlorinated Dioxins, Dibenzofurans and Biphenyls* (Volume 11) and *Indoor Air Contaminants* (Volume 12). Additional volumes planned will deal with collection, preparation and storage of biological samples; mineral fibres (asbestos); polymer process industries (formaldehyde, ethylene oxide, styrene, acrylonitrile, butadiene) and polycyclic aromatic hydrocarbons and their nitro-derivatives. As far as possible, they will reflect emphasis on mixtures of environmental carcinogens and the increasing reliance on biological monitoring for the enhancement of epidemiological assessments.

Lawrence Fishbein
Chairman, Editorial Board
(from 1983)

MEMBERS OF THE EDITORIAL BOARD

---

[1] Present address: ENVIRON Corporation, 1000 Potomac Street NW, Washington DC, USA.

MEMBERS OF THE REVIEW BOARD

---

[1] Present address: ENVIRON Corporation, 1000 Potomac Street NW, Washington DC, USA.

REVIEWERS

J. Angerer — Central Institute for Occupational Medicine, University of Hamburg, Hamburg, FRG

O. Axelson — Department of Occupational Medicine, University Hospital, Linköping, Sweden

M. Berlin — Monitoring and Assessment Research Centre, London, UK

R.H. Brown — Health and Safety Executive, The Occupational Medicine and Hygiene Laboratories, London, UK

J.P. Buchet — Industrial Toxicology Unit, Catholic University of Louvain, Brussels, Belgium

I.J. Flek — Institute of Hygiene and Epidemiology, Prague, Czechoslovakia

N.A. Leidel — National Institute for Occupational Safety and Health, Centers for Disease Control, Atlanta, GA, USA

G. Obe — Free University of Berlin, Institute of Genetics, Berlin (West), FRG

M. Risk — Environmental Health Research and Testing, Inc, Cincinnatti, OH, USA

B. Seifert — Institute for Water, Soil and Air Hygiene, Federal Health Office, Berlin-Dahlem, FRG

R. Snyder — Rutgers University, College of Pharmacy, Piscataway, NJ, USA

O. Vesterberg — Occupational Health Department, Chemistry Division, National Board of Occupational Safety and Health, Solna, Sweden

ACKNOWLEDGEMENTS

Contributions to Volume 10

We thank all the authors and reviewers who have contributed their time freely. We should also like to thank the following persons whose considerable efforts have greatly expedited publication of this volume: Dr W. Davis and his staff (technical editing), Dr A. MacKenzie Peers (copy and revising editor), Ms B. Dodet (compiling editor). The detailed advice of members of the Review Board, during and subsequent to the Review Board meeting in Stockholm, Sweden, has been most helpful. For secretarial assistance, we are grateful to M. Courcier and M. Wrisez (IARC).

BIOLOGICAL AND TOXICOLOGICAL EFFECTS

CHAPTER 1

CARCINOGENICITY OF BENZENE, TOLUENE AND XYLENE: EPIDEMIOLOGICAL AND EXPERIMENTAL EVIDENCE

A.J. McMichael

Department of Community Medicine
University of Adelaide
Adelaide, South Australia

INTRODUCTION

Benzene was first isolated in 1825, and commercially recovered from coal-tar-derived light oil in 1849 and from petroleum in 1941 (IARC, 1982). By the late 1950's, most commercial benzene was petroleum-derived.

Chronic human exposure[1] to benzene may result in adverse haematological effects, characterized by a variety of blood dyscrasias, including leucopenia, thrombocytopenia, pancytopenia and anaemia. Benzene is also considered to be a human carcinogen and is well established as a cause of leukaemia (IARC, 1982). It is recognized as being carcinogenic by the governments of Finland, the Federal Republic of Germany, Italy, Japan, Sweden, Switzerland and the U.S.A.

By comparison with benzene, there is no direct epidemiological evidence concerning the carcinogenicity of toluene and xylenes, and only limited experimental evidence from animal studies.

EVIDENCE OF BENZENE CARCINOGENICITY IN HUMANS

Leukaemia and other lympho-haematopoietic cancers: early studies

There have been many case reports, case series and epidemiological studies associating exposure to benzene with leukaemia in humans. However, very few of the studies have provided quantitative information about the relative risk of leukaemia under specified conditions of exposure.

---

[1]Exposure concentrations are given throughout in parts per million – ppm. To convert to ISO recommended units, for benzene, 1 ppm = 3.25 mg/m^3 ($\sim 20\,^{\circ}$C)

The first case report suggesting an association between exposure to benzene and leukaemia was given by Delore and Borgomano (1928). An acute lymphoblastic leukaemia was observed in a worker in France, who was exposed to benzene for five years. Since then, numerous reports describing leukaemia cases among persons exposed to benzene have appeared, predominantly from Italy, France and Turkey (Goldstein, 1983).

Several pioneering epidemiological studies investigating the relationship between exposure to benzene and leukaemia, as well as other lympho-haematopoietic cancers, were published in the mid-1970's. Aksoy published a number of reports on the risk of leukaemia among Istanbul shoe makers exposed to benzene-containing solvents (Aksoy *et al.*, 1972, 1974; Aksoy, 1980). He estimated that the annual crude incidence rate of leukaemia among the shoe makers was 13.5 per 100 000, compared with an overall annual incidence rate in the general population of 6 per 100 000.

Vigliani (1976), reviewing earlier studies (Vigliani & Saita, 1964), estimated the increase in risk of leukaemia to be 20-fold for workers exposed to benzene in shoe factories in Italy. As with Aksoy's studies, the apparent levels of exposure to benzene were predominantly within the 200–500 ppm range. However, these exposure data were too imprecise for further quantitative analysis.

Thorpe (1974) reported an epidemiological study of leukaemia incidence among workers from eight Esso Petroleum affiliates in Europe. Employees were divided into two groups: those with a potential exposure to 1% or more benzene over a five-year period and those not exposed or only occasionally exposed. Among the exposed, 8 leukaemia deaths were observed, compared to the expected 6.6, yielding an age-standardized mortality ratio (SMR) of 121 (not statistically significant). Among the non-exposed, the number of deaths observed was 10 and the expected figure was 16.7, the corresponding SMR being 60 (not statistically significant). These figures indicate that the employees exposed to benzene experienced an approximately two-fold risk of leukaemia when compared to non-exposed employees. No benzene exposure levels were available from the study.

Epidemiological studies enabling quantitative estimates of risk for leukaemia

The results of a U.S. National Institute of Occupational Safety and Health (NIOSH) study of 748 white male workers exposed to benzene during the manufacture of rubber hydrochloride have been published on three occasions (Infante *et al.*, 1977, 1979; Rinsky *et al.*, 1981). The first two papers were based on the results with 75% complete follow-up of vital status, while the Rinsky *et al.* (1981) paper was based on data with 98% complete follow-up. The findings were essentially the same in each of the three papers: there was a three-fold increase in the risk of death from lympho-haematopoietic cancers and an almost six-fold increase for leukaemia specifically (7 leukaemia deaths *versus* 1.25 expected). Among workers employed for more than 5 years, 5 had died from leukaemia, compared to 0.23 expected, indicating a 21-fold increase in risk.

Rinsky *et al.* (1981) devoted considerable discussion to the industrial hygiene measurements available for one of the two study locations in Ohio. However, the investigators made no link between the available benzene measurements and the

Table 1. Estimate of excess risk of leukaemia deaths per 1 000 workers exposed to benzene[a]

Number of years exposed	Exposure level			
	10 ppm		1 ppm	
	NIOSH study[b]	Dow study[c]	NIOSH study	Dow study
45[d]	44–152	48–136	5–16	5–15
30	30–104	32–93	3–11	3–10
15	15–54	16–48	1.5–5	2–5
5	5–18	5–16	0.5–2	0.5–2
1	1–4	1–3	0.1–0.4	0.1–0.3

[a] From White et al. (1982).
[b] Rinsky et al. (1981).
[c] Ott et al. (1978).
[d] 45 years = occupational lifetime.

employment histories of the individual cohort members. (Subsequently, Crump and Allen (1984) and Rinsky et al. (1985) did link these data in unpublished risk assessments. Cumulative benzene exposures of individual workers in this cohort were estimated from job-exposure matrices. This approach indicated a heightened, 45-fold, increase in risk of leukaemia in the highest cumulative exposure category (Rinsky et al., 1985). See also Appendix, p. 18.)

Ott et al. (1978) reported the mortality of a cohort of 594 Dow Chemical workers exposed to benzene in the production of chlorobenzol, alkyl benzene and ethyl cellulose from 1938 to 1970. Their mortality experience was observed from 1940 through 1973. With expected deaths based on U.S. white male mortality, no statistically significant increases were found in any cause of death for the cohort as a whole, even when mortality was analysed by estimated cumulative benzene dose (ppm-months) and latency. However, further review of the three cases of leukaemia showed all three to be myelocytic, with two being classified as acute. Based on incidence data reported in the U.S. Third National Cancer Survey, the expected incidence of myelocytic leukaemia was only 0.8 cases.

Because the Occupational Safety and Health Administration in the U.S.A. is legally required to consider quantitative risk assessments whenever possible from available data, such an assessment has been attempted (White et al., 1982) using the above-mentioned two cohort studies. Uncertainties regarding the levels and lengths of exposure to benzene were incorporated into the analysis and the results are shown in Table 1. Based on the one-hit model, and subject to the typical uncertainties of epidemiological data, the assessment indicates that a working lifetime exposure to benzene at an exposure level of 10 ppm poses a substantial excess risk of death from leukaemia.

White et al. (1982) selected the one-hit, or linear, model because the biological mechanism of benzene-induced leukaemia is not understood well enough to justify a more complicated model, and because information from epidemiological studies regarding the relative risks of leukaemia at different levels of exposure to benzene was

Table 2.   Analyses of relative risk and excess risk of death from leukaemia per 1 000 workers exposed to benzene for an occupational lifetime [a]

Authors	Relative risk	Estimated cohort exposure	Excess risk per 1 000 workers	Excess risk per 1 000 exposed to	
				10 ppm	1 ppm
Ott et al. (1978)	3.75	1–30 ppm for 8–9 years	72	24–720	2.4–72
Infante et al. (1977)	5.6	10–100 ppm, 8.5 years average	170	17–170	1.7–17
Rinsky et al. (1981)	21	10–100 ppm, $\geqslant$ 5 years exposure	140	14–140	1.4–14
Vigliani (1976)	20	200–500 ppm, 9 years average	475	9.5–23.8	1.0–2.4
Aksoy (1977)	25	150–210 ppm, 9.7 years average	534	25.4–35.6	2.5–3.6

[a] Table adapted from Infante and White (1985). Calculations in the last three columns were performed using the method applied by IARC (1982) to data from Infante et al. (1977) and Rinsky et al. (1981).

inadequate for testing more complex models. Furthermore, as Infante and White (1985) have subsequently noted, several indications of benzene toxicity to bone marrow and peripheral blood cells have demonstrated a linear dose-response relationship.

This linear, non-threshold model assumes that every increment of dose is accompanied by a commensurate increment in the excess cancer risk. The use of this toxicologically plausible model allows extrapolation of risks from relatively high dose levels, where cancer responses can be measured, to relatively low dose levels, where such risks are too small to be measured directly through animal or epidemiological studies (WHO, 1981).

The IARC (1982) also conducted a quantitative cancer risk assessment for benzene and leukaemia using the results of four studies (Vigliani, 1976; Aksoy, 1977; Ott et al., 1978; Rinsky et al., 1981). IARC assumed a linear dose-response relationship, with cumulative benzene dose predicting the relative risk of developing leukaemia. It also made slightly different assumptions from those of White et al. (1982) regarding the length of exposure for the NIOSH (Rinsky) and Dow (Ott) studies. For purposes of comparison with the estimations of White et al. (1982), a summary of the IARC (1982) assessment of benzene risk, with extrapolation to levels of 10 ppm and 1 ppm is shown in Table 2. The calculations in the last three columns were performed by Infante and White (1985), using the method applied by the IARC (1982) to the NIOSH study and taking account of the IARC's opinion that "risk calculations (should) reflect the degree of uncertainty in the estimates of dose rate . . . by citing upper and lower bounds of such estimates" (IARC, 1982). The estimated excess risks of leukaemia associated with a working lifetime (45 years) of exposure to 10 ppm and 1 ppm of benzene are similar in Tables 1 and 2.

Recognizing the need for further quantitative investigations into the relationship between benzene exposure and lymphatic and haematopoietic cancers, Wong (1983) carried out a large industry-wide mortality study of U.S. chemical workers occupationally exposed to benzene. The population in this historical cohort study consisted of 4 602 male chemical workers from seven plants, who were occupationally exposed to benzene for at least 6 months between 1946 and 1975, and a comparison group of 3 074 male chemical workers from the same plants who were employed for at least 6 months during the same period of time, but who were never occupationally exposed to benzene. Exposure to benzene was divided into two categories: continuous exposure and intermittent exposure. Continuously-exposed workers were classified according to both an eight-hour time-weighted average (TWA) and a peak exposure level, whereas intermittently-exposed workers were characterized by a peak exposure level only. The eight-hour TWA's were estimated by company industrial hygienists, using uniform criteria; nevertheless, it was not possible to quantify accurately the exposure of workers to benzene.

The major findings of this study were as follows. When compared to the U.S. population, the SMR's in the exposed group for all lymphatic and haematopoietic cancer combined, for leukaemia, and for non-Hodgkin's lymphoma (lymphosarcoma, reticulosarcoma and other lymphoma) were slightly, but not significantly, higher than the national norm. When the group with no occupational exposure was used for comparison, the exposed group (continuous and intermittent) experienced a lympho-haematopoietic cancer relative risk (RR) of 2.99 (borderline statistical significance). This excess was primarily due to seven leukaemia deaths in the exposed group, *versus* none in the comparison group.

For the continuously exposed group, the RR for lympho-haematopoietic cancer was 3.20 (p < 0.05). The association between exposure to benzene, and, specifically, leukaemia was of borderline significance when those exposed continuously and those exposed intermittently were grouped together, but the association between continuous exposure alone and leukaemia was statistically significant (p < 0.05). None of the seven leukaemia deaths was of the acute myelogenous cell type. The RR for non-Hodgkin's lymphoma among white males in the continuously exposed group was 5.02, but was not significant (p = 0.12).

Furthermore, the data demonstrated statistically significant dose-response relationships between the estimated cumulative exposure to benzene and mortality from all lympho-haematopoietic cancers combined and from leukaemia. Those chemical workers with a cumulative exposure of at least 720 ppm-months experienced an RR of 3.93 for lymphatic and haematopoietic cancer, when compared to the workers with no occupational exposure. However, as Wong (1983) acknowledges, the limitations in exposure estimates preclude useful dose-response analysis at low levels of exposure.

In a more recent attempt to derive quantitative risk assessments of leukaemia in subjects exposed to benzene, Crump and Allen (1984) used the data from Ott *et al.* (1978), Rinsky *et al.* (1981) and Wong (1983), along with animal experimental data from inhalation studies. The estimates of leukaemia risk derived by Crump and Allen (1984) from animal inhalation studies (Table 3), while quite consistent, are all considerably less than those made from human data (Table 2). Accepting the assumptions underlying these estimates, this indicates that rodents may be less susceptible than humans to benzene-induced leukaemia.

Table 3. Estimates[a] of lifetime human risk per 1 000 exposed persons[b] from animal inhalation studies[c]

Data set	Benzene air concentration (ppm)	Risk
All squamous-cell carcinomas, male rats, NTP (1984)	1	0.77
	10	7.65
All squamous-cell carcinomas, male mice NTP (1984)	1	2.01
	10	19.90
Leukaemia, both sexes, rats, Maltoni et al. (1983)	1	0.15
	10	1.46
Leukaemia, male mice, Goldstein et al. (1982)	1	0.04
	10	0.38

[a] Assuming risk to animals is the same as risk to humans when dose is measured in mg/kg body weight/day.
[b] Length of human exposure to benzene = 40 years.
[c] Table based on Crump and Allen (1984).

Crump and Allen (1984) consider that their estimates from human studies, based upon cumulative or weighted exposure, are the most reliable. The attendant estimates of additional leukaemia cases per 1 000 workers exposed to 10 ppm of benzene range from 0.5 to 2.6 cases from one year of exposure beginning at age 20, to 15 to 88 cases from 40 years of exposure. The "window exposure" variable (defined as a shorter-term exposure occurring at the putative, latency-related, cancer induction time) tends to give lower estimates than either weighted or cumulative exposure. However, Crump and Allen (1984) judge that the estimates based on either cumulative exposure or weighted exposure are preferable to those based on window exposure.

Non-linear models would predict about the same results as linear models at high doses (10 ppm for 40 years). A person exposed to 10 ppm for 40 years would attain a cumulative exposure of 400 ppm-years, which, in the Rinsky et al. (1981) cohort, would place him in a category for which a significant excess of leukaemia occurred. Indeed, the subsequent re-analysis by Rinsky et al. (1985) gave an estimated 45-fold increase in risk of leukaemia for that category of exposure. Thus, no extrapolation to low doses is required to estimate risk from lifetime occupational exposure to 10 ppm.

However, the assumption of linearity plays a more important role at lower exposure levels, and the estimates of risk are more uncertain. This is important, since, under the benzene exposure limit of 10 ppm prevailing in the U.S.A., the risks estimated from continuous exposure to 10 ppm represent a theoretical maximum, as it is unlikely that any current worker's exposure will approximate this if the 10 ppm standard is strictly enforced.

Crump and Allen (1984) point out that their estimates of risk from human data were limited to leukaemia, as this appeared to be the only type of cancer conclusively linked to exposure to benzene in humans. This approach could underestimate cancer risk if, in fact, benzene causes other cancers, as it does in rodents. The recent epidemiology literature (Decouflé *et al.*, 1983; Rinsky *et al.*, 1985) suggests that benzene exposure may also cause multiple myeloma in humans.

Other less quantitative or less specific studies

In a cohort study of 35 000 workers at 8 petroleum refineries in the U.K., the leukaemia SMR was found to be 94 (Rushton & Alderson, 1981a). Using data from this cohort study, 36 cases with leukaemia mentioned on the death certificate were the subject of a subsequent case-control study (Rushton & Alderson, 1981b). Benzene measurements were not available, but each worker was assigned, based on work histories, to either low, medium or high levels of exposure to benzene. A two-fold increase in risk was detected for workers with medium or high exposure, relative to those with low exposure to benzene, when length of service was taken into account. This two-fold increase was of borderline statistical significance (p = 0.05). There was no evidence that the risk increased with length of service.

Decouflé *et al.* (1983) conducted a historical cohort mortality study of 259 male employees of a chemical plant (converted from a petroleum refinery) where benzene was used in large quantities. Unfortunately, no quantitative measures of exposure were available from the plant. Four deaths from lympho-haematopoietic cancers were observed, when only 1.06 deaths were expected; the SMR of 377 was statistically significant. Three of these four deaths were from leukaemia: one was chronic lymphocytic, one acute monocytic and one acute myelomonocytic. This last leukaemia case also had a history of multiple myeloma. Since the fourth lympho-haematopoietic cancer death was due to multiple myeloma, the authors suggested a possible link between benzene and multiple myeloma.

A number of epidemiological studies have found significant mortality excess from leukaemia among workers exposed to solvents in the rubber industry. However, the relationship between this observed leukaemia excess and, specifically, benzene is less clear. In one cohort, benzene was not the predominant solvent used and the authors were hesitant in ascribing to benzene the sole responsibility for the excess of leukaemia (Monson & Nakano, 1976). In another cohort of rubber workers, the excess risk was limited to lymphocytic leukaemia and was not associated with either monocytic or myelocytic leukaemia (McMichael *et al.*, 1975, 1976; Wolf *et al.*, 1981). However, workers in this cohort were exposed to other solvents as well as benzene, although the latter often occurs as a contaminant of other solvents (e.g., petroleum naphtha).

To further investigate in this latter cohort the relationship between the observed excess of lymphocytic leukaemia and exposure to various solvents, Arp *et al.* (1983) examined the solvent exposure histories of 15 cases of lymphocytic leukaemia and 30 matched controls within this second cohort. An individual was classified as exposed to a solvent if the cumulative length of exposure exceeded 12 months. The relative risk estimates were elevated for exposure to benzene (RR = 4.50) and to other solvents (RR = 4.50). Neither finding reached statistical significance at the 0.05 level. A much more detailed analysis of this same population was reported by Wilcosky *et al.* (1984). Details of estimated individual exposure to each of 25 solvents were obtained. Lymphosarcoma and lymphatic leukaemia were strongly associated with exposure to carbon tetrachloride and carbon disulphide, whereas their association with benzene and xylene was of marginal statistical significance only.

Several epidemiological studies of petroleum refinery workers who are potentially exposed to petroleum products, including benzene, have also found an excess of lympho-haematopoietic cancers (Tabershaw/Cooper Associates, 1974; Thomas *et al.*, 1982; Hanis *et al.*, 1982). However, none of these refinery studies provided any direct link between the observed mortality excess in lympho-haematopoietic cancer and benzene exposure.

Evaluation of the epidemiological evidence

On the basis of these studies there is substantial epidemiological evidence that persons exposed to benzene (or an associated impurity) experience an elevated risk of certain types of lymphatic and haematopoietic cancer, particularly leukaemia. Reports providing such epidemiological evidence include those of Aksoy *et al.* (1974), Ott *et al.* (1978), Vianna and Polan (1979), Aksoy (1980), Rinsky *et al.* (1981), Rushton and Alderson (1981b), Decouflé *et al.* (1983) and Wong (1983). The most frequently reported form of leukaemia associated with benzene exposure is the acute myelocytic form. However, research on rubber workers (McMichael *et al.*, 1975, 1976) indicates that, in chronic low-level exposure situations, lymphocytic leukaemia may predominate. Perhaps this is a more likely manifestation of non-acute bone marrow insult. (Chronic forms of leukaemia are also less likely to be reported on death certificates as the underlying cause of death.)

On the other hand, there are reports indicating no increased risk of lympho-haematopoietic cancer as a result of benzene exposure. A recent cohort study (Tsai *et al.*, 1983) of 454 male refinery workers exposed to benzene during 1952 to 1978 at a Texas refinery did not find any lympho-haematopoietic cancer deaths; however, the cohort size was small and the statistical power to detect a modest risk in either lympho-haematopoietic cancer or leukaemia was limited. The case-control studies of lymphocytic leukaemia among rubber workers (Arp *et al.*, 1983; Wilcosky *et al.*, 1984) indicated that the lymphocytic leukaemia excess in the rubber industry came primarily from carbon tetrachloride and carbon disulfide, rather than from xylene or, even less likely, from benzene. The large mortality study of Thorpe (1974) of 38 000 petroleum workers potentially exposed to benzene has often been cited as showing no evidence of significant leukaemia excess as a result of exposure to benzene. This interpretation, however, ignores the comparison of the exposed workers with the control workers (from the same facilities, but not exposed to benzene); the exposed group had a two-fold risk for leukaemia relative to the non-exposed group.

There are a number of outstanding issues regarding the relationship between exposure to benzene and increased risk of lympho-haematopoietic cancers. First, none of the published studies provides adequate exposure information for satisfactory dose-response analysis. Second, the choice of an appropriate comparison is an important issue. In a number of studies, analyses based on comparisons with the general population failed to detect an increased risk for lympho-haematopoietic cancer or leukaemia. In the Thorpe (1974) study in Europe, the industry-wide study of refinery workers in the U.S.A. (Tabershaw/Cooper Associates, 1974) and the

Table 4.   Studies of chromosomal breakage in workers exposed to "low" atmospheric concentrations of benzene

Author	Level of exposure to benzene (TWA)			
Picciano[a] (1979)	Controls	1 ppm	1–2.5 ppm	2.5–10 ppm
	3% (workers)[b]	22%	26%	33%
Sarto et al.[c] (1984)	Range of short-term samples = 0.2–12.4 ppm			
	1.2% (cells)[b]	2.7%		

[a] Benzene measured in 8-h TWA's; chromosome breakage = breaks, dicentrics, translocations and exchange figures.
[b] % = % of workers with chromosome breakage.
[c] Benzene measured in 5- and 20-min samples.

cohort study of eight oil refineries in Britain (Rushton & Alderson, 1981a), the initial calculations of the leukaemia SMR, based on a comparison with the general population, revealed no significant excess. However, subsequent analyses that took account of variations in benzene exposure between categories of workers revealed positive associations with leukaemia. Third, although some studies (Aksoy, 1980; Ott et al., 1978; Rinsky et al., 1981) indicate that acute myelogenous leukaemia is the type frequently associated with benzene exposure, other reports show associations with different leukaemia cell types (Tabershaw/Cooper Associates, 1974; McMichael et al., 1976; Linos et al., 1980; Schottenfeld et al., 1981). The studies of Decouflé et al. (1983) and Rinsky et al. (1985) have also suggested an increased risk of multiple myeloma.

Mutagenicity and chromosomal effects in humans

Numerous studies have been carried out on the chromosomes of bone-marrow cells and peripheral lymphocytes from people known to have been exposed to benzene (Dean, 1978; Picciano, 1979; Watanabe et al., 1980; Sarto et al., 1984). The populations included in these studies fall into two general categories: (1) patients with either a current or a past history of benzene-induced blood dyscrasias ("benzene haemopathies"), often associated with extensive exposure to benzene; and (2) workers with known current or past exposure to benzene, but with no obvious clinical effects. In some of these studies, significant increases in chromosomal aberrations have been seen; in some cases these have persisted for years after cessation of exposure (IARC, 1982).

The findings from two studies are summarized in Table 4. Picciano (1979) reported that 52 workers exposed to average benzene concentrations below 10 ppm demonstrated a statistically significant two- to three-fold excess of chromosomal damage, compared to that observed among 44 unexposed workers. Furthermore, the percentage of workers exhibiting both chromosome breaks and marker chromosomes was 20, 25 and 32% for workers categorized as exposed to average benzene concentrations below 1, 1.0–2.5 and 2.5–10.0 ppm, respectively. Less than 3% of the unexposed workers exhibited both chromosome breaks and marker chromosomes. More recently, Sarto et al. (1984) have reported supportive, albeit weaker, evidence of chromosomal breaks in workers exposed to benzene.

Other cancers in humans

Although induction of types of cancers other than of the lympho-haematopoietic system has been suspected, these have not been adequately evaluated from epidemiological studies of workers exposed to benzene. The studies have not had sufficient statistical power to detect low excess relative risks. However, since 1978, experimental studies have demonstrated that benzene administered either by oral gavage or by inhalation induces cancer at multiple sites in experimental animals. This research is reviewed further on.

Possible carcinogenicity of toluene and xylene

No epidemiological studies of differentiated exposure to toluene or xylene have been reported. It is possible that some or all of the above-mentioned increased cancer risk associated with non-specific exposure to solvents is attributable to these, or other, non-benzene solvents. However, evidence of any such effect will be difficult to obtain, particularly since benzene occurs as an impurity in toluene and xylene.

ANIMAL EXPERIMENTAL STUDIES OF BENZENE

Carcinogenicity

Intragastric administration of benzene dissolved in pure olive oil to female rats induced Zymbal gland carcinomas, mammary gland carcinomas and leukaemia. With the exception of leukaemias in the high-dose group, no such tumours occurred in male rats (Maltoni & Scarnato, 1979).

Experimental studies of lifetime benzene inhalation at 300 ppm im mice show the widespread occurrence of anaemia, lymphocytopenia, neutrophilia and bone-marrow hypo- or hyperplasia (Snyder *et al.*, 1980). Statistically significant increases in the incidence of lympho-haematopoietic tumours (lymphocytic lymphoma, plasma-cytoma and myelogenous leukaemia) also occurred (Snyder *et al.*, 1978a, 1980). However, no such tumour occurred in similarly exposed (male) rats (Snyder *et al.*, 1978b).

Subsequent studies by Maltoni and co-workers have shown that benzene is a potent carcinogen in rats of both sexes, whether ingested or inhaled; benzene produces different types of tumours in different organs and is therefore a "multipotential carcinogen" (Maltoni *et al.*, 1985).

Since all the benzene inhalation studies reported to date entail concentrations in the 200–300 ppm range, there is no direct animal experimental evidence relating to low-concentration exposures that now typify human occupational exposures. Long-term carcinogenicity bioassays at 50, 25, 10, 5 and 1 ppm may therefore be helpful for scientific risk assessment in humans.

Chromosomal damage

An earlier comprehensive review of the experimental data (IARC, 1982) concluded that benzene does not induce specific gene mutations in bacterial test systems, in

Drosophila melanogaster, or in mammalian cells. However, there was evidence that benzene induces cytogenetic abnormalities (chromosomal aberrations in bone-marrow cells) (IARC, 1982). Furthermore, the micronucleus test in mice and rats has been consistently positive, and numerous studies have shown that exposure of experimental animals to benzene *in vivo* leads to the induction of chromosomal aberrations in bone-marrow cells (IARC, 1982).

While Van Raalte *et al.* (1984) have argued that only peak exposure to benzene above 100 ppm can cause leukaemia or bone marrow toxicity, the results of recent epidemiological and experimental research suggest otherwise. Several recent animal experimental studies have demonstrated adverse effects on chromosomes and bone marrow as a result of low-level exposure to benzene.

It has recently been demonstrated by Tice *et al.* (unpublished data quoted by Infante & White, 1985) that exposure to benzene at a concentration of 10 ppm in air, 6 h/day for 9 days, induces a significant increase in micronuclei (a measure of bone-marrow chromosomal damage) in peripheral blood cells of mice. Mice exposed to 28 ppm benzene for a total of only 4 h had a two-fold increase in sister chromatid exchanges (SCE) in bone-marrow cells. The effect on mouse bone-marrow cells increased linearly with increasing levels of 4-h benzene exposure, indicating a linear dose-response. Previously, Kligerman had reported that mice exposed to 10 ppm benzene by inhalation for only 6 h demonstrated a significant increase in SCE in peripheral blood lymphocytes and in micronuclei in bone-marrow erythrocytes (Kligerman *et al.,* 1983).

Gad-El-Karim *et al.* (1984) have reported a dose-response increase in micronuclei in bone-marrow erythrocytes of mice administered a total of two oral doses of benzene at concentrations as low as 8.8 mg/kg body weight. This dosage would be equivalent to two 8-h atmospheric exposures of approximately 6 ppm.

Collectively, these studies demonstrate chromosomal damage in bone-marrow cells as a result of the equivalent of one to several working day exposure to 10 ppm of benzene. They also demonstrate a linear dose-response for benzene exposure and chromosomal damage to both marrow and peripheral blood cells.

Since most leukaemias and related disorders in man seem to involve stem-cell anomalies, the response of haematopoietic stem cells was investigated by Baarson *et al.* (1984) who exposed mice by inhalation to 10 ppm benzene for 6 h/day, 5 days/week for 32, 66 and 178 days. Progenitor cells from the exposed mice showed markedly reduced abilities to form colonies, compared to cells from control mice.

In another recent study, short-term exposure (6 h/day for 6 days) to 10 ppm benzene in air significantly depressed mitogen-induced blastogenesis of both B- and T-lymphocytes in mice (Rosen *et al.,* 1984). The authors concluded that benzene exposure at or near 10 ppm may affect immune function.

Thus, less than one week of exposure to 10 ppm of benzene is associated with chromosomal damage to bone-marrow cells, significant depression of the bone marrow and disturbances of immune system function. Since most leukaemias and related disorders in man seem to involve stem-cell abnormalities and immune system deficiencies, these animal experimental findings may be highly relevant to leukaemia and exposure to benzene in humans. The findings provide further support for the conclusion that an elevated risk of a bone-marrow proliferative cancer (leukaemia) could be expected as a result of exposure to 10 ppm benzene (Infante & White, 1985).

ANIMAL EXPERIMENTAL STUDIES OF TOLUENE AND XYLENE

In a series of experiments, primarily directed at studying benzene carcinogenicity in rats, Maltoni *et al.* (1985) have also studied the effects of other benzene-correlated aromatics (toluene, xylene and ethyl-benzene). At high concentrations, toluene and xylene (and, to a lesser extent, ethyl-benzene) caused an increase in the total number of malignant tumours. The increase in tumour yield was approximately one-third that induced by an equal dose of benzene.

No other experimental data on this question appear to have been published.

SUMMARY

Benzene

The evidence for carcinogenicity of benzene in humans was evaluated by the IARC in 1982 as follows:

"It is established that human exposure to commercial benzene or benzene-containing mixtures can cause damage to the haematopoietic system, including pancytopenia. The relationship between benzene exposure and the development of acute myelogenous leukaemia has been established in epidemiological studies.

"Reports linking exposure to benzene with other malignancies were considered to be inadequate for evaluation.

"There is *sufficient evidence* that benzene is carcinogenic to man."

This evaluation now warrants some elaboration and updating. While the epidemiological evidence concerning benzene carcinogenicity is strongest for acute myelocytic leukaemia, there is some limited evidence of increased risks of chronic myeloid and chronic lymphocytic leukaemia. In addition, recent studies have suggested an increased risk of multiple myeloma, while others indicate a dose-related increase for total lymphatic and haematopoietic neoplasms. Corroborative evidence for such a generalized effect comes from experimental studies showing that exposure to benzene depresses all lympho-haematopoietic cell lines.

While only limited evidence of benzene carcinogenicity in experimental animals exists, the recent findings of the National Toxicology Program (NTP, 1984) in the U.S.A. and Maltoni *et al.* (1985) strongly indicate that benzene is an experimental carcinogen.

Toluene and xylene

While no direct human evidence is available, there is recent evidence of carcinogenicity of toluene and xylene at high concentrations in experimental animals. It should also be noted that any future epidemiological observations of cancer risks associated with toluene or xylene would have to take account of the suspected effects of benzene impurities.

REFERENCES

Aksoy, M. (1977) Leukemia in workers due to occupational exposure to benzene. *New Istanbul Contrib. clin. Sci., 12,* 3–14

Aksoy, M. (1980) Different types of malignancies due to occupational exposure to benzene: a review of recent observations in Turkey. *Environ. Res., 23,* 101–190

Aksoy, M., Dincol, K., Erdem, S. & Dincol, G. (1972) Acute leukemia due to chronic exposure to benzene. *Am. J. Med., 52,* 160–166

Aksoy, M., Erdem, S. & Dincol, G. (1974) Leukemia in shoe-workers exposed chronically to benzene. *Blood, 44,* 837–841

Arp, E.W., Wolf, P.H. & Checkoway, H. (1983) Lymphocytic leukaemia and exposures to benzene and other solvents in the rubber industry. *J. Occup Med., 25,* 598–602

Baarson, K.A., Snyder, C.A. & Albert, R.E. (1984) Repeated exposure of C57B1 mice to inhaled benzene at 10 ppm markedly depressed erythropoietic colony formation. *Toxicol. Lett., 20,* 337–342

Crump, K.S. & Allen, B.C. (1984) *Quantitative Estimates of Risk of Leukaemia from Occupational Exposure to Benzene.* Unpublished report prepared for U.S. Occupational Safety and Health Administration

Dean, B.J. (1978) Genetic toxicology of benzene, toluene, xylene and phenols. *Mutat. Res., 47,* 75–97

Decouflé, P., Blattner, W. & Blair, A. (1983) Mortality among chemical workers exposed to benzene and other agents. *Environ. Res., 30,* 16–25

Delore, P. & Borgomano, C. (1928) Acute leukemia following benzene poisoning. *J. Med. Lyon, 9,* 227–233

Gad-El-Karim, M.M., Harper, B.L. & Legator, M.S. (1984) Modifications in the myeloclastogenic effect of benzene in mice with toluene, phenobarbital, 3-methylcholanthene, Aroclor 1254 and SKF-525A. *Mutat. Res., 135,* 225–243

Goldstein, B. (1983) Benzene is still with us. *Am. J. Ind. Med., 4,* 585–587

Goldstein, B.D., Snyder, C.A., Laskin, S., Bromberg, I., Albert, R.E. & Nelson, N. (1982) Myelogenous leukaemia in rodents inhaling benzene. *Toxicol. Lett., 13,* 169–173

Hanis, N.M., Holmes, T.M., Shallenberger, L.G. & Jones, K.E. (1982) Epidemiology study of refinery and chemical plant workers. *J. Occup. Med., 24,* 203–212

IARC (1982) *IARC Monographs on the Evaluation of the Carcinogenic Risk of Chemicals to Humans, Vol. 29, Some Industrial Chemicals and Dyestuffs,* Lyon, International Agency for Research on Cancer, pp. 93–148

Infante, P. & White, M. (1985) Projections of leukemia risk associated with occupational exposure to benzene. *Am. J. Ind. Med., 7,* 403–413

Infante, P.F., Rinsky, R.A., Wagoner, J.K. & Young, R.J. (1977) Leukemia in benzene workers. *Lancet, 2,* 76–78

Infante, P.F., Rinsky, R.A., Wagoner, J.K. & Young, R.J. (1979) Leukemia in benzene workers. *J. Environ. Pathol. Toxicol., 2,* 251–257

Kligerman, A.D., Erexson, G.L. & Wilmer, J.L. (1983) Development of rodent peripheral blood lymphocyte culture systems to detect cytogenetic damage in vivo.

(Abstract) *Int. Symp. Sister Chromatid Exchange,* Brookhaven Natl. Lab., Dec. 1983

Linos, A., Kyle, R.A., O'Fallon, W.M. & Kurland, L.T. (1980) A case-control study of occupational exposures and leukemia. *Int. J. Epidemiol., 9,* 131–135

Maltoni, C. & Scarnato, C. (1979) First experimental demonstration of the carcinogenic effects of benzene. *Med. Lav., 5,* 352–357

Maltoni, C., Conti, B., Cotti, G. & Belpoggi, F. (1983) A multipotential carcinogen. Results of long-term bioassays performed at the Bologna Institute of Oncology. *Am. J. Ind. Med., 4,* 589–630

Maltoni, C., Conti, B., Cotti, G. & Belpoggi, F. (1985) Experimental studies on benzene carcinogenicity at the Bologna Institute of Oncology: current results and ongoing research. *Am. J. Ind. Med., 7,* 415–446

McMichael, A.J., Spirtas, R., Kupper, L.L. & Gamble, J.E. (1975) Solvent exposure among rubber workers: an epidemiological study. *J. Occup. Med., 17,* 234–239

McMichael, A.J., Spirtas, R., Gamble, J.R. & Tousey, P.M. (1976) Mortality among rubber-workers: relationship to specific jobs. *J. Occup. Med., 18,* 178–185

Monson, R.R. & Nakano, K.K. (1976) Mortality among rubber workers. I. White male union employees in Akron, Ohio. *Am. J. Epidemiol., 103,* 284–296

NTP (1984) National Toxicology Program. *Toxicology and carcinogenesis studies of benzene in F344/N rats and B6C3F mice (gavage studies).* NTP-83-072, NIH Publication 84-2545. U.S. Department of Health and Human Services

Ott, M.G., Townsend, J.C., Fishbeck, W.A. & Langner, R.A. (1978) Mortality among individuals occupationally exposed to benzene. *Arch. Environ. Health, 33,* 3–9

Picciano, D. (1979) Cytogenetic study of workers exposed to benzene. *Environ. Res., 19,* 33–38

Rinsky, R.A., Young, R.J. & Smith, A.B. (1981) Leukemia in benzene workers. *Am. J. Ind. Med., 2,* 217–45

Rinsky, R.A., Smith, A.B., Hornung, R., Filloon, T.G., Young, R.J., Okun, A.H. & Landrigan, P.J. (1985) *Benzene and leukemia: an epidemiologic risk assessment.* Unpublished report, U.S. Department of Health and Human Services, Public Health Service

Rosen, M.G., Snyder, C.A. & Albert, R.E. (1984) Depressions in B- and T-lymphocyte mitogen-induced blastogenesis in mice exposed to low concentrations of benzene. *Toxicol. Lett., 20,* 343–349

Rushton, L. & Alderson, M.R. (1981a) An epidemiological survey of eight oil refineries in Britain. *Br. J. Ind. Med., 38,* 225–234

Rushton, L. & Alderson, M.R. (1981b) A case-control study to investigate the association between exposure to benzene and deaths from leukemia in oil refinery workers. *Br. J. Cancer, 43,* 77–84

Sarto, F., Cominato, I., Pinton, A.M., Brovedani, P.G., Merler, E., Peruzzi, M., Bianchi, V. & Levis, A.G. (1984) A cytogenetic study of workers exposed to low concentrations of benzene. *Carcinogenesis, 5,* 827–832

Schottenfeld, D., Warshauer, M.E., Zauber, A.G., Meikle, J.G. & Hart, B.R. (1981) A prospective study of morbidity and mortality in petroleum industry employees in the United States – a preliminary report. In: *Quantification of Occupational Cancer (Banbury Report 9).* Cold Spring Harbor, NY, CSH Press, pp. 247–265

Snyder, CA., Goldstein, B.D., Sellakumar, A., Albert, R.E. & Laskin, S. (1978a) The toxicity of inhaled benzene (Abstract No. 106) *Toxicol. Appl. Pharmacol., 45,* 265

Snyder, C.A., Goldstein, B.D., Sellakumar, A., Wolman, S.R., Bromberg, I., Erlichman, M.N. & Laskin, S. (1978b) Hematotoxicity of inhaled benzene to Sprague-Dawley rats and AKR mice at 300 ppm. *J. Toxicol. Environ. Health, 4,* 605–618

Snyder, C.A., Goldstein, B.D., Sellakumar, A.R., Bromberg, I., Laskin, S. & Albert, R.E. (1980) The inhalation toxicology of benzene: incidence in hematopoietic neoplasms and hematotoxicity in AKR/J and C57BL/6J mice. *Toxicol. Appl. Pharmacol., 54,* 323–31

Tabershaw/Cooper Associates (1974) *A mortality study of petroleum refinery workers.* The American Petroleum Institute, Berkeley, California

Thomas, T.L., Waxweiler, R.J., Moure-Erasso, R., Itaya, S. & Fraumeni, J.F., Jr. (1982) Mortality patterns among workers in three Texas oil refineries. *J. Occup. Med., 24,* 135–141

Thorpe, J.J. (1974) Epidemiologic survey of leukemia in persons potentially exposed to benzene. *J. Occup. Med., 16,* 375–382.

Tsai, S.P., Wen, C.P., Weiss, N.S., Wong, O., McCellan, W.A. & Gibson, R.L. (1983) Retrospective mortality and medical surveillance studies of workers in benzene areas of refineries, *J. Occup. Med., 25,* 685–692

Van Raalte, H.G.S., Grasso P. & Irvine, D. (1984) Tackling a very difficult problem. Letter to the Editor. *Risk Anal., 4,* 1–8

Vianna, N.J. & Polan, A. (1979) Lymphomas and occupational benzene exposure. *Lancet,* 1394–1395

Vigliani, E.C. (1976) Leukemia associated with benzene exposure. *Ann. N.Y. Acad. Sci., 271,* 143–51

Vigliani, E.C. & Saita, G. (1964) Benzene and leukemia. *New Eng. J. Med., 271,* 872–876

Watanabe, T., Endo, A., Kato, Y., Shima, S., Watanabe, T. & Ikeda, M. (1980) Cytogenetics and cytokinctics of cultured lymphocytes from benzene-exposed workers. *Int. Arch. Occup. Environ. Health, 46,* 31–41

White, M., Infante, P. & Chu, K. (1982) A quantitative estimate of leukemia mortality associated with occupational exposure to benzene. *Risk Anal., 2,* 195–203

Wilcosky, T.C., Checkoway, H., Marshall, E.G. and Tyroler, H.A. (1984) Cancer mortality and solvent exposures in the rubber industry. *Am. Ind. Hyg. Assoc. J., 45,* 809–811

Wolf, P.H., Andjelkovich, D., Smith, A. & Tyroler, H. (1981) A case-control study of leukemia in the U.S. rubber industry. *J. Occup. Med., 23,* 103–108

Wong, O. (1983) *An industry-wide mortality study of chemical workers occupationally exposed to benzene.* Washington, D.C., Chemical Manufacturers Association, December, 1983

WHO (1981) *Environmental Health Criteria 18, Arsenic.* Geneva, World Health Organization, pp. 144–145

APPENDIX (added in proof)

The extended follow-up of the NIOSH cohort (Rinsky *et al.*, 1985) has now been published (Rinsky *et al.*, 1987)[1]. These data appear to provide a better basis for quantitative risk assessment than do earlier studies. The authors estimated the cumulative exposure of individual workers to benzene by use of a job-exposure matrix to link detailed job histories with industrial hygiene measurement (historical air sampling of benzene concentrations).

The overall SMR for leukaemia (9 deaths) in benzene-exposed workers was 337 (95% confidence interval, 154–641), and that for multiple myeloma (4 deaths) was 409 (110–1047).

For leukaemia, a dose-response relationship was evident, with SMRs increasing from 109 (2 cases) to 322 (2 cases), 1186 (2 cases) and 6637 (3 cases), with increases in cumulative benzene exposure from less than 40 ppm-years, to 40–199, 200–399 and 400 or more, respectively (400 ppm-years is equivalent to a mean annual exposure of 10 ppm over a 40-year working lifetime).

The authors concluded that an exponential function best described the dose-response relationship, and that a substantial decrease in the risk for death from leukaemia could therefore be achieved by lowering occupational exposure to benzene, including (importantly) exposure within the range 10 ppm–0.1 ppm.

---

[1] Rinsky, R.A., Smith, A.B., Hornung, R., Filloon, T.G., Young, R.J., Okun, A.H. & Landrigan, P.J. (1987) Benzene and leukaemia: an epidemiologic risk assessment. *New Engl. J. Med., 316,* 1044–1050

CHAPTER 2

GENETIC EFFECTS OF BENZENE, TOLUENE AND XYLENE

L. Fishbein[1]

Department of Health and Human Services
Food and Drug Administration
National Center for Toxicological Research
Jefferson, Arkansas 72079, USA

INTRODUCTION

Salient aspects of the genetic effects of benzene (Snyder & Kocsis, 1975; National Research Council, 1976; Dean, 1978, 1985a; Snyder *et al.,* 1980; IARC, 1982a,b; Van Raalte & Grasso, 1982; Fishbein, 1984a; Gad-El-Karim *et al.,* 1984, 1985; Goldstein, 1984; Styles & Richardson, 1984; Erexson *et al.,* 1985, 1986) and of toluene, xylenes and phenols (Dean, 1978, 1985a; Fishbein, 1984b, 1985) have recently been reported.

The haematopoietic toxicity of benzene is unique among the simple aromatic hydrocarbons. Benzene is directly associated with human cancers, leukaemias and lymphomas being the predominant neoplasias (Snyder & Kocsis, 1975; National Research Council, 1976; Vigliani, 1976; Vianna & Polan, 1979; Snyder *et al.,* 1980; Rinsky *et al.,* 1981; IARC, 1982a,b; Goldstein, 1984). In addition to haematopoietic neoplasms, including thymic lymphoma and leukaemias, observed in rodents exposed to benzene either by inhalation or gavage, other types of tumours have been found, such as Zymbal gland carcinomas, hepatocellular carcinomas and squamous-cell papillomas and squamous-cell carcinomas of the oral cavity (Snyder *et al.,* 1980; Goldstein *et al.,* 1982; Maltoni *et al.,* 1982, 1983, 1985; National Toxicology Program, 1984). The sensitivity of individuals to benzene exposure is extremely variable, and possible complicating factors such as age, immunocompetence and life-style are recognized (Snyder & Kocsis, 1975; IARC, 1982a; Maltoni *et al.,* 1983; Dean, 1985a; Erexson *et al.,* 1985).

---

[1] Present address: ENVIRON Corporation, 1000 Potomac Street NW, Washington DC, USA

Fig. 1. Schematic diagram of the known and proposed metabolism of benzene. The figure is a modified and composite representation of the metabolic pathways for benzene as reported by Rusch *et al.* (1977), Irons *et al.* (1981) and Sawahata *et al.* (1985)

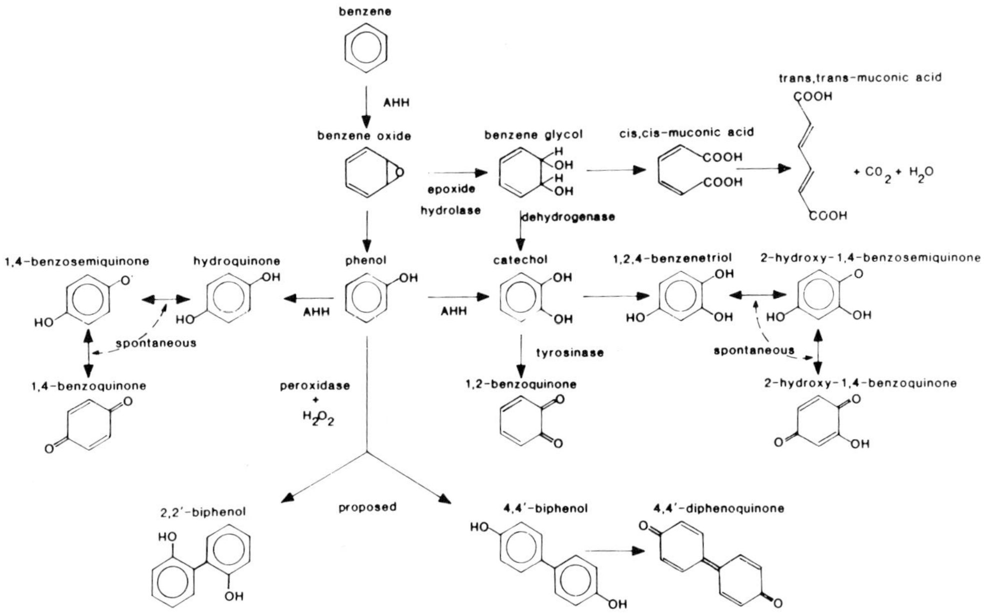

BENZENE

Metabolism

The haematopoietic toxicity (myelotoxicity) of benzene requires metabolism by host mono-oxygenases and associated enzymes, and the basic pathways of activation and conjugation have been described in several in-vivo and in-vitro systems (Snyder & Kocsis, 1975; Rusch *et al.*, 1977; Irons *et al.*, 1981, 1982; Erexson *et al.*, 1985; Gad-El-Karim *et al.*, 1985; Pellack-Walker *et al.*, 1985; Sawahata *et al.*, 1985). However, the *precise* mechanism(s) by which benzene causes its haematotoxicity, leukaemogenicity and clastogenicity are not completely understood (Harper *et al.*, 1984; Morimoto *et al.*, 1983). Figures 1 and 2 illustrate the known and proposed metabolic pathways for benzene (Erexson *et al.*, 1985; Pellack-Walker *et al.*, 1985). The initial step involves the cytochrome P-450 catalysed conversion of benzene in the liver to a benzene oxide intermediate which may spontaneously rearrange or be enzymatically hydrolysed (*via* epoxide hydrolase) to the major metabolite, phenol. Although most of the phenol is conjugated and excreted, further ring oxidation can form hydroquinone, which spontaneously oxidizes to 1,4-benzoquinone. In addition, benzene oxide is conjugated with glutathione by epoxide transferase to yield the inactivation product, phenylmercapturic acid. Lymphocytes could also convert benzene oxide to benzene glycol *via* the action of epoxide hydroxylase. Subsequent dehydrogenation of the glycol could then yield predominantly catechol, which upon

Fig. 2. Possible pathways for bioactivation of benzene *in vivo*

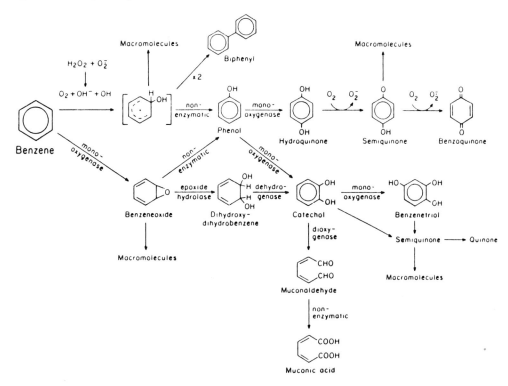

further oxidation forms *trans,trans*-muconic acid. Although a small amount of catechol is ring oxidized to 1,2,4-benzene triol, it is mostly conjugated and excreted (Erexson *et al.*, 1985). All of the hydroxylated metabolites have been detected in mammalian systems, following benzene exposure. And, as noted above, it is also possible for these hydroxylated metabolites to be oxidized to their corresponding quinones and semiquinone radicals, generating reactive oxygen species in the process (Greenlee *et al.*, 1981a,b; Pellack-Walker *et al.*, 1985).

Since benzene is metabolized primarily in the liver and the sites of toxicity are principally in the haematopoietic tissues, transport of benzene or its active metabolites by blood is required. It has been reported that further metabolism of benzene or its known metabolites can occur in the bone marrow (Irons *et al.*, 1980; Snyder *et al.*, 1982a,b). Bone-marrow homogenate (free of mature erythrocytes) in the presence of hydrogen peroxide or horse-radish peroxidase can metabolize phenol to 2,2′-biphenol, 4,4′-biphenol and 4,4′-diphenoquinone (Sawahata & Neal, 1982) (Figure 2).

Although epoxides are generally believed to be toxic and carcinogenic derivatives of aromatic hydrocarbons, many studies would suggest that benzene oxide is not the ultimate toxic metabolite of benzene. Much experimental evidence suggests that the toxicity of benzene, particularly its haematoxicity, is associated with the interaction of benzoquinones with cellular macromolecules. While it is not known which benzene metabolite causes the ultimate toxicity, it is known that hydroquinone and catechol concentrate in the bone marrow (Rickert *et al.*, 1979, 1981; Greenlee *et al.*, 1981a,b), where these metabolites may be further metabolized and affect blood-forming cells (Andrews *et al.*, 1979; Irons *et al.*, 1980, 1982; Bolcsak & Nerland, 1983; Johansson & Ingelman-Sundberg, 1983).

Benzene is preferentially cytotoxic to the maturing blood precursor cells within the bone marrow. Benzene cytotoxicity has been shown toward progenitor cells of the lymphocyte, erythrocyte, granulocyte and monocyte classes (Lee *et al.*, 1974; Tunek *et al.*, 1981; Pfeiffer & Irons, 1982). It is broadly acknowledged that the nature of the metabolite(s) of benzene responsible for its genotoxicity, haematoxicity and leukaemogenesis remains to be fully elucidated (Snyder & Kocsis, 1975; Lutz & Schlatter, 1977; Tunek *et al.*, 1978, 1980; Gill & Ahmed, 1981; Harper *et al.*, 1984; Goldstein, 1984; Dean, 1985a; Erexson *et al.*, 1985; Gad-El-Karim *et al.*, 1985; Kalf *et al.*, 1985; Pellack-Walker *et al.*, 1985).

Earlier studies of rodents injected with either [^{3}H]- or [^{14}C]benzene have shown that a metabolite(s) binds covalently to rat liver DNA (Lutz & Schlatter, 1977) and mitochondrial DNA from mouse liver and bone marrow (Gill & Ahmed, 1981; Kalf *et al.*, 1982). The metabolites of benzene are bound predominately to microsomal protein and, to a lesser extent, RNA, following the incubation of benzene with rat liver microsomes in the presence of a NADPH-generating system (Tunek *et al.*, 1978).

The chronic exposure of laboratory animals and man to benzene causes progressive degeneration of bone marrow and aplastic anaemia and may lead to leukaemia in man. These effects might result from covalent binding of one or more toxic metabolites of benzene to mitochondrial DNA (mt DNA) to produce damage leading to an inhibition of mitochondrial transcription and translation (Kalf *et al.*, 1985; Schwartz *et al.*, 1985). Changes in the mt DNA of bone-marrow stem cells have been found to correlate with the frequency of transformation of these cells to acute myelogenous leukaemia (Robberson *et al.*, 1981). Incubation of mitoplasts from rabbit bone-marrow cells with benzene metabolites resulted in a concentration-dependent inhibition of mitochondrial RNA synthesis and in covalent binding of activated metabolites of radio-labelled benzene to mt DNA *in vitro*. Elution profiles indicated that mt DNA contained seven deoxyguanosine adducts with benzene metabolites, including adducts of *p*-benzoquinone, hydroquinone, phenol and 1,2,4-benzenetriol with guanine (Kalf *et al.*, 1985). Although this study revealed the adducting of benzene metabolites to mitochondrial DNA, it could not be ascertained whether the inhibition of transcription by benzene results from the covalent binding of some metabolite to mt DNA and the subsequent impedance of the progress of RNA polymerase along the template, or from inactivation of RNA polymerase as a result of the binding of a metabolite to some sensitive site, e.g., sulfhydryl, on the enzyme (Kalf *et al.*, 1985).

p-Benzoquinone and hydroquinone (as well as 1,2,4-benzenetriol) were also shown to inhibit the activity of partially purified rat liver mt DNA polymerase gamma, using either activated calf thymus DNA or poly(nA).p(dt)$_{12-18}$ as primer/template, by a possible mechanism which involves a stable interaction of *p*-benzoquinone (or a semiquinone intermediate of hydroquinone, or a semiquinone intermediate of hydroquinone oxidation) with an essential sulfhydryl residue on mt DNA polymerase gamma (Schwartz *et al.*, 1985).

Recent studies of Pellack-Walker *et al.* (1985), in which the effects of benzene and its metabolites on the rate of DNA synthesis were measured in the mouse lymphoma cell line L5178YS, indicated a specific dose-response inhibition of DNA synthesis following exposure to catechol, hydroquinone, benzenetriol and benzoquinone. The irreversible inhibition of DNA synthesis following treatment with nontoxic concentrations of benzoquinone (the benzene metabolite with the greatest DNA-damaging potential) may represent irreparable DNA damage and hence this altered DNA might have significant implications for carcinogenesis and genotoxicity.

The inhibition of RNA synthesis and interleukin-2 production in lymphocytes in a dose-dependent manner *in vitro* by benzene and its metabolites, hydroquinone and *p*-benzoquinone, was recently reported (Post *et al.,* 1985). These studies are of importance, since T-lymphocytes are a potent source of factors that regulate haematopoiesis, and lymphocytopenia is an early and distinctive feature of benzene-induced aplastic anaemia (Irons & Moore, 1980; Goldstein, 1984).

Genotoxicity

Some of the evidence for the modifying effects of various inducers and inhibitors on different end-points of benzene toxicity and for benzene genotoxicity in various experimental systems can be considered contradictory and confusing (Dean, 1978, 1985a,b; Harper *et al.,* 1984; Styles & Richardson, 1984).

(a) Microbial systems

Benzene has consistently given negative results when tested in a variety of tester strains of *Salmonella typhimurium* (e.g., TA97, TA102, TM677) in over ten laboratories employing the conventional plate-incorporation assay, as well as pre-incubation protocols and a variety of microsomal activation systems (Dean, 1978, 1985a,b; Lebowitz *et al.,* 1979; Bartsch *et al.,* 1980; Nestmann *et al.,* 1980; Shimizu *et al.,* 1983; Venitt, 1985). This suggests that a liver microsomal activation system is unable to generate DNA-reactive metabolites and perhaps directs metabolism of benzene toward a predominance of non-covalent binding metabolites (Dean, 1985a). However, an isolated positive result has been reported using a sensitive microsuspension fluctuation assay; i.e., a significant increase in histidine revertants was found when benzene was tested against *S. typhimurium* TA100 with metabolic activation (McCarroll *et al.,* 1980). A positive *rec*-assay with *B. subtilis* has also been reported (McCarroll *et al.,* 1981a).

When tested in a comprehensive series of yeast assays as part of an International Collaborative Study (CSSTT) which employed 25 assays, benzene yielded variable and somewhat conflicting results. It appeared to give negative results for mitotic gene conversion and mitotic crossing-over, but induced gene mutations in yeast in the G6 and D61-M strains of *Saccharomyces cerevisiae* under certain experimental conditions (Dean, 1985a; Parry, 1985; Parry & Eckardt, 1985a). Benzene induced significant petite mutants in *S. cerevisiae* strain D5 under conditions optimizing metabolic activation (Ferguson, 1985) and increased mitotic gene conversion and point mutations in *S. cerevisiae* strain D7 (Parry & Eckardt, 1985b).

(b) Insect assays

Mutagenicity assays of benzene in *Drosophila* have also been found to give conflicting results (Nylander *et al.,* 1978; Kale & Baum, 1983; Dean, 1985a; Fujikawa *et al.,* 1985; Vogel, 1985a,b). Thus, benzene was clearly positive when examined in somatic mutation assays in *Drosophila* in a recent CSSTT collaborative study (Vogel, 1985a), while negative data were reported using an eye spot assay that detected only gene mutations and deletions (Fujikawa *et al.,* 1985), and equivocal results were found upon observation of wing spot changes that corresponded to chromosomal breakage, deletions and aneuploidy, gene mutations and mitotic recombination. These ambivalent results suggest that, while benzene is capable of inducing genetic changes in meiotic assays in *Drosophila,* the damage may be highly stage-specific and limited to particular genetic events (e.g., recombination or, possibly, aneuploidy in both meiosis and mitosis (Dean, 1985a)).

(c) Cultured mammalian cell assays

A large number of genotoxicity studies employing cultured mammalian cells have been reported for benzene. Although the majority of the published studies on the induction of unscheduled DNA synthesis suggest that benzene is unlikely to cause reparable DNA damage in primary rat hepatocytes (Probst *et al.,* 1981; Williams *et al.,* 1985) or in HeLa cells (Martin & Campbell, 1985; Barrett, 1985), one positive study has been reported in primary rat hepatocyte cultures (Glauert *et al.,* 1985).

Metaphase chromosome studies of the effect of benzene in cultured cells are also somewhat ambiguous (Dean, 1985a). Early in-vitro chromosome studies indicated no (Gerner-Smidt & Friedrich, 1978), or only slight (Dean, 1978), induction of chromatid breakage. In a recent CSSTT collaborative study (Ashby *et al.,* 1985), three of eight assays detected induction of chromatid aberrations (taking into account mitotic delay), while five were negative.

Chromosome aberrations have been detected in a human lymphocyte assay in the presence or absence of an S9 microsomal activation system, with benzene concentrations ranging from 9 to 88 µg/mL (Howard *et al.,* 1985). Structural aberrations have been observed in a Chinese hamster lung fibroblast assay (Ishidate & Sofuni, 1985), and both positive (Palitti *et al.,* 1985) and negative results have been obtained with benzene in Chinese hamster CHO cells. While no evidence of benzene-induced polyploidy in cultured cells has been found (Dean, 1985a,b), a significant induction of aneuploidy in Chinese hamster liver-cell cultures exposed to 62.5 µg/mL benzene has been reported (Danford, 1985). Dean (1985a) concluded that benzene is capable of inducing both structural chromosomal aberrations and aneuploidy in cultured cells when an appropriate protocol is employed.

A number of comprehensive studies of the effects of benzene and its metabolites on sister chromatid exchange (SCE) frequencies in cultured human lymphocytes have been reported (Morimoto & Wolff, 1980; Morimoto, 1983; Morimoto *et al.,* 1983; Erexson *et al.,* 1985). Morimoto and Wolff (1980) initially showed that, in the absence of an exogenous source of metabolizing enzymes, benzene failed to induce SCE in lymphocyte cultures, while catechol, hydroquinone and, to a lesser extent, phenol, induced SCE in phytohaemagglutinin-stimulated lymphocytes. Subsequent studies using 3-day cultures showed that rat liver S9 augmented SCE induction in human lymphocytes exposed to phenol, catechol and hydroquinone during a 2-hour pulse treatment at 40 to 42 h (Morimoto *et al.*, 1983), and that benzene induced SCE in human lymphocytes only after incubation of these cells in the presence of rat liver S9. It should also be noted that benzene failed to induce SCE in human peripheral lymphocytes in culture, with and without metabolic activation (Obe *et al.*, 1985). A recent study by Erexson *et al.* (1985) further elucidated SCE induction in human T-lymphocytes exposed to benzene and its metabolites *in vitro*. Benzene, phenol, catechol, 1,2,4-benzenetriol, hydroquinone and 1,4-benzoquinone induced significant concentration-related increases in the SCE frequency, decreases in mitotic indices and inhibition of cell cycle kinetics. Based on the slope of the linear regression curves for SCE induction, the relative potencies were as follows: catechol > 1,4-benzoquinone > hydroquinone > 1,2,4-benzenetriol > phenol > benzene, and catechol was approximately 221 times more active than benzene at the highest concentrations studied. While *trans,trans*-muconic acid had no significant effect on the cytogenetic parameters studied, 2,2′-biphenol induced a significant increase in SCE only at the highest concentration employed and 4,4′-biphenol showed a significant increase in SCE frequency that was not dose-related. Both of the isomeric biphenols also caused significant cell cycle delay and mitotic inhibition. These studies demonstrate that, in addition to phenol, di- and trihydroxy metabolites exhibit an important role in SCE induction and that, while benzene *per se* can induce SCE, it is possible as well that mononuclear leucocytes have a limited capability for activating benzene (Erexson *et al.*, 1985).

A recent CSSTT collaborative study (involving six separate studies) failed to reveal the induction of SCE in Chinese hamster CHO or V79 cells, both with and without S9, or in rat liver (RL4 cells) (Dean, 1985b).

Additionally, no convincing evidence has been reported to indicate that benzene could induce gene mutations in cultured mammalian cells in a CSSTT collaborative study (Garner, 1985) involving 15 separate studies including assays in mouse lymphoma L5178Y cells at the TK locus (seven studies), one assay at the ouabain locus in L5178Y cells, three assays of 6-thioguanine resistance in Chinese hamster V79 cells, studies of 6-thioguanine and ouabain resistance in CHO cells and the TK and HGPRT loci in human lymphocytes. However, weak positive responses were obtained when benzene was tested in the presence of metabolic activation for the induction of forward mutation at the thymidine kinase locus of L5178Y mouse lymphoma cells in culture (Oberly *et al.*, 1985). Benzene was also weakly positive when tested at two loci in human lymphoblast cell lines (Crespi *et al.*, 1985).

Neoplastic transformation studies of benzene in cultured cells have been rather limited (Amacher & Zelljadt, 1983; Dean, 1985a; McGregor & Ashby, 1985). In Syrian hamster embryo (SHE) cells, benzene significantly increased the incidence of cell clones with the classical morphology of neoplastic transformation (Amacher & Zelljadt, 1983). This was later confirmed in an IPCS Collaborative Study (CSSTT) (McGregor & Ashby, 1985). The CSSTT studies also involved the testing of benzene in transformation assays using Balb/c 3T3 mouse fibroblasts (negative), C3H10T1/2 mouse cells (equivocal results), Chinese hamster CHO cells (negative) and enhancement of viral (SA7) transformation in SHE cells (negative) (Dean, 1985a;

McGregor & Ashby, 1985). Only the Syrian hamster embryo (SHE) system, of all the commonly used assays for neoplastic transformation, gave reproducibly positive results. Dean (1985a) has noted that only the SHE assay employs primary cultures of embryonic material that retains a representative spectrum of endogenous metabolizing enzymes, in contrast to the other assays using established cell lines that require supplementary metabolic activation in the form of S9 liver microsomal fraction.

(d) Cytogenetic studies in animals

A large number of cytogenetic studies in rodents have been reported in an attempt to characterize the induction of chromosome aberrations and SCEs and their relationship to benzene metabolism under various conditions, including various dose regimens and routes of administration, periods of exposure and metabolic induction (Dean, 1978, 1985a; Meyne & Legator, 1980; Hite et al., 1980; Siou et al., 1982; Tice et al., 1980; Gad-El-Karim et al., 1984, 1985; Harper et al., 1984; Styles & Richardson, 1984; Erexson et al., 1986). Significant increases were found in the number of bone-marrow polychromatid erythrocytes (PCEs) and micronuclei (MN) in both male and female CD-1 mice given 125 mg benzene/kg per day by gavage and sacrificed 18 h after the second dose (Hite et al., 1980). Male CD-1 mice exhibited higher frequencies of chromosome aberrations and MN than females after exposure to 500 mg benzene/kg per day by gavage or i.p. injections at 24-h intervals for three consecutive days (Meyne & Legator, 1980). A significant increase in PCEs containing MN were found in male Swiss mice after two gavages of 25.6 mg benzene/kg per day at 24-h intervals (Siou et al., 1982). NMRI mice continuously exposed to 45 mg/m^3 benzene by inhalation for one to eight weeks showed a significant increase in PCEs containing MN (Toft et al., 1982)[1].

Significant increases in SCE have been found in the bone marrow of both male and female DBA/2 and C57B1/6 mice after a 4-h inhalation exposure to 90 mg/m^3 benzene (Tice et al., 1980). Evidence of a concentration-dependent increase of chromosome aberrations in bone marrow of male Wistar rats has been reported after inhalation exposure to benzene concentrations of 3, 32, 320 or 3 200 mg/m^3 for 6 h. Significant clastogenic effects were noted in rat bone-marrow cells at 320 and 3 200 mg/m^3, while at 32 mg/m^3 and 3 mg/m^3 there were no significant differences in the incidence of aberrant cells in treated animals compared with controls, although the levels were elevated and showed a dose-response (Styles & Richardson, 1984).

Erexson et al. (1986) reported that benzene can induce statistically significant cytogenetic effects in peripheral blood lymphocytes (PBLs), as well as PCEs and MN in both male DBA/2 mice and male Sprague-Dawley rats after a 6-h inhalation of benzene at low concentrations (e.g., 3 mg/m^3).

The greater sensitivity of male rodents to the clastogenic effects of benzene was further confirmed in CD-1 mice after two daily oral or i.p. benzene doses of 400 or 880 mg/kg (Gad-El-Karim et al., 1984, 1985). The incidences of PCEs with MN were found to be 4–6 times higher after oral than after i.p. benzene administration (Gad-El-

---

[1] 3.2 mg/m^3 benzene = 1 ppm (~ 20 °C)

Karim *et al.*, 1984). Later studies employing germ-free and conventional (non-germ-free) male CD-1 mice ruled out the possibility that the involvement of gut flora in benzene transformation was responsible for the above observation (Gad-El-Karim *et al.*, 1985). The myeloclastogenic effect of benzene (an agent which causes chromosomal breakage, including MN formation in the bone marrow; Gad-El-Karim *et al.*, 1984, 1985; Harper *et al.*, 1984) appears to be the earliest benzene-induced cellular damage in which chromosomal DNA is a primary critical target and which is readily quantified and antedates changes in peripheral blood counts (leucocytic, platelet counts, etc.). In studies focusing on the relation between the myeloclastogenicity of benzene and metabolism, it was noted that enhancement of chromosomal damage was affected by P-448 (e.g., 3-methylcholanthrene or β-naphthoflavone) rather than P-450 (e.g., phenobarbital) enzyme inducers. Hydroquinone, catechol and phenol do not possess any of the potent myeloclastogenicity of the parent compound, benzene, and it was postulated that benzene can induce its own metabolism (Gad-El-Karim *et al.*, 1985).

As noted above (Figures 1, 2), benzene is metabolized in mammals to phenol, hydroquinone, catechol, 1,2,4-benzenetriol and *p*-benzoquinone. The decreases in mitotic indices noted after the inhalation of benzene in the study of Erexson *et al.* (1986) might be attributed to the formation of hydroquinone and *p*-benzoquinone, metabolites which react with sulfhydryl groups of cytoskeletal proteins vital for blastogenesis (Irons & Neptun, 1980; Irons *et al.*, 1981; Pfeifer & Irons, 1981). Possibly a majority of the SCEs induced *in vivo* in the mouse B-lymphocytes and rat T-lymphocytes are caused by catechol, *p*-benzoquinone and 1,2,4-benzenetriol, compounds which are relatively efficient SCE inducers in cultured human T-lymphocytes exposed *in vitro* (Morimoto & Wolff, 1980; Erexson *et al.*, 1985). The data obtained in the recent study of Erexson *et al.* (1985) show parallel induction of SCE and micronuclei in both mice and rats, suggesting to the authors that a common benzene metabolite(s) might be involved. There are also reports showing that *p*-benzoquinone is negative in the *Drosophila* sex-linked recessive lethal mutation test and in the aberration test with human lymphocytes *in vitro* (Lüers & Obe, 1972).

Additionally, a number of studies support the hypothesis that micronuclei in bone-marrow PCEs are a result of chromosome breakage (or possibly non-disjunctional events) after exposure to benzene (Philip & Krogh Jensen, 1970; Dean, 1978; Anderson & Richardson, 1981; Styles & Richardson, 1984).

Although it is well established that exposure to benzene induces bone-marrow genotoxic damage, *less definitive* data are available concerning the effect of exposure frequency and duration on the genotoxic response *in vivo* (Styles & Richardson, 1984; Barale *et al.*, 1985; Dean, 1985a; Luke *et al.*, 1985). While single inhalation exposures are effective in producing clastogenic changes in rats (Styles & Richardson, 1984; Dean, 1985a; Erexson *et al.*, 1986), the opposite is true when repeated inhalation exposures are given (Dean, 1985a). Repeated exposure of rats to benzene over a period of five days did not increase the frequency of aberrations over that observed after a single exposure. In addition, the frequency of chromosome aberrations observed after a 2-h inhalation was significantly higher than that found after a 6-h exposure to the same concentration (Dean, 1985a). These data would suggest that repeated exposure of rats to benzene induces hepatic enzyme systems that reduce the generation of clastogenic metabolites from benzene in two to three weeks (Dean, 1985a). In contrast, studies of repeated exposure of mice to benzene inhalation (e.g., five days exposed, two days unexposed, three days exposed and four days unexposed) did not lead to a reduction in the generation of clastogenic metabolites (Luke *et al.*, 1985).

It has also been shown that intermittent exposures to benzene were more damaging than constant exposures (Tice *et al.*, 1984) and that less damage was induced with increasing duration of chronic exposure (Barale *et al.*, 1985). In the study of Barale *et al.* (1985), no evident toxic effects were noted during the chronic treatment of Swiss mice with benzene for up to 42 days, except for a decrease in body weight and in the PCEs:normochromatic erythrocytes ratio in males treated with benzene at the highest dose by gavage (0.500 mL/kg). A significant increase in MN was observed only after 21 days of treatment at the highest doses, and female animals were always less sensitive, a result consistent with previous findings in bone-marrow cells (Meyne & Legator, 1980; Siou *et al.*, 1981; Gad-El-Karim *et al.*, 1984). A steady-state frequency of MN appeared after 28 days in females, and later on in males, depending on the dose. A decline in MN frequency was also observed after longer periods and was postulated to be due to (a) selection of resistant cells, (b) a decreased ability to convert benzene to genotoxic metabolites, or (c) an increased ability to detoxify active benzene metabolites (Barale *et al.*, 1985).

(e) Cytogenetic studies in humans

Epidemiological studies have demonstrated that benzene is clastogenic in peripheral blood lymphocytes of occupationally exposed workers (IARC, 1982a,b). An extensive literature deals with the effects on bone-marrow cells or peripheral lymphocytes of individuals generally chronically exposed to relatively high concentrations of benzene vapour (Forni *et al.*, 1971a,b; Hartwich & Schwanitz, 1972; Erdogan & Aksoy, 1973; Khan & Khan, 1973; Funes-Cravioto *et al.*, 1977; Dean, 1978, 1985a; Picciano, 1979, 1980; Van den Berghe *et al.*, 1979; Watanabe *et al.*, 1980; Rinsky *et al.*, 1981; HSE, 1982; Van Raalte & Grasso, 1982). The populations included in these studies fall into two general categories; (a) patients with either a current or a past history of benzene-induced blood dyscrasias ("benzene haemopathies"), often associated with extensive exposure to benzene, and (b) workers with known current or past exposure to benzene, but with no obvious clinical effects (IARC, 1982a). In an assessment of the chromosomal effects of benzene in exposed individuals, IARC (1982a) concluded that "There is a clear correlation between exposure to benzene and the appearance of chromosomal aberrations in the bone marrow and peripheral lymphocytes of individuals exposed to high levels of benzene (> 100 ppm). Such levels of exposure usually lead to clinical symptoms of benzene-induced blood dyscrasias. These aberrations may persist for many years after exposure and after manifestations of haematotoxicity... Although aberrations have been reported following chronic exposures to as little as 10 ppm, this has not been a consistent finding. Environmental factors and exposure to other agents may have interacted with benzene in these studies of low exposure." (IARC, 1982a).

Dean (1985a) has noted that since the introduction of more stringent controls over industrial exposure to benzene, human chromosome studies have concentrated on establishing the cytogenetic consequences of low-level exposure to benzene and of occasional peak exposures. Additionally, the difficulties encountered in the interpretation of human chromosome studies with benzene (as well as other clastogens) are often cited and have necessitated the selection of a control population closely matched for sex, age, smoking habits and other contributing factors. The control population is sampled, cultured and analysed simultaneously with the exposed population, which is accurately described in terms of exposure (Archer, 1984; Dean, 1985a).

TOLUENE AND XYLENES

Toluene and the xylenes, like benzene, are produced in very large quantities and are employed in a wide variety of applications, primarily as solvents (frequently in admixture with benzene in the past) and in gasoline as part of the B-T-X component (benzene-toluene-xylene). It should be noted that benzene is a common contaminant of toluene. While highly purified toluene (reagent grade and nitration grade) contains less than 0.01% benzene, industrial grade and crude grade toluene (90–120 °C boiling range) can contain significant quantities of benzene (e.g., as much as 25%) and probably other hydrocarbons as well (Clement Associates, 1977a). For example, samples of commercial toluene (toluol) in the U.S.A. were stated to contain 2–10% of benzene in the 1940s (Wilson, 1943) and levels of 15% and 10% of benzene and xylene, respectively, were reported in samples of commercial toluene in the Federal Republic of Germany in the 1950s (Humperdinck, 1954). There is a broad potential for exposure to these aromatic hydrocarbons; exposure concerns both industrial workers in the production and use of these agents and the general public *via* vehicle exhausts, consumer products, etc.

Compared with benzene, very much less is known of the human health hazards, particularly the chronic and genotoxic effects, of either toluene or xylene or of the specific isomers, either separately or in admixture with other alkyl benzenes (Clement Associates, 1977a,b; WHO, 1981; NAS, 1982; Fishbein, 1984b, 1985). In contrast to the case of benzene, there are no epidemiological reports on the incidence of cancer following exposure to toluene or the xylenes *per se*. However, it should be noted that there are industrial occupations and settings (e.g., rubber and plastic industries) where mixed solvents, often including benzene, have been employed.

Metabolism

The biotransformation of toluene has been reviewed (Astrand, 1975; Angerer, 1979a,b; Cohr & Stokholm, 1979; Toftgard & Gustafsson, 1980; NAS, 1982; Lauwerys, 1983). The metabolism of toluene in mammals is illustrated in Figure 3 (Dean, 1978). Absorption of toluene results primarily from inhalation of its vapour, although significant amounts may be absorbed through the skin by contact with the liquid form. Approximately 15–20% of a dose of toluene is eliminated unchanged in

Fig. 3. Metabolism of toluene in mammals (Dean, 1978)

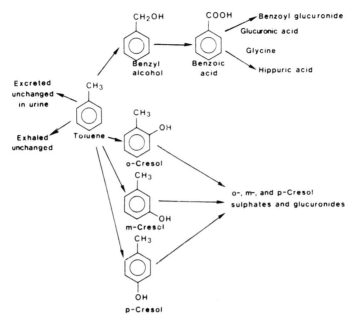

the expired air, and about 0.06% is excreted unchanged in the urine. The remainder is oxidized by transformation of the methyl radical into a carboxyl radical, which is mainly conjugated to produce hippuric acid. Toluene is transformed mainly in the microsomes of the liver parenchymal cells by oxidation in one of several positions. Less than 1% of the absorbed toluene is hydroxylated to *ortho-, meta-* and *para-*cresol, which are not normal constituents of urine (Woiwode *et al.,* 1979; WHO, 1981a; Lauwerys, 1983). This oxidation occurs *via* epoxide formation and is catalysed by the enzyme arylmono-oxygenase (Jerina *et al.,* 1968; Jerina & Daly, 1974). Phenolic derivatives are excreted in the urine as glucuronides and sulfates (Cohr & Stokholm, 1979). Toluene is known to alter the metabolism of other solvents. In rats, the biotransformation of benzene and styrene is suppressed by toluene (Ikeda *et al.,* 1972).

The metabolic scheme for the isomeric xylenes is illustrated in Figure 4 (Fishbein, 1985). The major pathway of biotransformation of xylene isomers in man and animals is *via* oxidation to the corresponding toluic acids (methyl benzoic acids), followed by conjugation, principally with glycine, to form *ortho-, meta-* and *para-*methylhippuric acids (toluric acids). Methylhippuric acids represent over 95% of the metabolized fraction of xylene (Ogata *et al.,* 1970; Flek & Sedivec, 1975) and their identification in urine provides an index of the amount of xylene absorbed. Hydroxylation of the aromatic ring, with the formation of xylenols (dimethylphenols), may also occur in man. However, the xylenols produced and excreted unchanged or as the glucuronic acid conjugates represent less than 20% of the amount of xylene absorbed (Riihimäki *et al.,* 1979; Sedivec & Flek, 1976a,b). The metabolism of xylene proceeds rapidly in

Fig. 4. Metabolic scheme for isomeric xylenes

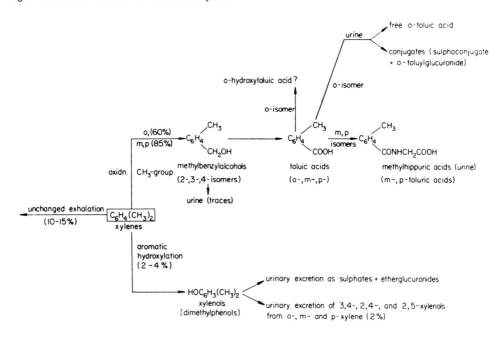

the liver *via* the microsomal oxidation mixed-function oxidase system, as well as *via* cytoplasmic dehydrogenases (Carlone & Fouts, 1974; Harper *et al.,* 1975).

Genotoxicity

(a) *Toluene*[1]

To date, short-term mutagenicity assays of toluene have been reported to be negative for mitotic mutation in *S. typhimurium* TA98, TA100, TA1535, TA1537 and TA1538, with and without metabolic activation (Litton Bionetics, Inc., 1978; Lebowitz *et al.,* 1979; Nestmann *et al.,* 1980; Bos *et al.,* 1981; Haworth *et al.,* 1983), for mitotic gene conversion in *S. cerevisiae* D4 (Litton Bionetics, Inc., 1978), in the microsuspension assay for DNA damage in appropriate strains of *Escherichia coli* and *Bacillus subtilis* (McCarroll *et al.,* 1981a,b), for specific locus forward mutation induction in the L5178Y thymidine kinase lymphoma cell assay (Litton Bionetics, Inc., 1978) and in the sex-linked recessive lethal mutation test in *Drosophila melanogaster* (Donner *et al.,* 1981).

There was no evidence of induction of chromosome aberrations in bone marrow of male Wistar rats after inhalation of 1 150 mg/m³ toluene (6/h for 24 h, 5 days/week) for 15 weeks. Although an increase in SCE was observed in bone-marrow cells

_____

[1] 3.8 mg/m³ toluene ≃ 1 ppm.

cultured from animals after 11 and 13 weeks of exposure, this had returned to control levels after 15 weeks (Donner *et al.*, 1981).

A daily subcutaneous injection of toluene (0.8–1.0(g/kg)/day) for 12 days caused an increased frequency (13.7%) of chromosome damage in the bone-marrow cells of rats, compared to a frequency of 4.2% in a control group. Chromatid gaps were the most common changes detected in bone-marrow cells from toluene-treated rats (Lyapkalo, 1973). Recent studies, however, have failed to confirm the findings of Dobrokhotov (1972) and Lyapkalo (1973) of an induction of chromosome aberrations in rat bone marrow after toluene exposure by either injection or inhalation. For example, CD-1 mice treated by gavage or i.p. with 0.86 or 1.72 g/kg redistilled toluene on each of two successive days did not exhibit clastogenic activity in the examined bone-marrow cells (Gad-El-Karim *et al.*, 1984).

Chromosome aberrations in rats were measured after an inhalation exposure for four hours daily for three months to air containing 610 mg/m^3 of toluene or 610 mg/m^3 of toluene plus 300 mg/m^3 benzene. During this exposure, the percentage of metaphases with damaged chromosomes in the bone marrow of rats increased gradually to 21.56% (toluene) and 41.21% (toluene plus benzene), compared to 4.02% in controls. Additionally, toluene and the mixture of toluene and benzene caused leukosis (Dobrokhotov & Enikeev, 1977). In a 12-day study it was estimated that toluene administered subcutaneously to rats in doses of 0.8 g/kg per day induced the same frequency of chromosome damage as did benzene in doses of 0.2 g/kg per day (Dobrokhotov, 1972).

The effects of toluene (as well as the isomeric xylenes and ethylbenzene) on the induction of MN in bone-marrow PCEs of mice were most recently investigated by Mohtashamipur *et al.* (1985) employing male NMRI mice. Each compound was administered i.p. (two identical doses, 24 h apart). Increased formation of MN within PCEs of femoral bone marrow 30 h after the first injection was considered to be due to the clastogenic effect of the test compound. (MN are chromosomal fragments that are not included in the daughter nuclei during maturation of erythroblasts to erythrocytes in the bone marrow, but can also originate from whole chromosomes.) Of the chemicals tested, only toluene gave a dose-dependent increase in the frequency of PCEs with MN when tested at levels of 2×0.12 to 2×0.50 mL/kg body weight. This genotoxicity was confirmed in analogous studies in male B6C3F1 mice.

Although the clastogenic effects of benzene and toluene were reported to be additive when inhaled simultaneously, as noted above (Dobrokhotov, 1972; Dobrokhotov & Enikeev, 1976), Gad-El-Karim *et al.* (1984) and Tice *et al.* (1980) found that toluene (which showed no clastogenic activity *per se*) antagonized the clastogenic activity of benzene when the mixture was administered to mice by inhalation.

Conflicting cytogenic observations have been reported for humans exposed to toluene. For example, Forni *et al.* (1971b) were unable to detect a significant increase in chromosome aberrations in 24 workers exposed to toluene for periods up to 15 years. Atmospheric concentrations during the period were generally close to the maximum allowable concentration of 760 mg/m^3, although workers were occasionally exposed to much higher concentrations. In some of these analyses, however, the blood was cultured for 72 h, making any firm conclusion difficult. The purity of toluene was not mentioned in those studies which reported toluene-induced myelotoxicity (Cohr & Stokholm, 1979).

Funes-Cravioto *et al.* (1977) observed an excess of lymphocyte chromosome aberrations (chromatid and isochromatid breaks) in 14 workers exposed only to toluene in a rotogravure printing factory, compared with controls. However, it was noted that the exposure background of this group may not have been well documented and hence a significant excess of chromosome aberrations could have been due to exposure to chemicals other than toluene (Mäki-Paakkanen *et al.*, 1980).

In a more recent study, peripheral blood lymphocytes from 32 male rotogravure workers exposed daily to toluene were examined for chromosome aberrations and SCE. Although neither of these parameters differed significantly from the corresponding frequencies in 15 unexposed control subjects, a significant increase in SCE was observed among smokers, both exposed and occupationally unexposed, compared to non-smoking referents (Mäki-Paakkanen *et al.*, 1980).

Haglund *et al.* (1980) reported chromosome analyses from paint-industry workers exposed to a mixture of organic solvents (mainly containing xylene or toluene). The frequency of structural chromosome aberrations in five workers with the highest exposure (toluene concentration > 100 mg/m^3) was found to be no different from that of their matched controls.

Bauchinger *et al.* (1982) reported cytogenetic analyses in peripheral lymphocytes from 20 male workers exposed only to toluene in a rotogravure plant for more than 16 years. Compared with a group of 24 unexposed controls, significantly higher yields of chromatid breaks, chromatid exchanges and gaps were observed. The number of SCEs was significantly increased in smoking and non-smoking toluene-exposed workers, compared with the corresponding control groups. These studies suggested that toluene or its metabolites (Dean, 1978) may induce a weak clastogenic effect in human lymphocytes *in vivo*. The observed chromosome changes in the study of Bauchinger *et al.* (1982) were of the chromatid types (breaks and exchanges) and the results further suggested an additive effect of smoking and toluene exposure on SCE frequency.

A recent study of Schmid *et al.* (1985) was carried out to determine whether recovery of chromosomal changes can be observed after cessation of toluene exposure. Chromosome analyses were determined in peripheral lymphocytes of 27 workers exposed to toluene in a rotogravure plant. At the time of blood sampling, none of the workers had been exposed to toluene for at least four months and some for as long as five years. Up to two years after cessation of exposure to toluene, a higher incidence of chromatid aberrations could be observed than in controls. After longer post-exposure periods, the aberration yields could no longer be distinguished from background levels. No differences were found in SCE frequencies of smoking or non-smoking workers, after toluene exposure, compared with the corresponding controls.

(b) Xylenes

Most studies of the xylenes have failed to disclose mutagenic activity. Xylene (nature of the isomer unspecified) was not mutagenic when tested in a battery of short-term tests including (1) gene mutation in *Salmonella typhimurium* TA98, TA100, TA1535, TA1537 and TA1538, with and without metabolic activation; (2) specific locus forward mutation induction in the L5178Y thymidine kinase mouse lymphoma cell assay, and (3) a test for mitotic gene conversion in yeast *Saccharomyces cerevisiae* D4. Additionally, xylene did not produce significant increases in chromosome aberrations in rat bone-marrow cells at levels of 0.044, 0.147 and 0.444 mg/kg body weight (Litton Bionetics, Inc., 1978).

In more recent studies (Bos *et al.*, 1981), *o-*, *m-* and *p*-xylene, as well as *o*-methylbenzyl alcohol and *o*-methylbenzyl sulfate, were found to be nonmutagenic when tested in *Salmonella typhimurium* strains TA1535, TA1537, TA1538, TA98 and TA100, either with or without metabolic activation by an S9 mix derived from the livers of rats, either untreated or induced with Aroclor 1254. Additionally, all these compounds, at concentrations ranging from 10^{-7} to 10^{-3} mol/L, did not evoke DNA excision repair in suspensions of freshly isolated rat hepatocytes (Bos *et al.*, 1981). Mixed isomers of xylene were found to lack mutagenic activity when tested in various *S. typhimurium* tester strains (Lebowitz *et al.*, 1979). Additionally, the xylene isomers were negative when tested in the mouse lymphoma L5178Y thymidine kinase forward mutation assay and when tested for chromosome damage in bone-marrow cells of rats after i.p. dosing with xylene.

Technical-grade xylol was inactive in the *E. coli* and *B. subtilis* DNA repair microsuspension assays (McCarroll *et al.*, 1981a,b). Technical-grade xylene (containing 18.3% ethylbenzene) caused recessive lethals ($0.01 < p < 0.05$) in *Drosophila*, while neither the pure isomers nor ethylbenzene caused an increase above the spontaneous recessive lethal frequency (Donner *et al.*, 1980).

No additional clastogenic effects were noted (when compared with control animals) when rats were exposed to atmospheric xylene (mixed isomers) at 1 320 mg/m^3, 6 h/day, 5 days a week for 9, 14 and 18 weeks (Donner *et al.*, 1980).

Gerner-Smidt and Friedrich (1978) found no increase either in the frequency of SCE or in the number of structural chromosomal aberrations in human lymphocytes *in vitro*. However, in these studies, it should also be noted that xylene and toluene, when given at the same concentrations (w/v) as benzene, inhibited cell growth, whereas benzene did not. These results, and those of Nomiyama (1964, 1965) and Boutwell (1967), suggest that the direct toxicity of xylene and toluene seems to be higher than that of benzene, whereas the metabolites of benzene are more toxic than the metabolites of the other two solvents.

GENOTOXICITY OF METABOLITES OF BENZENE, TOLUENE AND XYLENE

Metabolites of benzene

The metabolites of benzene (Figures 1 and 2) have been more extensively investigated than those of the two other aromatic hydrocarbons, in an attempt to further delineate the clastogenicity of benzene.

Conflicting data have been reported for the mutagenicity of phenol. While the earliest study (Demerec *et al.*, 1951) considered phenol to be mutagenic in the *E. coli*

B/Sd-4 assay and later studies reported the induction of mutations in *S. typhimurium* TA1538 in the presence of rat liver microsomal activation (Gocke *et al.,* 1981), a complete absence of mutagenic activity in the *Salmonella* assay using strains TA1535, TA1537, TA98 and TA100 was reported by Haworth *et al.* (1983), whose observations suggest that phenol is metabolized to a frameshift mutagen that is specifically active in strain TA1538. Phenol was inactive in *Drosophila* and in micronuclei production in mouse bone marrow (Gocke *et al.,* 1981). However, phenol induced a small increase in SCE in cultured human lymphocytes at a growth-inhibitory concentration of 10^{-3} mol/L (94 µg/mL) without metabolic activation. The incidence of SCE induction by this concentration of phenol was enhanced following S9 microsomal activation by Aroclor-induced rat liver (Morimoto & Wolff, 1980), suggesting that phenol is metabolized to DNA reactants (Morimoto & Wolff, 1980; Dean, 1985a). A significant increase in chromatid aberrations in mouse spermatogonia and primary spermatocytes following oral exposure to phenol has been reported (Bulsiewicz, 1977).

Although hydroquinone has been reported to be inactive in the *Salmonella*/microsomal assay by Haworth *et al.* (1983), Gocke *et al.* (1981) found a dose-related increase in mutations in strain TA1535 in the *absence* of metabolic activation, whereas the presence of S9 activation eliminated mutagenic activity. Hydroquinone induced SCE in cultured human lymphocytes in the absence of exogenous activation, and the incidence of SCE was increased by the incorporation of 3% S9 mixture (Morimoto *et al.,* 1983). Erexson *et al.* (1985), as noted earlier, reported that the metabolites of benzene (catechol, 1,4-benzoquinone, hydroquinone and 1,2,4-benzenetriol) induced significant concentration-related increases in SCE frequency, decreases in mitotic indices and inhibition of cell cycle kinetics in cultured human lymphocytes. Hydroquinone was also shown to induce micronuclei and to reduce cellularity in mouse bone marrow after repeated subcutaneous injections (Gocke *et al.,* 1981; Tunek *et al.,* 1982).

Catechol has been found to be inactive when examined in *Salmonella* tester strains TA1535, TA1537, TA98 and TA100 (Haworth *et al.,* 1983). It induced SCE in cultured human lymphocytes, both in the absence and presence of metabolic activation (Morimoto *et al.,* 1983). Erexson *et al.* (1985) found catechol to be the most potent of the benzene metabolites in the induction of SCEs in cultured human peripheral T-lymphocytes (see BENZENE, *Genotoxicity,* part *(c)*). Catechol did not induce micronuclei in mouse bone marrow (Tunek *et al.,* 1982).

Quinone metabolites formed by the oxidation of catechol and hydroquinone are toxic to lymphoid cells and bone marrow (Irons *et al.,* 1981; Pfeifer & Irons, 1981, 1982; Wierda & Irons, 1982). Quinones and semiquinones have been suggested to be the ultimate reactive metabolites of benzene in the liver (Tunek *et al.,* 1980), in human lymphocytes (Morimoto, 1983; Morimoto *et al.,* 1983) and in rabbit bone-marrow nuclei (Post *et al.,* 1985).

Metabolites of toluene and xylene

The metabolic pathways for toluene and xylene are illustrated in Figures 3 and 4, respectively. The isomeric cresols have been shown to induce anaphase aberrations and mitotic spindle anomalies in *Allium cepa* root tips (Sharma & Gosh, 1965) but were inactive when tested in *Salmonella*/microsomal assays (Nestmann *et al.*, 1980; Haworth *et al.*, 1983). In the study of Haworth *et al.* (1983), *ortho*-cresol was cytotoxic to most *Salmonella* strains when tested at 33 µg/plate, while the *meta* and *para* isomers were toxic at above 333 µg/plate.

Of the three isomers of cresol examined for the induction of SCE in cultured human fibroblasts and in various cells in DBA/2 mice at concentrations up to 30 mmol/L (3.2 µg/mL), only the *ortho* isomer was found to cause a small increase in SCE when cultures were treated at the 8 mmol/L level. All of the isomers of cresol were found to be cytotoxic above the 8 mmol/L level (Cheng & Kligerman, 1984).

No indication of SCE induction was found in bone marrow, alveolar macrophages or regenerating liver cells of male DBA/2 mice after single i.p. doses of 200 mg/kg *ortho*- or *meta*-cresol or 75 mg/kg *para*-cresol (Cheng & Kligerman, 1984).

The non-mutagenicity of *o*-methylbenzyl alcohol and *o*-methylbenzyl sulfate (metabolites of the xylenes) in various *Salmonella* tester strains, with and without metabolic activation, as well as in DNA excision repair assays in rat hepatocytes (Bos *et al.*, 1981) has been cited earlier.

REFERENCES

Amacher, D.E. & Zelljadt, J. (1983) The morphological transformation of Syrian hamster embryo cells by chemicals reportedly nonmutagenic to *Salmonella typhimurium*. *Carcinogenesis*, **4**, 291–295

Anderson, D. & Richardson, C.R. (1981) Issues relevant to the assessment of chemically induced chromosome damage in vivo and their relationship to chemical mutagenesis. *Mutat. Res.*, **90**, 261–272

Andrews, L.S., Sesame, H.A. & Gillette, J.R. (1979) ³H-Benzene metabolism in rabbit bone marrow. *Life Sci.*, **25**, 567–572

Angerer, J. (1979a) Chronische Lösungsmittelbelastung am Arbeitsplatz. V. Chromatographische Methoden zur Bestimmung von Phenolen im Harn. *Int. Arch. Occup. Environ. Health*, **42**, 257–268

Angerer, J. (1979b) Occupational chronic exposure to organic solvents. VII. Metabolism of toluene in man. *Int. Arch. Occup. Environ. Health*, **43**, 63–67

Archer, P. (1984) Some statistical and methodologic issues in cytogenic testing. In: Omenn, G.S. & Gelboin, H.V., eds, *Genetic Variability in Response to Chemical Exposure*, Cold Spring Harbor, NY, CSH Press, pp. 369–376

Ashby, J., de Serres, F.J., Draper, M., Ishidate, M., Jr, Margolin, B.J., Matter, B.E. & Shelby, M.D., eds (1985) *Evaluation of Short-term Tests for Carcinogens: Report on the International Program on Chemical Safety Collaborative Study on in vitro Assays*, Amsterdam, Elsevier

Astrand, I. (1975) Uptake of solvents in the blood and tissues of man: a review. *Scand. J. Work Environ. Health*, **1**, 199–218

Barale, R., Giorgelli, F., Migliore, L., Ciranni, R., Casini, D., Zucconi, D. & Loprieno, N. (1985) Benzene induces micronuclei in circulating erythrocytes of chronically treated mice. *Mutat. Res.*, **144**, 193–196

Barrett, R.H. (1985) Assays for unscheduled DNA synthesis in HeLa 53 cells. In: Ashby, J., de Serres, F.J., Draper, M., Ishidate, M., Jr, Margolin, B.H., Matter, B.E. & Shelby, M.D., eds, *Progress in Mutation Research,* Vol. 5, Amsterdam, Elsevier, pp. 347–352

Bartsch, H., Malaveille, C., Camus, A.M., Martel-Planche, G., Brun, G., Hautfeuille, A., Sabadie, N., Barbin, A., Kuroki, T., Drevon, C., Piccoli, C. & Montesano, R. (1980) Validation and comparative studies on 180 chemicals with *S. typhimurium* strains and V79 Chinese hamster cells in the presence of various metabolising systems. *Mutat. Res., 76,* 1–50

Bauchinger, M., Schmid, E., Dresp, J., Kolin-Gerresheim, J., Hauf, R. & Suhr, E. (1982) Chromosome changes in lymphocytes after occupational exposure to toluene. *Mutat. Res., 102,* 439–445

Bolcsak, L.E. & Nerland, D.E. (1983) Inhibition of erythropoiesis by benzene and benzene metabolites. *Toxicol. Appl. Pharmacol., 69,* 363–368

Bos, R.P., Brouns, R.M.E., van Doorn, R., Theuws, J.L.G. & Henderson, P.Th. (1981) Non-mutagenicity of toluene, *o-, m-* and *p*-xylene, *o*-methylbenzylalcohol and *o*-methylbenzylsulphate in the Ames assay. *Mutat. Res., 88,* 273–297

Boutwell, R.K. (1967) Phenolic compounds as tumour promoting agents. In: Finkle, B.J. & Runeckle V.C., eds, *Phenolic Compounds and Metabolic Regulation,* New York, Appleton-Century-Crofts, pp. 120–141

Bulsiewicz, H. (1977) The influence of phenol on chromosomes in mice (*Mus musculus*) in the process of spermatogenesis. *Folia Morphol. (Warsaw), 36,* 13–22

Carlone, M.F. & Fouts, J.R. (1974) In vitro metabolism of *p*-xylene by rabbit lung and liver. *Xenobiotica, 4,* 705

Cheng, M. & Kligerman, A.D. (1984) Evaluation of the genotoxicity of cresols using sister chromatid exchanges (SCE). *Mutat. Res., 137,* 51–55

Clement Associates (1977a) Toluene. In: *Information Dossiers on Substances Designated by TSCA Interagency Testing Committee (October, 1977).* Contract NSF-C-ENV-77-15417, Washington DC, December

Clement Associates (1977b) Xylenes. In: *Information Dossiers on Substances Designated by TSCA Interagency Testing Committee (October, 1977).* Contract NSF-C-ENV-77-15417, Washington DC, December

Cohr, K.H. & Stokholm, J. (1979) Toluene: a toxicological review. *Scand. J. Work Environ. Health, 5,* 71–90

Crespi, C.L., Ryan, C.G., Seixas, G.M., Turner, T.R. & Penman, B.W. (1985) Tests for mutagenic activity using mutation assays at two loci in the human lymphoblast cell lines TK 6 and AHH-1. In: Ashby, J., de Serres, F.J., Draper, M., Ishidate, M., Jr, Margolin, B.H., Matter, B.E. & Shelby, M.D., eds, *Progress in Mutation Research,* Vol. 5, Amsterdam, Elsevier, pp. 497–516

Danford, N.D. (1985) Tests for chromosome aberrations and aneuploidy in the Chinese hamster fibroblast cell line CH1-L. In: Ashby, J., de Serres, F.J., Draper, M., Ishidate, M., Jr, Margolin, B.H., Matter, B.E. & Shelby, M.D., eds, *Progress in Mutation Research,* Vol. 5, Amsterdam, Elsevier, pp. 397–411

Dean, B.J. (1978) Genetic toxicology of benzene, toluene, xylenes and phenols. *Mutat Res., 47,* 75–97

Dean, B.J. (1985a) Recent findings on the genetic toxicology of benzene, toluene, xylenes and phenols. *Mutat. Res., 154,* 153–181

Dean, B.J. (1985b) Summary report on the performance of cytogenetic assays in cultured mammalian cells. In: Ashby, J., de Serres, F.J., Draper, M., Ishidate, M., Jr, Margolin, B.H., Matter, B.E. & Shelby, M.D., eds, *Progress in Mutation Research,* Vol. *5,* Amsterdam, Elsevier, pp. 69–83

Demerec, M., Bertani, G. & Flint, J. (1951) A survey of chemicals for mutagenic activity in *E. coli. Am. Nat., 85,* 119–136

Dobrokhotov, V.B. (1972) The mutagenic effect of benzol and toluol under experimental conditions. *Gig. Sanit., 37,* 36–39

Dobrokhotov, V.B. & Enikeev, M.I. (1976) The mutagenic action of benzol, toluol and a mixture of these hydrocarbons in a chronic test. *Gig. Sanit., 41,* 32–34

Dobrokhotov, V.B. & Enikeev, M.I. (1977) Mutagenic effect of benzene, toluene and a mixture of these hydrocarbons in a chronic experiment. *Gig. Sanit., 42,* 32–34 (*Chem. Abstr., 86* (1977) 84355F)

Donner, M., Mäki-Paakkanen, J., Norppa, H., Sorsa, M. & Vainio, H. (1980) Genetic toxicology of xylenes. *Mutat. Res., 74,* 171–172

Donner, M., Husgafvel-Pursiainen, K., Mäki-Paakkanen, J., Sorsa, M. & Vainio, H. (1981) Genetic effects of in-vivo exposure to toluene. *Mutat. Res. 85,* 293–294

Erdogan, G. & Aksoy, M. (1973) Cytogenetic studies in thirteen patients with pancytopenia and leukemia associated with long-term exposure to benzene. *New Istanbul Contr. Clin. Sci., 10,* 230–247

Erexson, G.L., Wilmer, J.L. & Kligerman, A.D. (1985) Sister chromatid exchange induction in human lymphocytes exposed to benzene and its metabolites in vitro. *Cancer Res., 45,* 2471–2477

Erexson, G.L., Wilmer, J.L., Steinhagen, W.H. & Kligerman, A.D. (1986) Induction of cytogenic damage in rodents after short-term inhalation of benzene. *Environ. Mutagenesis, 8,* 29–40

Ferguson, L.R. (1985) Petite mutagenesis in *Saccharomyces cerevisiae* strain D$_5$. In: Ashby, J., de Serres, F.J., Draper, M., Ishidate, M., Jr, Margolin, B.H., Matter, B.E. & Shelby, M.D., eds, *Progress in Mutation Research,* Vol. *5,* Amsterdam, Elsevier, pp. 225–234

Fishbein, L. (1984a) An overview of environmental and toxicological aspects of aromatic hydrocarbons. I. Benzene. *Sci. Total Environ., 40,* 189–218

Fishbein, L. (1984b) An overview of environmental and toxicological aspects of aromatic hydrocarbons. II. Toluene. *Sci. Total Environ., 42,* 267–288

Fishbein, L. (1985) An overview of environmental and toxicological aspects of aromatic hydrocarbons. III. Xylene. *Sci. Total Environ., 43,* 165–183

Flek, J. & Sedivec, V. (1975) Metabolism of isomeric xylene in man. *Prac. Lek., 27,* 9–16

Forni, A.M., Cappellini, A., Pacifico, E. & Vigliani, E.C. (1971a) Chromosome changes and their evolution in subjects with past exposure to benzene. *Arch. Environ. Health, 23,* 385–391

Forni, A., Pacifico, E. & Limonta, A. (1971b) Chromosome studies in workers exposed to benzene or toluene or both. *Arch. Environ. Health, 22,* 373–378

Fujikawa, K., Ryo, H. & Kondo, S. (1985) The Drosophila gene mutation and small deletion assay using the *zeste-white* somatic eye colour system. In: Ashby, J., de Serres, F.J., Draper, M., Ishidate, M., Jr, Margolin, B.H., Matter, B.E. & Shelby, M.D., eds, *Progress in Mutation Research,* Vol. *5,* Amsterdam, Elsevier, pp. 319–324

Funes-Cravioto, F., Kolmodin-Hedman, B., Lindsten, J., Nordenskjold, M., Zapata-Gayon, C., Lambert, B., Norberg, E., Olin, R. & Svensson, A. (1977) Chromosome aberrations and sister chromatid exchanges in workers in chemical laboratories and a rotoprinting factory and in children of women laboratory workers. *Lancet, ii,* 322

Gad-El-Karim, M.M., Harper, B.L. & Legator, M.S. (1984) Modifications in the myeloclastogenic effect of benzene in mice with toluene, phenobarbital, 3-methyl-cholanthrene, Aroclor 1254 and SKF-525A. *Mutat. Res., 135,* 225–243

Gad-El-Karim, M.M., Ramanujam, S., Ahmed, A.E. & Legator, M.S. (1985) Benzene myeloclastogenicity: a function of its metabolism. *Am. J. Ind. Med., 7,* 475–484

Garner, R.C. (1985) Summary report on the performance of gene mutation assays in mammalian cells in culture. In: Ashby, J., de Serres, F.J., Draper, M., Ishidate, M., Jr, Margolin, B.H., Matter, B.E. & Shelby, M.D., eds, *Progress in Mutation Research,* Vol. *5,* Amsterdam, Elsevier, pp. 85–94

Gerner-Smidt, P. & Friedrich, U. (1978) The mutagenic effect of benzene, toluene and xylene studied by the SCE technique. *Mutat. Res., 58,* 313–316

Gill, D.P. & Ahmed, A.E. (1981) Covalent binding of ^{14}C-benzene to cellular organelles and bone-marrow nucleic acids. *Biochem. Pharmacol., 30,* 1127–1131

Glauert, H.P., Kennan, W.S., Sattler, G.L. & Pitot, H.C. (1985) Assays to measure the induction of unscheduled DNA synthesis in cultured hepatocytes. In: Ashby, J., de Serres, F.J., Draper, M., Ishidate, M., Jr, Margolin, B.H., Matter, B.E. & Shelby, M.D., eds, *Progress in Mutation Research,* Vol. *5,* Amsterdam, Elsevier, pp. 371–379

Gocke, E., King, M.T., Cekhart, K. & Wild, D. (1981) Mutagenicity of cosmetic ingredients licensed by the European Communities. *Mutat. Res., 90,* 91–109

Goldstein, B.D. (1984) Clinical hematotoxicity of benzene, In: Mehlman, M.A., ed., *Carcinogenicity and Toxicity of Benzene,* Princeton, NJ, Princeton Scientific Publishers, pp. 51–61

Goldstein, B.D., Snyder, C.A. & Larkin, S. (1982) Myelogenous leukemia in rodents inhaling benzene. *Toxicol. Lett., 13,* 169–173

Greenlee, W.F., Gross, E.A. & Irons, R.D. (1981a) Relationship between benzene toxicity and the disposition of ^{14}C-labeled benzene metabolites in the rat. *Chem.-Biol. Interact., 33,* 345–360

Greenlee, W.F., Sun, J.D. & Bus, J.S. (1981b) A proposed mechanism for benzene toxicity: formation of reactive intermediates for polyphenol metabolites. *Toxicol. Appl. Pharmacol., 58,* 187–195

Haglund, U., Lundberg, J. & Zech, L. (1980) Chromosome aberrations and sister chromatid exchanges in Swedish paint industry workers. *Scand. J. Work Environ. Health, 6,* 291–298

Harper, B.L., Ramanujam, S., Gad-El-Karim, M.M. & Legator, M.S. (1984) The influence of simple aromatics on benzene clastogenicity. *Mutat. Res., 128,* 105–114

Harper, C., Drew, R.T. & Fouts, J.R. (1975) In: Jollow, D.J., Kocsis, J.J., Snyder, R. & Vainio, H., eds, *Biological Reactive Intermediates,* London, Plenum Press, pp. 302–311

Hartwich, G. & Schwanitz, G. (1972) Chromosome studies after chronic benzol exposure. *Dtsch. Med. Wochenschr., 77,* 149–155

Haworth, S., Lawler, T., Mortelsmans, K., Speck, W. & Zeiger, E. (1983) Salmonella mutagenicity test results for 250 chemicals. *Environ. Mutagenesis, 5,* 3–142

Hite, M., Pecharo, M., Smith, I. & Thornton, S. (1980) The effect of benzene in the micronucleus test. *Mutat. Res., 77,* 149–155

Howard, C.A., Sheldon, T. & Richardson, C.R. (1985) Chromosomal analysis of human lymphocytes exposed in vitro to five chemicals. In: Ashby, J., de Serres, F.J., Draper, M., Ishidate, M., Jr, Margolin, B.H., Matter, B.E. & Shelby, M.D., eds, *Progress in Mutation Research,* Vol. 5, Amsterdam, Elsevier, pp. 457–467

HSE (1982) *Toxicity Review – Benzene,* London, Her Majesty's Stationery Office

Humperdinck, J. (1954) Besondere Form der Knochenmarkschädigung bei einem Tiefdrucker. *Berufsgenossensch,* p. 89

IARC (1982a) *IARC Monographs on the Evaluation of the Carcinogenic Risk of Chemicals to Humans,* Vol. 29, *Some Industrial Chemicals and Dyestuffs,* Lyon, International Agency for Research on Cancer, pp. 93–148

IARC (1982b) *IARC Monographs on the Evaluation of the Carcinogenic Risk of Chemicals to Humans,* Suppl. 4, *Chemicals, Industrial Processes and Industries Associated with Cancer in Humans. IARC Monographs, Volumes 1 to 29,* Lyon, International Agency for Research on Cancer, pp. 56–57

Ikeda, M., Ohtsuji, H. & Imamura, T. (1972) In vivo suppression of benzene and styrene oxidation by co-administered toluene in rats and effects of phenobarbitol. *Xenobiotica, 2,* 101

Irons, R.D. & Moore, B.J. (1980) Effect of short-term benzene administration on circulating lymphocyte subpopulations in the rabbit: evidence of a selective B-lymphocyte sensitivity. *Res. Commun. Chem. Pathol. Pharmacol., 27,* 147–155

Irons, R.D. & Neptun, D.A. (1980) Effects of the principal hydroxymetabolites of benzene on microtubule polymerization. *Arch. Toxicol., 45,* 297–305

Irons, R.D., Dent, J.G., Baker, T.S. & Rickert, D.E. (1980) Benzene is metabolized and covalently bound in bone marrow in situ. *Chem.-Biol. Interact., 30,* 241–245

Irons, R.D., Neptun, D.A. & Pfeifer, R.W. (1981) Inhibition of lymphocyte transformation and microtubule assembly by quinone metabolites of benzene: evidence for a common mechanism. *J. Reticuloendothel. Soc., 30,* 359–371

Irons, R.D., Greenlee, W.F., Wierda, D. & Bus, J.S. (1982) Relationship between benzene metabolism and toxicity: a proposed mechanism for the formation of reactive intermediates from polyphenol metabolites. In: Snyder, R., Parke, D.V., Kocsis, J.J., Jollow, D.J., Gibson, G.G. & Witmer, C.M., eds, *Biological Reactive Intermediates – II,* New York, Plenum Press, pp. 229–243

Ishidate M., Jr & Sofuni, T. (1985) The in vitro chromosome aberration test using Chinese hamster lung (CHL) fibroblast cells in culture. In: Ashby, J., de Serres, F.J., Draper, M., Ishidate, M., Jr, Margolin, B.H., Matter, B.E. & Shelby, M.D., eds, *Progress in Mutation Research,* Vol. 5, Amsterdam, Elsevier, pp. 427–432

Jerina, D.M. & Daly, J.W. (1974) Arene oxides: a new aspect of drug metabolism. *Science, 185*, 573–582

Jerina, D.M., Daly, J.W. & Witkop, B. (1968) The role of arene oxide-oxepin systems in the metabolism of aromatic substrates. II. Synthesis of 3,4-toluene-4-^{2}H oxide and subsequent "NIH shift" to 4-hydroxy toluene-3-^{2}H. *J. Am. chem. Soc., 90*, 6523–6525

Johansson, I. & Ingelman-Sundberg, M. (1983) Radical-mediated, cytochrome P-450 dependent metabolic activation of benzene in microsomes and reconstituted enzyme systems from rabbit liver. *J. Biol. Chem., 258*, 7311–7316

Kale, P.G. & Baum, J.W. (1983) Genetic effects of benzene in *Drosophila melanogaster* males. *Mutagenesis, 5*, 223–226

Kalf, G.F., Rushmore, T. & Snyder, R. (1982) Benzene inhibits RNA synthesis in mitochondria from liver and bone marrow. *Chem.-Biol. Interact., 42*, 353–370

Kalf, G.F., Snyder, R. & Rushmore, T.H. (1985) Inhibition of RNA synthesis by benzene metabolites and their covalent binding to DNA in rabbit bone marrow mitochondria in vitro. *Am. J. Ind. Med., 7*, 485–492

Khan, J. & Khan, M.H. (1973) Cytogenetic studies following chronic exposure to benzene. *Arch. Toxicol., 31*, 39–49

Lauwerys, R.R. (1983) *Industrial Chemical Exposure Guidelines for Biological Monitoring,* Davis, CA, Biomedical Publications

Lebowitz, H., Brusick, D., Matheson, D., Jagannath, D.R., Reed, M., Goode, S. & Roy, G. (1979) Commonly used fuels and solvents evaluated in a battery of short-term bioassays. *Environ. Mutagenesis, 1*, 172–173

Lee, F.W., Kocsis, J.J. & Snyder, R. (1974) Acute effect of benzene on ^{59}Fe incorporation into circulating erythrocytes. *Toxicol. Appl. Pharmacol., 27*, 431–436

Litton Bionetics, Inc. (1978) *Mutagenicity Evaluation of Toluene. Final Report Submitted to the American Petroleum Institute,* Washington, DC, LBI Project No. 20847, Kensington, MD, May

Lüers, H. & Obe, G. (1972) Zur Frage einer möglichen mutagenen Wirksamkeit von p-Benzochinon. *Mutat. Res., 15*, 77–80

Luke, C.A., Tice, R.R. & Drew, R.T. (1985) Duration and regimen induced micronuclei in the peripheral blood of mice exposed chronically to benzene. *Environ. Mutagenesis, 7*, Suppl. 3, 29

Lutz, W.K. & Schlatter, C.H. (1977) Mechanism of the carcinogenic action of benzene: irreversible binding to rat liver DNA. *Chem.-Biol. Interact., 18*, 241–245

Lyapkalo, A.A. (1973) Genetic activity of benzene and toluene. *Gig. Tr. Prof. Zabol., 17*, 24–28

Mäki-Paakkanen, J., Husgafvel-Pursiainen, K., Kalliomaki, P.L., Tuominen, J. & Sorsa, M. (1980) Toluene-exposed workers and chromosome aberrations. *J. Toxicol. Environ. Health, 6*, 775–781

Maltoni, C., Cotti, G., Valgimigli, L. & Mandrioli, A. (1982) Zymbal gland carcinomas in rats following exposure to benzene by inhalation. *Am. J. Ind. Med., 3*, 11–16.

Maltoni, C., Conti, B. & Cotti, G. (1983) Benzene: a multipotential carcinogen. Results of long-term bioassays performed at the Bologna Institute of Oncology. *Am. J. Ind. Med., 4*, 589–630

Maltoni, C., Conti, B., Cotti, G. & Belpoggi, F. (1985) Experimental studies on benzene carcinogenicity at the Bologna Institute of Oncology: current results on ongoing research. *Am. J. Ind. Med., 7,* 415–446

Martin, C.N. & Campbell, J. (1985) Tests for the induction of unscheduled DNA synthesis in HeLa cells. In: Ashby, J., de Serres, F.J., Draper, M., Ishidate, M., Jr, Margolin, B.H., Matter, B.E. & Shelby, M.D., eds, *Progress in Mutation Research,* Vol. *5,* Amsterdam, Elsevier, pp. 375–379

McCarroll, N.E., Piper, C.E. & Keech, B.H. (1980) Bacterial microsuspension assays with benzene and other organic solvents. *Environ. Mutagenesis, 2,* 281–282

McCarroll, N.E., Keech, B.H. & Piper, C.E. (1981a) A microsuspension adaptation of the *Bacillus subtilis* 'rec' assay. *Environ. Mutagenesis, 3,* 607–616

McCarroll, N.E., Piper, C.E. & Keech, B.H. (1981b) An *E. coli* microsuspension assay for the detection of DNA damage induced by direct-acting agents and promutagens. *Environ. Mutagenesis, 3,* 429–444

McGregor, D. & Ashby, J. (1985) Summary report on the performance of the cell transformation assays. In: Ashby, J., de Serres, F.J., Draper, M., Ishidate, M., Jr, Margolin, B.H., Matter, B.E. & Shelby, M.D., eds, *Progress in Mutation Research,* Vol. *5,* Amsterdam, Elsevier, pp. 103–115

Meyne, J. & Legator, M.S. (1980) Sex-related differences in cytogenetic effects of benzene in the bone marrow of Swiss mice. *Environ. Mutagenesis, 2,* 43–50

Mohtashamipur, E., Norpoth, K., Woelke, U. & Huber, P. (1985) Effects of ethylbenzene, toluene and xylene on the induction of micronuclei in bone marrow polychromatic erythrocytes in mice. *Arch. Toxicol., 58,* 106–109

Morimoto, K. (1983) Induction of sister chromatid exchanges and cell division delays in human lymphocytes by microsomal activation of benzene. *Cancer Res., 43,* 1330–1334

Morimoto, K. & Wolff, S. (1980) Increase of sister chromatid exchanges and perturbations of cell division kinetics in human lymphocytes by benzene metabolites. *Cancer Res., 40,* 1189–1193

Morimoto, K., Wolff, S. & Koizumi, A. (1983) Induction of sister-chromatid exchanges in human lymphocytes by microsomal activation of benzene metabolites. *Mutat. Res., 119,* 355–360

NAS (1982) *Alkylbenzenes,* Washington DC, National Academy of Sciences

National Research Council (1976) *Health Effects of Benzene: A Review,* Washington DC, National Academy of Sciences

National Toxicology Program (1984) *Technical Report on the Toxicology and Carcinogenesis Studies of Benzene (CAS No. 71-43-2) in F344/N Rats and B6C3F-1 Mice (Gavage Studies), NTP-TR-289,* Bethesda, MD, National Institute of Health

Nestmann, R.R., Lee, E.G.-H., Matula, T.I., Douglas, G.R. & Mueller, J.C. (1980) Mutagenicity of constituents identified in pulp and paper mill effluents using the Salmonella/mammalian-microsome assay. *Mutat. Res., 79,* 203–212

Nomiyama, K. (1964) Benzene poisoning. *Bull. Tokyo Med. Dent. Univ., 11,* 297–312

Nomiyama, K. (1965) Toxicity of benzene metabolites to hemopoiesis. *Ind. Health (Japan), 3,* 53–57

Nylander, P.O., Olofsson, H., Rasmuson, B. & Svahlin, H. (1978) Mutagenic effects of petrol in *Drosophila melanogaster*. I. Effects of benzene and 1,2-dichloroethane. *Mutat. Res., 57*, 163–167

Obe, G., Hille, A., Jonas, R., Schmidt, S. & Thenhaus, U. (1985) Tests for the induction of sister-chromatid exchanges in human peripheral lymphocytes in culture. In: Ashby., J., de Serres, F.J., Draper, M., Ishidate, M., Jr, Margolin, B.H., Matter, B.E. & Shelby, M.D., eds, *Progress in Mutation Research, Vol. 5*, Amsterdam, Elsevier, pp. 439–450

Oberly, T.J., Bewsey, B.J. & Probst, G.S. (1985) Tests for the induction of forward mutation at the thymidine kinase locus of L5178Y mouse lymphoma cells in culture. In: Ashby, J., de Serres, F.J., Draper, M., Ishidate, M., Jr, Margolin, B.H., Matter, B.E. & Shelby, M.D., eds, *Progress in Mutation Research, Vol. 5*, Amsterdam, Elsevier, pp. 569–576

Ogata, M., Tomokuni, K. & Takatsuka, Y. (1970) Urinary excretion of hippuric acid and *m*- or *p*-methyl hippuric acid in the urine of workers exposed to vapors of toluene and *m*- or *p*-xylene as a test of exposure. *Br. J. Ind. Med., 27*, 43

Palitti, F., Fiore, M., De Silva, R., Tanzarella, C., Ricordi, R., Forster, R., Mosesso, P., Astolfi, S. & Loprieno, N. (1985) Chromosome aberration assays of 5 chemicals in Chinese hamster cells in vitro. In: Ashby, J., de Serres, F.J., Draper, M., Ishidate, M., Jr, Margolin, B.H., Matter, B.E. & Shelby, M.D., eds, *Progress in Mutation Research, Vol. 5*, Amsterdam, Elsevier, pp. 443–450

Parry, J.M. (1985) Summary report on the performance of the yeast and Aspergillus assays. In: Ashby, J., de Serres, F.J., Draper, M., Ishidate, M., Jr, Margolin, B.H., Matter, B.E. & Shelby, M.D., eds, *Progress in Mutation Research, Vol. 5*, Amsterdam, Elsevier, pp. 25–46

Parry, J.M. & Eckardt, F. (1985a) The induction of mitotic aneuploidy, point mutation and mitotic crossing-over in the yeast, *Saccharomyces cerevisiae* strains D61-M and D6, In: Ashby, J., de Serres, F.J., Draper, M., Ishidate, M., Jr, Margolin, B.H., Matter, B.E. & Shelby, M.D., eds, *Progress in Mutation Research, Vol. 5*, Amsterdam, Elsevier, pp. 261–269

Parry, J.M. & Eckhardt, F. (1985b) The detection of mitotic gene conversion, point mutation and mitotic segregation using the yeast *Saccharomyces cerevisiae* strain D7. In: Ashby, J., de Serres, F.J., Draper, M., Ishidate, M., Jr, Margolin, B.H., Matter, B.E. & Shelby, M.D., eds, *Progress in Mutation Research, Vol. 5*, Elsevier, Amsterdam, pp. 270–277

Pellack-Walker, P., Walker, J.K., Evans, H.H. & Blumer, J.L. (1985) Relationship between the oxidation potential of benzene metabolites and their inhibitory effect on DNA synthesis in L5178YS cells. *Mol. Pharmacol., 28*, 560–566

Pfeifer, R.W. & Irons, R.D. (1981) Inhibition of lectin-stimulated lymphocyte agglutination and mitogenesis by hydroquinone: reactivity with intracellular sulfhydryl groups. *Exp. Mol. Pathol., 35*, 189–198

Pfeifer, R.W. & Irons, R.D. (1982) Effects of benzene metabolites on photohemagglutinin-stimulated lymphoporesis in rat bone marrow. *J. Reticuloendothel. Soc., 31*, 155–170

Philip, P. & Krogh Jensen, M. (1970) Benzene induced chromosome abnormalities in rat bone marrow cells. *Acta Pathol. Microbiol. Scand.* A, *78*, 489–490

Picciano, D.J. (1979) Cytogenic study of workers exposed to benzene. *Environ. Res.,* **19,** 33–38

Picciano, D.J. (1980) Monitoring industrial populations by cytogenetic procedures. In: Infante, P.F. & Legator, M.S., eds, *Proceedings of a Workshop on Methodology for Assessing Reproductive Hazards in the Workplace,* Washington DC, US Government Printing Office, pp. 293–306

Post, G.B., Snyder, R. & Kalf, B.F. (1985) Inhibition of RNA synthesis and interleukin-2 production in lymphocytes in vitro by benzene and its metabolites, hydroquinone and *p*-benzoquinone. *Toxicol. Lett.,* **29,** 161–167

Probst, G.S., McMahon, R.E., Holl, L.E., Thompson, C.Z., Epp, J.K. & Neal, S.B. (1981) Chemically-induced DNA synthesis in primary rat hepatocyte cultures: a comparison with bacterial mutagenicity using 218 compounds. *Environ. Mutagenesis, 3,* 11–32

Rickert, D.E., Baker, T.S., Bus, J.S., Barrow, C.S. & Irons, R.D. (1979) Benzene disposition in the rat after exposure by inhalation. *Toxicol. Appl. Pharmacol.,* **49,** 417–423

Rickert, D.E., Baker, T.S. & Chism, J.P. (1981) Analytical approaches to the study of the disposition of myelotoxic agents. *Environ. Health Perspect.,* **39,** 5–10

Riihimäki, V., Pfaffli, P., Savolainen, K. & Pekari, K. (1979) Kinetics of *m*-xylene in man. General features of absorption, distribution, biotransformation and excretion in repetitive inhalation exposure. *Scand. J. Work Environ. Health, 5,* 217–231

Rinsky, R.A., Young, R.J. & Smith, A.B. (1981) Leukemia in benzene workers. *Am. J. Ind. Med., 2,* 217–245

Robberson, D.L., Gay, M.D. & Wilkins, C.E. (1981) Genetically altered human mitochondrial DNA and a cytoplasmic view of malignant transformation. In: Arrighs, F.E., Rao, P.N. & Stubblefield, E., eds, *Genes, Chromosomes and Neoplasia,* New York, Raven Press, pp. 125–156

Rusch, G.M., Leong, B.K.J. & Laskin, S. (1977) Benzene metabolism. *J. Toxicol. Environ. Health, 2* (Suppl.), 23–36

Sawahata, T. & Neal, R.A. (1982) Horseradish peroxidase-mediated oxidation of phenol. *Biochem. Biophys. Res. Commun., 109,* 988–994

Sawahata, T., Rickert, D.E. & Greenlee, W.F. (1985) Metabolism of benzene and its metabolites in bone marrow. In: Irons, R.D., ed., *Toxicology of the Blood,* New York, Raven Press, pp. 41–48

Schmid, E., Bauchinger, M. & Hauf, R. (1985) Chromosome changes in time in lymphocytes after occupational exposure to toluene. *Mutat. Res., 142,* 37–39

Schwartz, C.S., Snyder, R. & Kalf, G.F. (1985) The inhibition of mitochondrial DNA replication in vitro by the metabolites of benzene, hydroquinone and *p*-benzoquinone. *Chem. Biol. Interact., 53,* 327–350

Sedivec, V. & Flek, J. (1976a) The absorption, metabolism and excretion of xylenes in man. *Int. Arch. Occup. Environ. Health, 37,* 205–217

Sedivec, V. & Flek, J. (1976b) Exposure test for xylenes. *Int. Arch. Occup. Environ. Health, 37,* 219–232

Sharma, A.K. & Gosh, S. (1965) Chemical basis of the action of cresols and nitrophenols on chromosomes. *Nucleus (Calcutta), 8,* 183–190

Shimizu, M., Yasui, Y. & Matsumoto, N. (1983) Structural specificity of aromatic compounds with special reference to mutagenic activity in *Salmonella typhimurium:* a series of chloro- or fluoro-nitrobenzene derivatives. *Mutat. Res., 116,* 217–238

Siou, G., Conan, L. & El Haitem, M. (1981) Evaluation of the clastogenic action of benzene by oral administration with two cytogenetic techniques in mouse and Chinese hamster. *Mutat. Res., 90,* 273–278

Siou, G., Conan, L. & Haitem, M. (1982) Comparative study of the effect of the carcinogens benzene and methyl methane sulfonate on the mouse and Chinese hamster. *Environ. Qual. Life, 15,* 353–359

Snyder, C.A., Goldstein, B.D., Sellakumar, A.R., Bromberg, I., Laskin, S. & Albert, R.E. (1980) The inhalation toxicology of benzene: incidence of hematopoietic neoplasms and hematotoxicity in AKR/J and C57BL/6J mice. *Toxicol. Appl. Pharmacol., 54,* 323–331

Snyder, R. & Kocsis, J.J. (1975) Current concepts of chronic benzene toxicity. *CRC Crit. Rev. Toxicol., 3,* 265–288

Snyder, R., Longacre, S.C., Witmer, C.M. & Kocsis, J.J. (1982a) Metabolic correlates of benzene toxicity. In: Snyder, R., Parke, D.V., Kocsis, J.J., Jollow, D.J., Gibson, G. & Witmer, C.M., eds, *Biological Reactive Intermediates,* New York, Plenum Press, pp. 245–256

Snyder, R., Sammett, D., Witmer, C. & Kocsis, J.J. (1982b) An overview of the problem of benzene toxicity and some recent data on the relationship of benzene metabolism to benzene toxicity. *Environ. Sci. Res., 25,* 225–240

Styles, J.A. & Richardson, C.R. (1984) Cytogenetic effects of benzene: dosimetric studies on rats exposed to benzene vapour. *Mutat. Res., 135,* 203–209

Tice, R.R., Costa, D.L. & Drew, R.T. (1980) Cytogenetic effects of benzene in murine bone marrow: induction of sister chromatid exchanges, chromosomal aberrations and cellular proliferation inhibition in DBA/2 mice. *Proc. Natl. Acad. Sci. USA, 4,* 2148–2152

Tice, R.R., Sawey, M.J., Drew, R.T. & Cronkite, E.P. (1984) Benzene-induced, micronuclei in the peripheral blood of mice: a retrospective analysis. *Environ. Mutagenesis, 6,* 421

Toft, K., Olofsson, T., Tunek, A. & Berlin, M. (1982) Toxic effects on mouse bone-marrow caused by inhalation of benzene. *Arch. Toxicol., 51,* 295–302

Toftgard, R. & Gustafsson, J.A. (1980) Biotransformation of organic solvents. A review. *Scand. J. Work Environ. Health, 6,* 1–18

Tunek, A., Platt, K.L., Bentley, P. & Oesch, F. (1978) Microsomal metabolism of benzene to species irreversibly binding to microsomal protein and effects of modification of this metabolism. *Mol. Pharmacol., 14,* 920–929

Tunek, A., Platt, K.L., Przybyski, M. & Oesch, F. (1980) Multi-step metabolic activation of benzene. Effect of superoxide dismutase on covalent binding to microsomal macromolecules, and identification of glutathione conjugates using high-pressure liquid chromatography and field desorption spectrometry. *Chem.-Biol. Interact., 33,* 1–17

Tunek, A., Olofsson, T. & Berlin, M. (1981) Toxic effects of benzene and benzene metabolites on granulopoietic stem cells and bone marrow cellularity in mice. *Toxicol. Appl. Pharmacol., 59,* 149–156

Tunek, A., Högstedt, B. & Olofsson, T. (1982) Mechanism of benzene toxicity. Effects of benzene and benzene metabolites on bone marrow cellularity, number of granulopoietic stem cells and frequency of micronuclei in mice. *Chem.-Biol. Interact., 39,* 129–138

Van den Berghe, H., Louwagie, A., Broeckaert-van Orshoren, A., David, G. & Verwilghen, R. (1979) Chromosome analysis in two unusual malignant blood disorders presumably induced by benzene. *Blood, 53,* 558

Van Raalte, H.G.S. & Grasso, P. (1982) Hematological, myelotoxic, clastogenic, carcinogenic and leukemogenic effects of benzene. *Regul. Toxicol. Pharmacol., 2,* 153–176

Venitt, S. (1985) Summary report of the performance of the bacterial mutation assays. In: Ashby, J., de Serres, F.J., Draper, M., Ishidate, M., Jr, Margolin, B.H., Matter, B.E. & Shelby, M.D., eds, *Progress in Mutation Research,* Vol. *5,* Amsterdam, Elsevier, pp. 11–23

Vianna, N.J. & Polan, A. (1979) Lymphomas and occupational benzene exposure. *Lancet, i,* 1394–1395

Vigliani, E.C. (1976) Leukemia associated with benzene exposure. *Ann. N.Y. Acad. Sci., 271,* 134–151

Vogel, E.W. (1985a) Summary report on the performance of the Drosophila assays. In: Ashby, J., de Serres, F.J., Draper, M., Ishidate, M., Jr, Margolin, B.H., Matter, B.E. & Shelby, M.D., eds, *Progress in Mutation Research,* Vol. *5,* Amsterdam, Elsevier, pp. 47–57

Vogel, E.W. (1985b) The Drosophila somatic recombination and mutation assay using the white-coral somatic eye colour system. In: Ashby, J., de Serres, F.J., Draper, M., Ishidate, M., Jr, Margolin, B.H., Matter, B.E. & Shelby, M.D., eds, *Progress in Mutation Research,* Vol. *5,* Amsterdam, Elsevier, pp. 313–317

Watanabe, T., Endo, A., Kato, Y., Shima, S., Watanabe, T. & Ikeda, M. (1980) Cytogenetics and cytokinetics of cultured lymphocytes from benzene-exposed workers. *Int. Arch. Occup. Environ. Health, 46,* 31–41

WHO (1981a) *Recommended health based limits in occupational exposure to selected organic solvents.* WHO Technical Reports Series No. 664. Geneva, World Health Organization, pp. 7–24

WHO (1981b) Xylene, In: *Recommended health based limits in occupational exposure to selected organic solvents.* WHO Technical Report Series No. 664. Geneva, World Health Organization, pp. 25–38

Wierda, D. & Irons, R.D. (1982) Hydroquinone and catechol reduce the frequency of progenitor B and lymphocytes in mouse spleen and bone marrow. *Immunopharmacology, 4,* 41–54

Williams, G.M., Tong, C. & Brat, S.V. (1985) Tests with the rat hepatocyte primary culture/DNA repair test. In: Ashby, J., de Serres, F.J., Draper, M., Ishidate, M., Jr, Margolin, B.H., Matter, B.E. & Shelby, M.D., eds, *Progress in Mutation Research,* Vol. *5,* Amsterdam, Elsevier, pp. 341–345

Wilson, R.H. (1943) Toluene poisoning. *J. Am. Med. Assoc., 123,* 1106

Woiwode, W.R., Wordarz, K. & Weichardt, H. (1979) Metabolism of toluene in man: gas chromatographic determination of *o-, m-* and *p-*cresol in urine. *Arch. Toxicol., 43,* 93–98

CHAPTER 3

TOXICOKINETICS OF BENZENE, TOLUENE AND XYLENES

A. Sato

Department of Environmental Health
Medical University of Yamanashi
Tamaho, Yamanashi 409-38
Japan

PHARMACOKINETIC PRINCIPLES FOR BENZENE, TOLUENE AND XYLENES

A biologically toxic substance elicits its action by binding to biological membranes, enzymes, DNA, etc., in the target tissue. The kind of toxicity it produces depends on the type of macromolecule with which it or its metabolites associate, but the intensity and duration of the toxic response are mainly dependent on the extent of association, which is determined by the concentration of the chemical or its metabolites at the site of action (Levy & Gibaldi, 1972; Gillette *et al.*, 1974). The kinetics of absorption, distribution, metabolism and excretion is therefore a very important aspect of the toxicology of foreign chemicals.

Benzene, toluene and xylenes are highly volatile and thus enter a living body chiefly through the respiratory route, with some of the absorbed fractions being excreted into expired air. The amount entering the body through the skin is considerable when the skin is directly in contact with the solvents in liquid form (Dutkiewicz & Tyras, 1968a,b; Engstrom *et al.*, 1977; Lauwerys *et al.*, 1978; Sato & Nakajima, 1978), but is negligible when the skin is exposed to air containing solvent vapours, absorption then amounting in most cases to less than 5% of that entering through the lungs (Piotrowski, 1967; Riihimäki & Pfaffli, 1978).

Figure 1 illustrates the pharmacokinetics of organic solvent vapours (Sato *et al.*, 1974a). When inhaled, the vapours in lung alveoli diffuse into the blood according to Henry's law. They are transported throughout the body by the circulatory system and distributed among the various body tissues. Some portion of the vapours is enzymatically transformed into metabolites with polar functions and finally excreted into the urine, after conjugation with glucuronic acid, sulfuric acid or glycine. Some fractions of the vapours return to the lungs *via* the venous blood and contribute to the equilibration process occurring at the alveoli. During inhalation (saturation

Fig. 1. Factors affecting pharmacokinetic processes involving organic solvent vapours in a living body
(Sato *et al.*, 1972, 1974a)

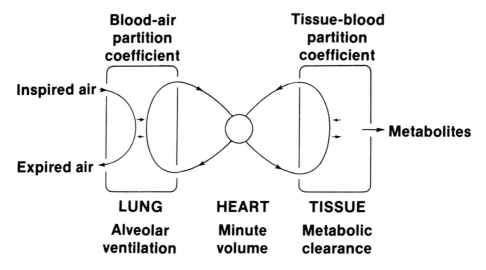

process), the alveolar, arterial, tissue and venous tensions gradually rise towards eventual equilibrium throughout the body. When a vapour is removed from the inspired air (desaturation process), the reverse occurs and the tensions gradually fall to zero.

The most important factor governing the pulmonary absorption or excretion is the partition coefficient between air and blood, which is defined as the concentration ratio of a vapour between blood and air at a defined temperature, and is numerically equal to the Ostwald solubility coefficient at that temperature (Larson, 1963; Åstrand, 1975; Sato & Nakajima, 1979a). A vapour with a high partition coefficient enters the body easily and achieves a high level of accumulation in the body because of its slow elimination from the lungs. A vapour with a low coefficient, on the contrary, cannot stay long in the body because of its rapid elimination into the expired air. Table 1 shows partition coefficients of benzene, toluene and xylenes between air and blood (Sato & Nakajima, 1979b). Their water/air, oil/air, oil/water and oil/blood partition coefficients are also shown in the table, together with other chemical and physical properties, as reference data. The blood/air partition coefficients increase in the order benzene < toluene < xylenes. It can be predicted that, if air containing these three solvent vapours at the same concentrations is inhaled, the eventual equilibrium concentration in the body will be in the order xylenes > toluene > benzene (Sato & Nakajima, 1977).

The amount of vapour taken up by various body tissues depends on the affinity of each vapour for each tissue. Table 2 shows the partition coefficients of benzene, toluene and *m*-xylene for a variety of body tissues of rabbits (Sato *et al.*, 1974a,b). The coefficients for each solvent range from 1 to 3 for all tissues other than adipose tissue and bone marrow. The values for fat tissue are extraordinarily high, being 20 to 30 times as high as those for the other tissues. The difference in solubility among triolein,

Table 1. Partition coefficients of benzene, toluene and xylenes for water, blood and oil

	Benzene	Toluene	o-Xylene	m-Xylene	p-Xylene
Molecular weight[a]	78.11	92.14	106.17	106.17	106.17
Density (20/4 °C)[a]	0.8787	0.8669	0.8802	0.8642	0.8611
Melting point (°C)[a]	5.5	−95	−25.18	−47.87	13.26
Boiling point (°C)[a]	80.10	110.62	144.41	139.10	138.35
Flash point (°C)[a]	−11	4.4	32	29	27
Vapour pressure (mm Hg)[a]	100	28.7	6.8	8.3	8.9
	(26.1 °C)	(25 °C)	(25 °C)	(25 °C)	(25 °C)
Partition coefficient[b]					
Water/air	2.78	2.23	2.63	1.66	1.57
Blood/air	7.8	15.6	31.1	26.4	37.6
Oil/air	492	1 471	4 360	3 842	3 694
Oil/water	177	659	1 658	2 314	2 353
Oil/blood	63	94	140	146	98

[a]Sandmeyer (1981). [b]Sato & Nakajima (1979b).

Table 2. Partition coefficients of benzene, toluene and m-xylene for body fluids and tissues of rabbits (Sato et al., 1974a,b)

	System[a]	Benzene	Toluene	m-Xylene
A	Blood	10.7	17.0	37.4
	Plasma	5.5	10.4	20.7
B	Liver	1.6	2.6	3.0
	Kidney	1.1	1.5	1.7
	Brain, whole	1.9	3.1	3.3
	Lung	1.3	1.9	2.1
	Heart	1.4	2.1	2.1
	Muscle, femoral	1.1	1.2	1.6
	Bone marrow	16.2	35.4	41.7
	Fat, retroperitoneal	58.5	113.2	145.8
C	Lecithin	196.4	608.8	1 799.8
	Triolein	535.7	1 726.5	4 621.4
	Cholesterol	21.0	53.0	118.2
	Cholesterol oleate	83.7	266.0	820.9
	Human fat, peritoneal	406.2	1 296.1	3 604.7
	Human blood[b]	7.8	14.7	29.0

[a]A: Fluid/air partition coefficients. B: Tissue/blood partition coefficients. C: Material/air partition coefficients
[b]From Sato et al. (1972).

lecithin and cholesterol clearly shows that the lipid content in the form of neutral fat is a primary determinant for the level of solubility; small changes in lipid content in any tissue are presumed to alter significantly the value of the partition coefficient for that tissue. It must therefore be remembered that tissue/blood partition coefficients vary according to age, weight, sex, nutritional status and physical condition, since fat content varies as a result of these factors.

As absorbed organic solvents are transported chiefly *via* the blood stream, blood flow (perfusion rate) is another determinant of the distribution of vapours in each tissue. In most pharmacokinetic models proposed so far, the whole body is generally divided into three tissue groups, depending on the solubility in the tissues and the rate of perfusion (Eger, 1963; Sato *et al.,* 1974a; Fiserova-Bergerova, 1983). About 75% of the cardiac output is delivered to a group of tissues comprising less than one tenth of the total body volume. This group is designated as the vessel-rich tissue group, or VRG. As mentioned above, the partition coefficients of benzene, toluene and xylenes into these tissues are in the range 1–3. The muscle group, or MG, consisting of muscles and skin, occupies 50% of the body volume and receives 18% of the cardiac output at rest. The partition coefficient for the MG is as low as 1–2. Fat tissues (including white bone marrow), which comprise roughly 20% of the body volume and receive only 5% of the cardiac output, are grouped into the third tissue group (FG), because most of the organic solvents have a very high affinity for these tissues. The basic features of this model are presented in Figure 2.

This three-compartment model has made it possible to express the transfer of organic solvents in three exponential forms: for the saturation process,

$$C = A_1(1 - e^{-\alpha_1 t}) + A_2(1 - e^{-\alpha_2 t}) + A_3(1 - e^{-\alpha_3 t}),$$

and for desaturation,

$$C = B_1 e^{-\alpha_1 \tau} + B_2 e^{-\alpha_2 \tau} + B_3 e^{-\alpha_3 \tau},$$

where C is the concentration in the VRG, i.e., the concentration in the blood; A_i and B_i ($i = 1$–3) are the constants determined by the initial conditions; t is the time elapsing after the start of inhalation; τ is the time after the cessation of inhalation; and α_i is the rate constant (Sato *et al.,* 1974a). Strictly speaking, in addition to the three tissue groups in the model, there exists a fourth tissue group which is composed of bones (not marrow), teeth, tendons, ligaments, contents of the alimentary canal and so on. Because of its relative avascularity, however, the absorption into, distribution in and elimination from the tissues in this group are considered to be far slower than those in VRG, MG and FG (Eger, 1963).

When organic solvent vapours are inhaled, the VRG is first filled up quickly, since its volume is small compared with the overwhelmingly large volume of blood perfusing the tissues. Then, the MG is filled up gradually until it reaches an apparent equilibrium with the VRG, and, finally, the FG is filled at a very slow rate. The desaturation process also proceeds in a three-exponential step, which is a reflected image of the saturation process. When the vapour is removed from the air being inhaled, it quickly disappears from the VRG through metabolic degradation and pulmonary exhalation. When the concentration in the VRG falls below that in the MG, the vapour in the MG will be transported to the VRG and will be eliminated therefrom. After a sufficient time has elapsed, the FG will become the only reservoir of the vapour and the mobilization rate from the FG will limit the overall rate of elimination.

Body fat therefore plays a major role in the pharmacokinetics of benzene, toluene and xylene. Body fat content is not the same in males and females, and this difference

Fig. 2. A three-compartment model for transfer of organic solvent vapours in a living body. VRG, vessel-rich tissue group, 8 L; MG, muscle group (muscle and skin) 30 L; FG, fat group (fat tissue and yellow bone marrow) 10 L; f, blood flow through each tissue group (f_1, 4.5 L/min, f_2, 1.1 L/min, and f_3, 0.3 L/min)

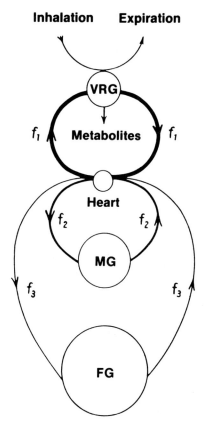

may affect the disposition of these fat-soluble substances. Indeed, a kinetic study has revealed that the rate of benzene elimination is slower in females than in males. The slower elimination in females is primarily due to the bulky distribution of body fat tissue (Sato *et al.*, 1975). Females are said to be more susceptible to benzene intoxication (Browning, 1965a). The difference in body fat content between the sexes may account for the sex-related difference in susceptibility to benzene toxicity.

Clearly, any physiological or environmental factor that alters respiratory and cardiovascular functions has a profound effect on the uptake, distribution and elimination of volatile substances. Physical activity is one of the most important factors (Åstrand, 1983). Alveolar ventilation during exercise can increase to as much as 10 times that at rest. Cardiac output also increases, although to a rather small extent compared with the alveolar ventilation. Physical exercise can also change the distribution of blood flow to each tissue: it increases the perfusion through muscles and adipose tissue, on the one hand, and reduces the flow through regions such as the

Table 3. Respiratory and metabolic clearances of benzene, toluene and *m*-xylene[a]

Substance	Respiratory clearance L/h (%)	Metabolic clearance L/h (%)
Benzene	43 (36)	75 (64)
Toluene	22 (18)	100 (82)
m-Xylene	13 (10)	116 (90)

[a] The clearances were calculated using the blood/air partition coefficients (Table 1) and the rates of metabolism *in vitro* (Nakajima & Sato, 1979), according to the method of Sato *et al.* (1977). Alveolar ventilation was assumed to be 336 L/h.

splanchnic area (hepato-portal) and kidneys (Åstrand, 1983). The blood flow through fat tissue considerably increases during exercise: the mean blood flow for a male with 10 kg of body fat is 0.15 L/min at rest, but increases to 0.45 to 0.7 mL/min during light to moderate physical work (Bülow & Madsen, 1976). This increase in perfusion, in conjunction with an increase in alveolar ventilation, during exercise markedly enhances the uptake of volatile, lipophilic substances in fat tissue. An experiment conducted on young male volunteers who inhaled air containing 300 mg/m^3 (80 ppm) of toluene for 2 h clearly shows this. The peak concentration in subcutaneous fat was approximately 1.3 mg/kg at rest, whereas the concentration reached during exercise was as high as 11.5 mg/kg (Carlsson & Ljungquist, 1982). In contrast, physical exercise reduces blood flow through the liver, where metabolic degradation of foreign chemicals takes place: the blood flow can drop to 20% of the flow in a resting condition (Rowell *et al.,* 1964). Thus, strenuous exercise can result in reduced availability of the chemicals to metabolic clearance. However, the effect of physical activity on clearance has not been quantitatively assessed.

Metabolic transformation is the most important pathway by which a living system eliminates absorbed benzene, toluene and xylenes: about 60% of the benzene disappears from the body by way of metabolic clearance, and 80 to 90% of both toluene and xylene are reported to disappear through this route (Table 3).

With respect to their toxicity, the metabolism of chemical substances is important in two respects. First, metabolism plays a decisive role in determining the biological half-lives of the substances. Second, biotransformation sometimes results in the production of highly-reactive intermediates which can bind covalently to critical components of the target cell and cause irreversible damage. The toxicity of organic solvents can be divided into two categories: parent compound-induced toxicity, e.g., narcotic action, which is a toxicity common to most of the fat-soluble volatile hydrocarbons (structure-nonspecific toxicity), and metabolite-mediated toxicity (structure-specific toxicity).

In the former case, metabolism or biotransformation accelerates the removal of toxic agents from the target organ; thus it always results in detoxication. In the latter case, biotransformation results in the formation of toxic metabolites; hence the reaction is called bioactivation or biotoxification. Fig. 3 illustrates the fate of organic

Fig. 3. General reactions of organic solvent vapours absorbed in a living body; k_i is the rate constant for each step

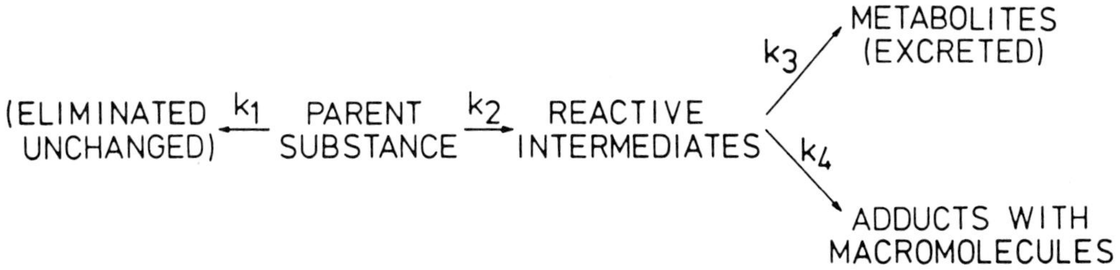

Fig. 4. A scheme of benzene metabolism (Nakajima et al., 1985a)

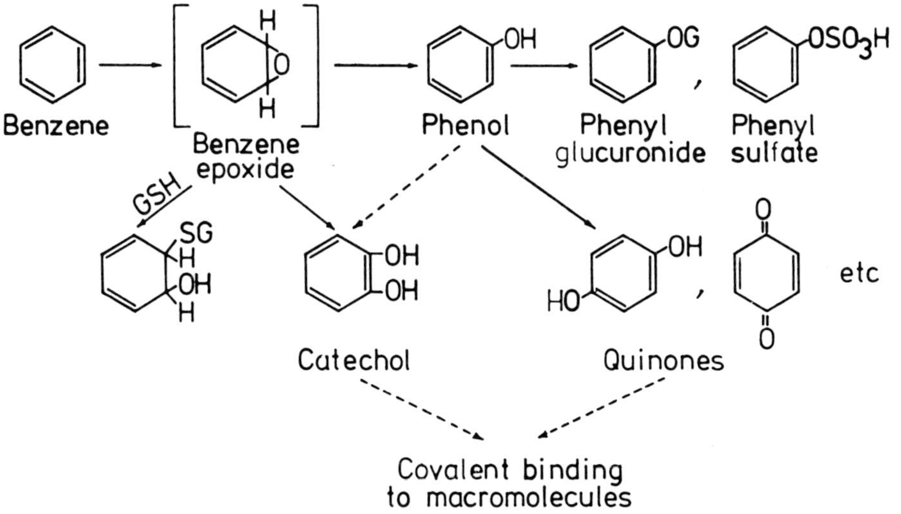

solvents absorbed in the body. The step with rate constant k_2 is a degradation reaction (phase 1 reaction) that requires energy to cleave chemical bonds: thus it is considered to be a rate-limiting step in the overall metabolism of organic solvents. The step with k_3 is a so-called phase 2 reaction or conjugation reaction, which is normally considered to be a detoxication process, and the resultant conjugates are excreted in urine. The enzymes in charge of the degradation reaction are cytochrome P-450-related monooxygenases, which are localized at the smooth endoplasmic reticulum and are called mixed-function oxidases.

Fig. 4 shows a scheme of benzene metabolism (Nakajima et al., 1985a). The pathway from benzene to benzene epoxide is a cytochrome P-450-dependent degradation and constitutes a rate-limiting step in the overall metabolism of benzene. The major part of benzene epoxide is non-enzymatically rearranged into phenol (Parke & Williams, 1953a), part of which is further metabolized via cytochrome P-450-dependent reactions into quinones (Sawahata & Neal, 1983; Nakajima et al., 1985b); the remainder undergoes conjugation reactions to be excreted in urine (Parke

& Williams, 1953b). Benzene has long been known to cause haematopoietic toxicity, i.e., aplastic anaemia and leukaemia. This toxicity is suggested to be mediated not by benzene itself, but by its metabolite(s) (Snyder & Kocsis, 1975). Recent studies suggest that not benzene epoxide, a metabolite once assumed to be responsible for benzene toxicity, but hydroquinone, catechol or their subsequent metabolites may mediate the toxicity (Tunek *et al.*, 1978; Rickert *et al.*, 1979; Tunek *et al.*, 1980). Whether the ultimate toxicant is produced in the liver (Snyder *et al.*, 1967; Gonasun *et al.*, 1973), where the enzymes responsible for the metabolism exist in abundance, or in the bone marrow (Andrews *et al.*, 1979), a postulated site of action of benzene, remains to be determined. The fact that partial hepatectomy, which decreased benzene metabolism by 70%, protected rats from benzene haematotoxicity led Sammett *et al.* (1979) to postulate that hepatic metabolism plays a critical role in producing toxicity: a metabolite is first formed in the liver, then transported to bone marrow, eliciting the toxic effect directly or after being further converted to more reactive metabolites.

Toluene is first transformed to benzoic acid (side-chain hydroxylation), then undergoes conjugation with glycine to form hippuric acid, which is excreted in urine. Small amounts of benzoic acid (less than 20%) may be conjugated with glucuronic acid. Minor amounts of absorbed toluene (less than 1%) undergo ring hydroxylation to form *o*- and *p*-cresols, which are excreted in urine as sulfate or glucuronide conjugates (ACGIH, 1984).

A major metabolic pathway for xylenes is hydroxylation of a methyl function to form methyl benzoic acid, which is conjugated with glycine and excreted in the urine as the respective methyl hippuric acid. Ring hydroxylation of xylenes to corresponding xylenols constitutes a minor metabolic pathway for xylenes (less than 2%) (ACGIH, 1984).

With regard to benzene and its homologues, only benzene is known to cause irreversible damage to the haematopoietic system, although earlier investigators reported that the haematopoietic disorder was also caused by toluene or xylene exposure (Ferguson *et al.*, 1933; Adler-Herzmark, 1933; Greenburg *et al.*, 1942). It would seem, however, that various degrees of benzene impurity in toluene and xylene employed in earlier studies were responsible for the reported haematopoietic disorder (Browning, 1965b). The side chain of the benzene ring is more subject to enzymic attack than the ring itself (Sato & Nakajima, 1979c). Toluene and xylenes quickly undergo side-chain hydroxylation to form less toxic benzoic acids. This is why the pure methyl- or dimethylbenzenes cause no haematopoietic deviations. As mentioned above, a small portion of toluene and xylenes is thought to be transformed into cresols and xylenols, respectively, *via* epoxidation of the benzene ring (Daly *et al.*, 1968; Bakke & Scheline, 1970; Kaubisch *et al.*, 1972; Angerer, 1979; Pfaffli *et al.*, 1979). Thus, the idea that the epoxide formation has some relevance to the haematotoxicity reportedly caused by these methylbenzenes cannot be totally discounted.

When more than one chemical enters a living body at the same time, interactions such as absorption, excretion, metabolism, protein binding and subcellular localization may take place at various sites. An experimental study revealed that the simultaneous presence of benzene and toluene did not affect their solubilities in blood or their binding with bovine serum albumin, suggesting that absorption and distribution may be unaffected by their simultaneous presence. *In vivo* and *in vitro*, however, toluene is a competitive inhibitor of benzene metabolism, and benzene competitively inhibits side-chain hydroxylation of toluene (Sato & Nakajima, 1979c). In accordance with this, several investigators have demonstrated that coadministration of toluene with benzene protects animals from benzene-induced haematotoxicity (Ikeda *et al.*, 1972; Andrews *et al.*, 1977; Tunek *et al.*, 1981, 1982).

DIETARY AND ETHANOL-INDUCED ALTERATION OF METABOLISM OF BENZENE, TOLUENE AND XYLENES

The metabolism of foreign chemicals, and consequently their toxicity, is altered by many environmental factors, among which diet is undoubtedly of prime importance (Sato & Nakajima, 1984). The following paragraphs deal with the effects of dietary manipulation and ethanol ingestion on the metabolism of benzene, toluene and xylenes.

One-day food deprivation accelerates the rat liver metabolism of 21 aromatic or chlorinated volatile hydrocarbons, including benzene, toluene and xylenes (Nakajima & Sato, 1979). The food deprivation caused no change in microsomal protein or cytochrome P-450 contents. The liver weight itself decreased by about 20%, and thus the amount of the protein or cytochrome per liver, i.e., the amount per rat, decreased. It is remarkable that the increase in metabolic rate was still noted even when expressed in terms of whole liver, regardless of its diminished size. This increase was confirmed to occur in both in-vitro and in-vivo systems. Fasting over a period of two to three days did not augment the increase caused by a one-day fast: overnight fasting most effectively enhanced the hepatic metabolism.

Food restriction increased the rate of in-vitro toluene metabolism almost linearly with decrease in food intake (Nakajima *et al.*, 1982), suggesting that the amount of food consumed on the day before toxicity testing can affect the metabolism of a variety of organic solvents and modify the toxicity. Dietary regimen thus needs to be standardized in the toxicological evaluation of benzene, toluene and xylenes.

The general belief so far has been that protein is the most important nutrient in regulating metabolism and toxicity of chemical substances (Campbell & Hayes, 1974; Campbell, 1978). It is known that a diet rich in protein can exacerbate carbon tetrachloride- or *N*-nitrosodimethylamine-induced hepatotoxicity by accelerating transformation of these chemicals to their respective reactive intermediates (McLean & McLean, 1966, 1969). In past experiments, however, protein content in the diet was varied at the expense of carbohydrates to make the diet isocaloric. A high-protein diet was another term for a low-carbohydrate diet, and a low-protein diet contained excessive amounts of carbohydrate. The metabolism study of Nakajima *et al.* (1982) has clearly demonstrated that it is dietary carbohydrate, not protein or fat, that regulates the hepatic metabolism of various hydrocarbons, including benzene, toluene and probably xylenes. The rate of metabolism increased linearly with decreasing carbohydrate intake, independently of protein or fat intake. One-day feeding of rats with a carbohydrate-free diet containing adequate amounts of protein, fat and other nutrients greatly enhanced the metabolism. The enhancement was almost comparable to that achieved by one-day complete food deprivation.

Ethanol administration exerts dual effects on the metabolism of volatile hydrocarbons, i.e., inhibition and stimulation (Sato et al., 1981). Which one is predominant seems to depend on the time elapsed after ethanol ingestion. At first, when ethanol occurs in the body at high concentrations, it preferentially acts as an inhibitor. On the contrary, when ethanol is disappearing from the body, i.e., 16 to 18 h after ingestion, the metabolism-enhancing effect makes its full appearance, while the inhibitory effect is minimized.

It is remarkable that the greatly-enhanced metabolism of volatile hydrocarbons following a three-week daily ethanol consumption returned almost to the normal level after a one-day withdrawal of ethanol (Sato et al., 1980). An acute dose of ethanol, 4 g/kg, eventually increased the hepatic metabolism of toluene about two-fold, but the effect disappeared 24 h after ethanol administration. Altogether, it can be said that recently-ingested ethanol pays an important part in enhancing the metabolism of these hydrocarbons.

A single dose of ethanol which induced enhanced metabolism increased neither the microsomal protein nor cytochrome P-450 content of rat liver (Sato et al., 1981). Prolonged administration of ethanol produced only a slight increase in these enzymic parameters (Sato et al., 1980). These findings give us the impression that ethanol-induced alteration of the metabolism of volatile hydrocarbons may be different from the enzyme induction produced by well-known enzyme inducers, such as phenobarbital (PB), but may resemble the effect of food deprivation or lowered carbohydrate intake.

Dietary carbohydrate intake level at the time of ethanol ingestion has a marked influence on the metabolism-enhancing effect of ethanol (Sato et al., 1983). A combination of ethanol with a carbohydrate-deficient diet quite markedly enhanced the metabolism of benzene and toluene, compared to a combination of ethanol with a high-carbohydrate diet (Fig. 5). In addition, only when ethanol was consumed with a low-carbohydrate diet, were liver microsomal protein and cytochrome P-450 contents significantly increased. The synergistic effects of ethanol ingestion and lowered carbohydrate intake are particularly interesting because, when drinking alcoholic beverages, moderate consumption of carbohydrates is often recommended because ethanol is a much better energy source (7 kcal/g) than carbohydrate (4 kcal/g).

As mentioned above, it is clear that food deprivation-, lowered carbohydrate intake- and ethanol-induced acceleration of volatile hydrocarbon metabolism differs from enzyme induction following PB, polychlorinated biphenyl (PCB) or 3-methylcholanthrene (MC) treatment. PB and PCB induced remarkable increases in microsomal protein and cytochrome P-450 contents, but caused no increase in the metabolism of benzene. (Both treatments, however, markedly increased the metabolism of toluene, whereas MC had no effect on the metabolism of either benzene or toluene; Sato & Nakajima, 1985.) Since both PB and PCB increased the microsomal protein and cytochrome P-450 contents, the rate of benzene metabolism per unit concentration of these parameters fell below that obtained with the liver of control (untreated) rats, suggesting that the major form of PB- or PCB-induced isozymes may have low affinity for benzene (Fig. 6).

Fig. 5. Metabolic rates for benzene and toluene in rats given 2.82 g of ethanol every day for 3 weeks in combination with a basal diet (A), a low-fat diet (B) and a low-carbohydrate diet (C). Diets A – ethanol, B + ethanol, and C + ethanol were each isocaloric. Ethanol added to Diet A was consumed as supplementary calories. Rats were given 80 mL of each liquid diet daily at 4 pm and were killed for metabolism assay at 10 am on the day after the last feeding (Sato *et al.*, 1983)

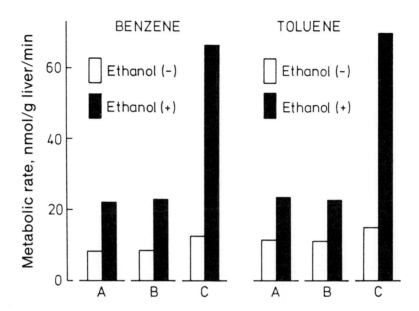

Conflicting results have been reported concerning the effect of PB treatment on the metabolism of benzene. Many investigators have found that benzene hydroxylase activity was increased by treating animals with PB (Snyder *et al.*, 1967; Drew & Fouts, 1974; Gut, 1976; Tunek & Oesch, 1979), but others (Gonasun *et al.*, 1973; Sato & Nakajima, 1985) have reported a negative effect. This apparent discrepancy may be due to differences in the substrate concentrations employed; for example, Sato & Nakajima (1985), who reported a "negative" effect, used a benzene concentration of 35.3 μmol/L, while much higher concentrations (2.3 to 4.5 mmol/L) were employed in one study where a "positive" effect was found (Snyder *et al.*, 1967).

Post and Snyder (1983) were the first to demonstrate that two distinct forms of isozymes metabolize benzene; one form is active at all substrate concentrations and the other preferentially acts in microsomes from PB-treated rats at benzene concentrations above 0.8 mmol/L. The most recent study of Sato's group (Nakajima *et al.*, 1987) has shown that a liver microsomal preparation from normally fed rats contains two forms of isozymes with different k_m values toward benzene. The isozyme with a k_m of 0.01 mmol/L disappeared following one-day food deprivation, but the deprivation increased the activity (V_{max}) of the other isozyme having a k_m of 0.1 mmol/L. Ethanol treatment markedly increased the activity of both the normally existing isozymes. In addition to these two naturally-occurring isozymes, PB treatment induced the synthesis of another isozyme with a high k_m value of 4.5 mmol/L, which was almost unidentifiable in microsomes from control (untreated)

Fig. 6. Metabolism of benzene and toluene by liver microsomal enzymes of rats maintained on various dietary regimens. Rats were fed daily at 4 pm and killed for metabolism assay at 10 am on the day after the last feeding (Sato & Nakajima, 1985). A, moderate-carbohydrate diet (basal diet); B, low-carbohydrate diet; C, basal diet + 2.0 g ethanol per day for 3 weeks; D, low-carbohydrate diet + 2.0 g ethanol per day for 3 weeks; E, basal diet + 80 mg/kg phenobarbital per day for 3 days; F, basal diet + a single dose (500 mg/kg) of polychlorinated biphenyl; G, basal diet + 20 mg/kg 3-methylcholanthrene per day for 3 days; H, rats on the basal diet were deprived of food on the day before killing

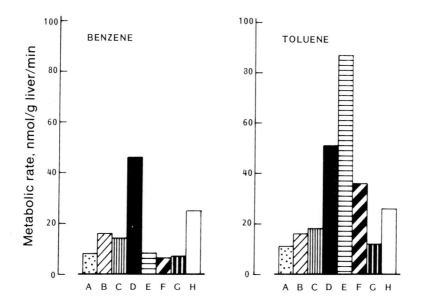

rats. Accordingly, food deprivation and ethanol consumption increased the metabolism of benzene at various substrate concentrations, whereas PB treatment did not increase it until the benzene concentration was as high as 2.26 mmol/L.

An isozyme of cytochrome P-450 with physicochemical and catalytic properties distinct from that induced by PB or MC has been isolated and purified from liver of ethanol-treated animals (Comai & Gaylor, 1973; Ohnishi & Lieber, 1977; Koop *et al.,* 1982). A series of metabolism studies conducted by Sato and coworkers suggests that ethanol, especially when administered concomitantly with a low-carbohydrate diet, may induce a form of cytochrome P-450 which is catalytically active for the metabolism of volatile hydrocarbons, including benzene, toluene and xylenes (Sato *et al.,* 1983; Sato & Nakajima, 1985; Nakajima *et al.,* 1985a, 1987). Similarly, food deprivation or restricted carbohydrate intake may stimulate the synthesis of a certain species of isozyme having a specifically high activity for volatile hydrocarbons (Tu & Yang, 1983) or may stimulate the enzyme activity by a modification of the membrane environment, or by displacing other endogenous or exogenous substrates already bound to the enzymes (Ioannides & Parke, 1973). However, food deprivation or ethanol consumption did not affect the hepatic metabolism of polycyclic aromatic hydrocarbons, such as 3,4-benzopyrene and 7,12-dimethylbenzanthracene (Sato *et al.*, 1986). The effect seems to be limited to chemicals characterized by volatility and low molecular weight.

It is well known that PB, PCB or MC treatment enhances the activity of enzymes involved in phase 2 reactions, such as glucuronyl transferase and glutathione *S*-transferase (Bock *et al.*, 1973; Vainio, 1974; Kaplowitz *et al.*, 1975; Thompson *et al.*, 1982). However, food deprivation, restricted carbohydrate intake or ethanol administration produced no significant effect on the activity of these enzymes (Sato & Nakajima, 1985). Therefore, changes in nutrition or ethanol consumption, which accelerate phase 1 metabolism of benzene (bioactivation) but do not affect phase 2 reactions (detoxication), may lead more directly to an increase in covalent binding to macromolecules than would PB treatment, which enhances the phase 2 reactions with little or no influence on the phase 1 reaction. In fact, ethanol administration aggravated benzene-induced haematotoxicity (Snyder *et al.*, 1980; Baarson *et al.*, 1982; Nakajima *et al.*, 1985a), whereas PB treatment protected animals from the toxicity (Ikeda & Ohtsuji, 1971; Mitchell, 1971; Gill *et al.*, 1979; Nakajima *et al.*, 1985a). However, the influence of food restriction may be more complicated because the restriction reduces the body fat content and therefore affects the pharmacokinetic profile of highly lipophilic substances like benzene. Benzene disappeared more quickly from the body of food-restricted rats than from the body of normally-fed rats, which may account for the prevention of benzene toxicity by food restriction (Sato *et al.*, 1975).

REFERENCES

ACGIH (1984) ACGIH transactions 1984. *Ann. Am. Conf. Gov. Ind. Hyg., 11,* 103–128

Adler-Herzmark, J. (1933) Periodische Untersuchung von Arbeitern. III. Periodische Untersuchungen von Wiener Arbeitern, die mit benzol-, toluol- und xylolhaltigen Materialien beschäftigt sind. *Arch. Gewerbepathol. Gewerbehyg., 4,* 486–490

Andrews, L.S., Lee, E.W., Witmer, C.M., Kocsis, J.J. & Snyder, R. (1977) Effects of toluene on the metabolism, disposition and hemopoietic toxicity of ³H-benzene. *Biochem. Pharmacol., 26,* 293–300

Andrews, L.S., Sasame, H.A. & Gillette, J.R. (1979) ³H-Benzene metabolism in rabbit bone marrow. *Life Sci., 25,* 567–572

Angerer, J. (1979) Occupational chronic exposure to organic solvents. VII. Metabolism of toluene in man. *Int. Arch. Occup. Environ. Health, 43,* 63–67

Åstrand, I. (1975) Uptake of solvent in the blood and tissues of man. A review. *Scand. J. Work Environ. Health, 1,* 199–218

Åstrand, I. (1983) Effect of physical exercise on uptake, distribution and elimination of vapors in man. In: Fiserova-Bergerova, V., ed., *Modeling of Inhalation Exposure to Vapors: Uptake, Distribution, and Elimination,* Vol. 2, Boca Raton, FL, CRC Press, pp. 107–130

Baarson, K.A., Snyder, C.A., Green, J.D., Sellakumar, A., Goldstein, B.D. & Albert, R.E. (1982) The hematotoxic effects of inhaled benzene on peripheral blood, bone marrow, and spleen cells are increased by ingested ethanol. *Toxicol. Appl. Pharmacol., 64,* 393–404

Bakke, O.M. & Scheline, R.R. (1970) Hydroxylation of aromatic hydrocarbons in the rat. *Toxicol. Appl. Pharmacol., 16,* 691–700

Bock, K.W., Frohling, W., Remmer, H. & Rexer, B. (1973) Effects of phenobarbital and 3-methylcholanthrene on substrate specificity of rat liver microsomal UDP-glucuronyltransferase. *Biochem. Biophys. Acta, 327,* 46–56

Browning, E. (1965a) *Toxicity and Metabolism of Industrial Solvents,* Amsterdam, Elsevier, pp. 3–31

Browning, E. (1965b) *Toxicity and Metabolism of Industrial Solvents,* Amsterdam, Elsevier, pp. 66–129

Bülow, J. & Madsen, J. (1976) Adipose tissue blood flow during prolonged, heavy exercise. *Pflügers Arch. Ges. Physiol., 363,* 231–234

Campbell, T.C. (1978) Effects of dietary protein on drug metabolism. In: Hathcock, J.N. & Coon, J., eds, *Nutrition and Drug Interactions,* New York, Academic Press, pp. 409–422

Campbell, T.C. & Hayes, J.R. (1974) Role of nutrition in the drug-metabolizing enzyme system. *Pharmacol. Rev., 26,* 171–197

Carlsson, A. & Ljungquist, E. (1982) Exposure to toluene. Concentration in subcutaneous adipose tissue. *Scand. J. Work Environ. Health, 8,* 56–62

Comai, K. & Gaylor, J.L. (1973) Existence and separation of three forms of cytochrome P-450 from rat liver microsomes. *J. Biol. Chem., 248,* 4947–4955

Daly, J., Jerina, D.M. & Witkop, B. (1968) Migration of deuterium during hydroxylation of aromatic substrates by liver microsomes. I. Influence of ring substituents. *Arch. Biochem. Biophys., 128,* 517–527

Drew, R.T. & Fouts, J.R. (1974) The lack of effects of pretreatment with phenobarbital and chlorpromazine on the acute toxicity of benzene in rats. *Toxicol. Appl. Pharmacol., 27,* 183–193

Dutkiewicz, T. & Tyras, H. (1968a) Skin absorption of toluene, styrene, and xylene by man. *Br. J. Ind. Med., 25,* 243

Dutkiewicz, T. & Tyras, H. (1968b) The quantitative estimation of toluene skin absorption in man. *Arch. Gewerbepathol. Gewerbehyg., 24,* 253–257

Eger, E.I., II (1963) A mathematical model of uptake and distribution. In: Papper, E.M. & Kitz, R.J., eds, *Uptake and Distribution of Anesthetic Agents,* New York, McGraw-Hill, pp. 72–87

Engstrom, K., Husman, K. & Riihimaki, V. (1977) Percutaneous absorption of *m*-xylene in man. *Int. Arch. Occup. Environ. Health, 39,* 181–189

Ferguson, T., Harvey, W.F. & Hamilton, T.D. (1933) An inquiry into the relative toxicity of benzene and toluene. *Ind. Hyg., 33,* 547–575

Fiserova-Bergerova, V. (1983) Physiological models for pulmonary administration and elimination of inert vapors and gases. In: Fiserova-Bergerova, V., ed., *Modeling of Inhalation Exposure to Vapors: Uptake, Distribution, and Elimination,* Vol. 1, Boca Raton, FL, CRC Press, pp. 73–100

Gill, D.P., Kempen, R.R., Nash, J.B. & Ellis, S. (1979) Modifications of benzene myelotoxicity and metabolism by phenobarbital, SKF-525A, and 3-methyl-cholanthrene. *Life Sci., 25,* 1633–1640

Gillette, J.R., Mitchell, J.R. & Brodie, B.B. (1974) Biochemical mechanisms of drug toxicity. *Ann. Rev. Pharmacol., 14,* 271–288

Gonasun, L.M., Witmer, C., Kocsis, J.J. & Snyder, R. (1973) Benzene metabolism in mouse liver microsomes. *Toxicol. Appl. Pharmacol., 26,* 398–406

Greenburg, L., Mayers, M.R., Heimann, H. & Moskowitz, S. (1942) The effects of exposure to toluene in industry. *J. Am. med. Assoc., 118,* 573–578

Gut, I. (1976) Effect of phenobarbital treatment on *in vitro* enzyme kinetics and *in vivo* biotransformation of benzene in the rat. *Arch. Toxicol., 35,* 195–206

Ikeda, M. & Ohtsuji, H. (1971) Phenobarbital-induced protection against toxicity of toluene and benzene in the rat. *Toxicol. Appl. Pharmacol., 20,* 30–43

Ikeda, M., Ohtsuji, H. & Imamura, T. (1972) *In vivo* suppression of benzene and styrene oxidation by co-administered toluene in rats and effects of phenobarbital. *Xenobiotica, 2,* 101–106

Ioannides, C. & Parke, D.V. (1973) The effect of ethanol administration on drug oxidations and possible mechanism of ethanol-barbiturate interactions. *Biochem. Soc. Trans., 1,* 716–720

Kaplowitz, N., Kuhlenkamp, J. & Clifton, G. (1975) Drug induction of hepatic glutathione-S-transferases in male and female rats. *Biochem. J., 146,* 351–356

Kaubisch, N., Daly, J.W. & Jerina, D.M. (1972) Arene oxides as intermediates in the oxidative metabolism of aromatic compounds. Isomerization of methyl-substituted arene oxides. *Biochemistry, 11,* 3080–3088

Koop, D.R., Morgan, E.T., Tarr, G.E. & Coon, M.J. (1982) Purification and characterization of a unique isozyme of cytochrome P-450 from liver microsomes of ethanol-treated rabbits. *J. Biol. Chem., 257,* 8472–8480

Larson, C.P., Jr (1963) Solubility and partition coefficients. In: Papper, E.M. & Kitz, R.J., eds, *Uptake and Distribution of Anesthetic Agents,* New York, McGraw-Hill, pp. 5–16

Lauwerys, R.R., Dath, T., Lachapelle, J.M., Buchet, J.P. & Roels, H. (1978) The influence of two barrier creams on the percutaneous absorption of *m*-xylene in man. *J. Occup. Med., 20,* 17–20

Levy, G. & Gibaldi, M. (1972) Pharmacokinetics of drug action. *Ann. Rev. Pharmacol., 12,* 85–98

McLean, A.E.M. & McLean, E.K. (1966) The effect of diet and 1,1,1-trichloro-2,2-bis-(*p*-chlorophenyl)ethane (DDT) on microsomal hydroxylating enzymes and on sensitivity of rats to carbon tetrachloride poisoning. *Biochem. J., 100,* 564–571

McLean, A.E.M. & McLean, E.K. (1969) Diet and toxicity. *Br. Med. Bull., 25,* 278–281

Mitchell, J.R. (1971) Mechanism of benzene-induced aplastic anemia. *Fed. Proc., 30,* 2044

Nakajima, T. & Sato, A. (1979) Enhanced activity of liver drug-metabolizing enzymes for aromatic and chlorinated hydrocarbons following food deprivation. *Toxicol. Appl. Pharmacol., 50,* 549–556

Nakajima, T., Koyama, Y. & Sato, A. (1982) Dietary modification of metabolism and toxicity of chemical substances — with special reference to carbohydrate. *Biochem. Pharmacol., 31,* 1005–1011

Nakajima, T., Okuyama, S., Yonekura, I. & Sato, A. (1985a) Effects of ethanol and phenobarbital administration on the metabolism and toxicity of benzene. *Chem.-Biol. Interact., 55,* 23–38

Nakajima, T., Yonekura, I. & Sato, A. (1985b) A simple method to evaluate liver microsomal enzyme activity for phenol metabolism with a high-performance liquid chromatograph. *Toxicol. Lett., 29,* 11–15

Nakajima, T., Okino, T. & Sato, A. (1987) Kinetic studies on benzene metabolism in rat liver – possible presence of three forms of benzene metabolizing enzymes in the liver. *Biochem. Pharmacol., 36,* 2799–2804

Ohnishi, K. & Lieber, C.S. (1977) Reconstitution of the microsomal ethanol-oxidizing system. Qualitative and quantitative changes of cytochrome P-450 after chronic ethanol consumption. *J. Biol. Chem., 252,* 7124–7131

Parke, D.V. & Williams, R.T. (1953a) Studies in detoxication. 49. The metabolism of benzene containing [^{14}C]benzene. *Biochem. J., 54,* 231–238

Parke, D.V. & Williams, R.T. (1953b) Studies in detoxication. 54. The metabolism of benzene. (a) The formation of phenylglucuronide and phenylsulfuric acid from [^{14}C]benzene. (b) The metabolism of [^{14}C]phenol. *Biochem. J., 55,* 337–340

Pfaffli, P., Savalainen, H., Kalliomaki, P.L. & Kalliokoski, P. (1979) Urinary *o*-cresol in toluene exposure. *Scand. J. Work Environ. Health, 5,* 286–289

Piotrowski, J.K. (1967) Quantitative estimate of the absorption of toluene in people. *Med. Pracy., 18,* 214–223

Post, G.B. & Snyder, R. (1983) Effects of enzyme induction on microsomal benzene metabolism. *J. Toxicol. Environ. Health, 11,* 811–825

Rickert, D.E., Baker, T.S., Bus, J.S., Barrow, C.S. & Irons, R.D. (1979) Benzene disposition in the rat after exposure by inhalation. *Toxicol. Appl. Pharmacol., 49,* 417–423

Riihimäki, V. & Pfaffli, P. (1978) Percutaneous absorption of solvent vapors in man. *Scand. J. Work Environ. Health, 4,* 73–85

Rowell, L.B., Blackman, J.R. & Bruce, R.A. (1964) Indocyanine green clearance and estimated hepatic blood flow during mild to maximal exercise in upright man. *J. Clin. Invest., 43,* 1677

Sammett, D., Lee, E.W., Kocsis, J.J. & Snyder, R. (1979) Partial hepatectomy reduces both metabolism and toxicity of benzene. *J. Toxicol. Environ. Health, 5,* 785–792

Sandmeyer, E.E. (1981) Aromatic hydrocarbons. In: Clayton, G.D. & Clayton, F.E., eds., *Patty's Industrial Hygiene and Toxicology,* Vol. 2B, New York, John Wiley & Sons, pp. 3253–3431

Sato, A. & Nakajima, T. (1977) Relationship between partition coefficients and biologic actions of some aromatic hydrocarbons. *Jpn. J. Ind. Health, 19,* 194–195

Sato, A. & Nakajima, T. (1978) Differences following skin or inhalation exposure in the absorption and excretion kinetics of trichloroethylene and toluene. *Br. J. Ind. Med., 35,* 43–49

Sato, A. & Nakajima, T. (1979a) A structure-activity relationship of some chlorinated hydrocarbons. *Arch. Environ. Health, 34,* 69–75

Sato, A. & Nakajima, T. (1979b) Partition coefficients of some aromatic hydrocarbons and ketones in water, blood and oil. *Br. J. Ind. Med., 36,* 231–234

Sato, A. & Nakajima, T. (1979c) Dose-dependent metabolic interaction between benzene and toluene *in vivo* and *in vitro. Toxicol. Appl. Pharmacol., 48,* 249–256

Sato, A. & Nakajima, T. (1984) Dietary carbohydrate- and ethanol-induced alteration of the metabolism and toxicity of chemical substances. *Nutr. Cancer, 6,* 121–132

Sato, A. & Nakajima, T. (1985) Enhanced metabolism of volatile hydrocarbons in rat liver following food deprivation, restricted carbohydrate intake, and administration of ethanol, phenobarbital, polychlorinated biphenyl and 3-methyl-cholanthrene: a comparative study. *Xenobiotica, 15,* 67–75

Sato, A., Fujiwara, Y. & Hirosawa, K. (1972) Solubility of benzene, toluene and *m*-xylene in blood. *Jpn. J. Ind. Health, 14,* 3–8

Sato, A., Nakajima, T., Fujiwara, Y. & Hirosawa, K. (1974a) Pharmacokinetics of benzene and toluene. *Int. Arch. Arbeitsmed., 33,* 169–182

Sato, A., Fujiwara, Y. & Nakajima, T. (1974b) Solubility of benzene, toluene and *m*-xylene in various body fluids and tissues of rabbits. *Jpn. J. Ind. Health, 16,* 30–31

Sato, A., Nakajima, T., Fujiwara, Y. & Murayama, N. (1975) Kinetic studies on sex difference in susceptibility to chronic benzene intoxication – with special reference to body fat content. *Br. J. Ind. Med., 32,* 321–328

Sato, A., Nakajima, T., Fujiwara, Y. & Murayama, N. (1977) A pharmacokinetic model to study the excretion of trichloroethylene and its metabolites after an inhalation exposure. *Br. J. Ind. Med., 34,* 56–63

Sato, A., Nakajima, T. & Koyama, Y. (1980) Effects of chronic ethanol consumption on hepatic metabolism of aromatic and chlorinated hydrocarbons in rats. *Br. J. Ind. Med., 37,* 382–386

Sato, A., Nakajima, T. & Koyama, Y. (1981) Dose-related effects of a single dose of ethanol on the metabolism in rat liver of some aromatic and chlorinated hydrocarbons. *Toxicol. Appl. Pharmacol., 60,* 8–15

Sato, A., Nakajima, T. & Koyama, Y. (1983) Interaction between ethanol and carbohydrate on the metabolism in rat liver of aromatic and chlorinated hydrocarbons. *Toxicol. Appl. Pharmacol., 68,* 242–249

Sato, A., Yonekura, I., Nakajima, T., Ohta, S., Shirai, T. & Ito, N. (1986) Augmentation of ethanol-induced enhancement of dimethylnitrosamine and diethylnitrosamine metabolism by lowered carbohydrate intake. *Jpn. J. Cancer Res., 77,* 125–130

Sawahata, T. & Neal, R.A. (1983) Biotransformation of phenol to hydroquinone and catechol by rat liver microsomes. *Mol. Pharmacol., 23,* 453–460

Snyder, C.A., Baarson, K.A., Goldstein, B.D. & Albert, R.E. (1980) Ingestion of ethanol increases the hematotoxicity of inhaled benzene in C57B1 mice. *Bull. Environ. Contam. Toxicol., 27,* 175–180

Snyder, R. & Kocsis, J.J. (1975) Current concepts of chronic benzene toxicity. *CRC Crit. Rev. Toxicol., 3,* 265–288

Snyder, R., Uzuki, F., Gonasun, L.M., Bromfeld, E. & Wells, A. (1967) The metabolism of benzene *in vitro. Toxicol. Appl. Pharmacol., 11,* 346–360

Thompson, T.N., Watkins, J.B., Gregus, Z. & Klaassen, C.D. (1982) Effect of microsomal enzyme inducers on the soluble enzymes of hepatic phase II biotransformation. *Toxicol. Appl. Pharmacol., 66,* 400–408

Tu, Y.Y. & Yang, C.S. (1983) High-affinity nitrosamine dealkylase system in rat liver microsomes and its induction by fasting. *Cancer Res., 43,* 623–629

Tunek, A. & Oesch, F. (1979) Unique behavior of benzene mono-oxygenase: activation by detergent and different properties of benzene- and phenobarbital-induced mono-oxygenase activities. *Biochem. Pharmacol, 28,* 3425–3429

Tunek, A., Platt, K.L., Bentley, P. & Oesch, F. (1978) Microsomal metabolism of benzene to species irreversibly binding to microsomal protein and effects of modifications of this metabolism. *Mol. Pharmacol., 14,* 920–929

Tunek, A., Platt, K.L., Przybylski, M. & Oesch, F. (1980) Multistep metabolic activation of benzene. Effect of superoxide dismutase on covalent binding to microsomal macromolecules, and identification of glutathione conjugates using high pressure liquid chromatography, and field desorption mass spectrometry. *Chem.-Biol. Interact., 33,* 1–17

Tunek, A., Oloffsson, T. & Berlin, M. (1981) Toxic effects of benzene and benzene metabolites on granulopoietic stem cells and bone marrow cellularity in mice. *Toxicol. Appl. Pharmacol. 59,* 149–156

Tunek, A., Högstedt, B. & Olofsson, T. (1982) Mechanism of benzene toxicity. Effects of benzene and benzene metabolites on bone marrow cellularity, number of granulopoietic stem cells and frequency of micronuclei in mice. *Chem.-Biol. Interact., 39,* 129–138

Vainio, H. (1974) Enhancement of microsomal drug oxidation and glucuronidation in rat liver by an environmental chemical, polychlorinated biphenyl. *Chem.-Biol. Interact., 9,* 379–387

OCCURRENCE

CHAPTER 4

BENZENE: USES, OCCURRENCE AND EXPOSURE

L. Fishbein[1]

Department of Health and Human Services
Food and Drug Administration
National Center for Toxicological Research
Jefferson, AR 72079, USA

INTRODUCTION

The aromatic hydrocarbons, primarily benzene, toluene, the xylenes, ethyl benzene, styrene, cumene and the halogenated benzenes are among the most important volatile aromatic compounds of commercial and environmental significance (IARC, 1979, 1982a; Merian, 1982; Merian & Zander, 1982; Fishbein, 1984, 1985a,b,c).

The pre-eminent role of benzene in environmental health, with regard to the scope of its production, use, occurrence, dispersion, human toxicity (primarily carcinogenicity) and considerations of occupational standard settings, has spawned a voluminous and burgeoning literature (ILO, 1971a,b; Snyder & Kocsis, 1975; OSHA, 1977, 1978; Goldstein *et al.*, 1978; Environmental Protection Agency, 1978; Cheremisinoff & Morresi, 1979; Lauwerys, 1979; Berlin *et al.*, 1980; DGMK, 1980; IAES/SECOTOX, 1980; NIOSH, 1980; Mehlman *et al.*, 1980; Watanabe *et al.*, 1980; Rinsky *et al.*, 1981; IARC, 1982a,b; Korte & Klein, 1982; Van Raalte & Grasso, 1982; Arp, *et al.*, 1983; Infante & White, 1983; Maltoni *et al.*, 1983; Mehlman, 1983; Berlin & Tunek, 1984; Fishbein, 1984; Aksoy, 1985; Berlin, 1985; Dean, 1985; Holmberg & Lundberg, 1985; Infante & White, 1985; Maltoni *et al.*, 1985; Runion & Scott, 1985).

PRODUCTION AND USE

Benzene is produced in enormous quantities, primarily in the U.S.A., Europe and Japan, with Canada and South America contributing considerable additional production. The U.S.A., western Europe and Japan together accounted for more than 75% of worldwide capacity for the production of benzene at the end of 1981 (SRI

---

[1]Present address: ENVIRON Corporation, 1000 Potomac Street NW, Washington DC, USA.

International, 1983a,b). The U.S. production of all grades of benzene by 33 companies at over 50 locations in 1980 totalled approximately 1 563 million gallons (5 217 thousand tonnes) (U.S. International Trade Commission, 1981). Approximately 4.12 million tonnes were produced in the U.S.A. in 1983 and 4.47 million tonnes in 1984, ranking benzene 16th in importance among the chemicals produced in the U.S.A. in those years (Webber, 1985). Although some recent forecasts suggested increasing market demands for benzene at approximately 3 to 5% annually (NTP, 1983a,b; Tobin, 1985), benzene production in 1985 was predicted to be approximately the same as in 1984 (i.e., 4.47 million tonnes), which represents approximately 55% of production capacity in the U.S.A. (Anon., 1985a).

In 1979, 31 U.S. companies produced 5.44 million tonnes of 1° and 2° benzene (which includes refined, nitration and industrial grades). It was estimated that almost as much additional benzene was produced in 1979 and 1980, but was not isolated from the various streams (catalytic reformate in oil refining, pyrolysis gasoline (pygas) in olefins plants, etc.) and was used for fuel purposes (IARC, 1982a). It was estimated that the U.S. production *capacity* for all grades of benzene by 36 producers at 54 locations in 1982–1984 totalled 2 406 thousand tonnes (SRI International, 1983a; Anon., 1985a).

Production of benzene in western Europe in 1979 was estimated at 4 800 thousand tonnes. It is produced by 66 companies in western European countries, the major producers being the U.K. (9 producers), the Federal Republic of Germany (16) and The Netherlands (4). The annual production capacity of benzene in 1980 was estimated to have been at least 6 877 thousand tonnes (IARC, 1982a). The production of benzene in 1984 was estimated to have been as follows (in thousands of tonnes): France, 609; Italy, 555; United Kingdom, 804; and Federal Republic of Germany, 1 430 (Anon., 1985b). Recent production of benzene by COMECON countries was estimated to have been as follows (in thousands of tonnes): USSR, 1 538 (1977); Czechoslovakia, 195 (1979); Romania, 162 (1979); Bulgaria, 61 (1979); Hungary, 34 (1979) and Poland, 15 (1979) (IARC, 1982a).

Approximately 2 170 thousand tonnes of benzene were produced in Japan in 1979 and the combined annual production capacity of 22 Japanese producers in 1980 was estimated to have been 2 882 thousand tonnes (IARC, 1982a). World production of benzene in 1977 was estimated to have been over 12 million tonnes, making it the fourth or fifth largest volume organic chemical produced on a worldwide basis (IARC, 1982a). Global annual production of benzene has recently been estimated at 14 million tonnes. It is thus in the range of 10% of the total annual global production of organic chemicals (Korte & Klein, 1982). In 1982, excess world benzene capacity reached 44% of total installed capacity and is projected to decline to only 23% by 1989; hence world benzene consumption is expected to grow somewhat faster in the future than during the past decade, projected at a rate of approximately 3.0% per year (Tobin, 1985).

Benzene was first isolated in 1825 by Faraday from a liquid condensed by compressing oil gas. In 1845, Hoffman found benzene in light oil derived from coal-tar and the commercial recovery of benzene from this source was further developed and described by Mansfield in 1849. Discovery of benzene in coal gas after 1876 initiated the recovery of coal gas light oil as a source of benzene. Although petroleum was known to contain benzene, its recovery was not undertaken on a commercial scale until about 1941 (Purcell, 1978; IARC, 1982a,b). It is one of the principal components of the light oil recovered from coal carbonization gases, the composition of the light oil depending primarily upon carbonization temperature. Light oil is usually more than 80% aromatic and less than 5% unsaturated. The yield of light oil from coke ovens producing furnace coke is approximately 13–17 L/tonne of coal carbonized. Light oil is now recovered from coal gases by continuous counter-current absorption in a high boiling liquid form, which is stripped by steam distillation (Purcell, 1978).

Until several years following World War II, benzene was principally produced commercially in the U.S.A. from coal, and until about 1960 coal was the source material for almost all of the benzene produced in Europe. Petroleum benzene was first produced in Europe by the United Kingdom in 1952, in France in 1958, in the Federal Republic of Germany in 1961 and in Italy in about 1962. The principal sources of Japanese benzene were coal-based until 1967. Major eastern European producers of benzene (e.g., German Democratic Republic, USSR) are believed currently to be producing benzene from petroleum feedstocks. It is anticipated that the major oil exporting countries, particularly Saudi Arabia, will produce and export significant amounts of benzene in the near future, along with other basic petrochemicals (Purcell, 1978).

The major commercial routes for obtaining benzene from petroleum sources include refinery streams (primarily catalytic reformate), pyrolysis gasoline and toluene dealkylation. In catalytic reforming, a low-sulfur naphtha-range petroleum fraction is catalytically reformed (using principally platinum or palladium dehydrocyclization catalysts) to produce a high-octane product for use in gasoline blending. Benzene and other aromatic hydrocarbons can be removed from the reformate by solvent extraction and fractional distillation of the extract to produce pure compounds. The production of benzene by reforming-separation processes is associated with the production of toluene and xylene (BTX plants). The relative production of the various hydrocarbons is a function of the feedstock, reactor conditions, catalyst and principally of the boiling range of the product fraction subjected to solvent extraction (Purcell, 1978).

A significant quantity of benzene is commercially obtained from pyrolysis gasoline (pygas; dripolene) in olefin plants as a by-product of the manufacture of ethylene or propylene by cracking naphtha or gas oil. This is a significant source of benzene if the feedstock is a naphtha gas oil or a similar heavy hydrocarbon. Aromatic compounds are recovered from the liquid by-product (pyrolysis gasoline) by partial hydrogenation, desulfurization, hydrocracking, hydrodealkylation and distillation (Purcell, 1978).

More recently, benzene has been produced from toluene by transalkylation (also called disproportionation). Since raw material costs make benzene produced by this route more expensive than that from other sources, the economic attractiveness of toluene dealkylation is sensitive to the relative prices of benzene and toluene. Many toluene dealkylation units produce benzene for in-house consumption or from captive toluene supplies not needed for gasoline (Purcell, 1978; Anon., 1980).

Catalytic reforming was the source of approximately 44–55% of the benzene produced in the U.S.A. in the period 1978–1981. In contrast to pygas, only 45% of the potentially obtainable benzene was extracted from catalytic reformate in the U.S.A. in 1981, the remainder going into the gasoline pool with toluene hydroalkylation providing almost 25% of the benzene supply in 1981. Historically, about 25–30% of benzene production is usually from dealkylation. This source is the "swing" supply of benzene and is an effective means of balancing supply and demand. Most of the remaining benzene supply is derived from light oil, a steel manufacturing by-product that is rich in benzene (SRI International, 1983b). In western Europe and Japan, the largest current source of benzene is pyrolysis gasoline (a by-product of ethylene manufacture), which accounts for 55% and 50%, respectively, of benzene capacity in those regions, with coke-oven operations providing less than 10% of production and the remainder approximately evenly divided between catalytic reformate and toluene hydrodealkylation (IARC, 1982a; SRI International, 1983b). The major impurities in commercial benzene are toluene and the xylenes, although the commercial grade of benzene can also be contaminated with phenol, thiophene, carbon disulfide, acetonitrile and pyridine.

Benzene is presently utilized principally as an intermediate in the manufacture of other chemicals, and as a solvent to increase the octane rating of unleaded gasoline. Industrial uses of benzene have included preparation of derivatives, such as polymers, detergents, pesticides and intermediates in the chemical and pharmaceutical industries (approximately 95% of demand in the U.S.A.), preparation of chlorinated solvents, extraction and rectification, uses in the rubber industry, in cements and adhesives, as a component of inks in the printing industry, as a coatings thinner and as a degreasing and cleaning agent (Brief *et al.,* 1980). Figure 1 indicates some products derived from benzene (Purcell, 1978). Benzene consumption and the flow of benzene through the U.S.A. is illustrated in Figure 2 (Cheremisinoff & Morresi, 1979), and Figure 3 depicts the commercial uses of the nitrobenzene derivative of benzene (Cheremisinoff & Morresi, 1979).

Apparent consumption of benzene in the U.S.A. grew at an average annual rate of 8.5% from 1955 through 1974. From 1974 to 1979, growth slowed to 2% annually. Consumption peaked in 1979 and has declined by an average 7.5–8.0% annually from 1979 through 1981. Worldwide, benzene demand is dominated by the production of three derivatives, i.e., ethylbenzene, cumene and cyclohexane. The largest chemical outlet for benzene is in the production of ethylbenzene, almost all of which is consumed for styrene manufacture and which accounted for more than 50% of benzene demand in the U.S.A. in 1981. Cumene/phenol production was the second largest outlet, followed by cyclohexane (SRI International, 1983b).

About 90–93% of benzene produced in the U.S.A. in 1978 was consumed as follows: ethylbenzene/styrene, over 50%; cumene/phenol, approximately 20%; cyclohexane, 15–16%; nitrobenzene/aniline, 4–5%; and maleic anhydride, chlorobenzenes, detergent alkylate (dodecyl benzene) and other uses, 2.5–3.0% each (Cheremisinoff & Morresi, 1979; IARC, 1982a). In 1984, the major consumption pattern for benzene was ethylbenzene, 50%; cumene, 20%; cyclohexane, 15%; and aniline, 5%; the major end uses were styrenic plastics, 35%; phenolic resin, 20% and nylons, 15% (Anon., 1985a).

It is anticipated that all U.S. capability for the production of maleic anhydride will be based on less expensive *n*-butane feedstock before 1986 (SRI International, 1983b).

Fig. 1. Some products derived from benzene (Purcell, 1978)

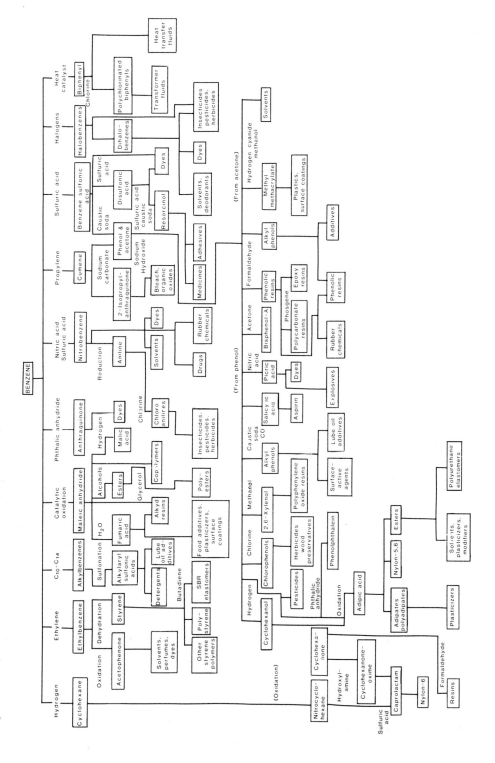

Fig. 2. Flow of benzene through the U.S.A. and benzene consumption (estimated usage in million gallons) (Cheremisinoff & Morresi, 1979)

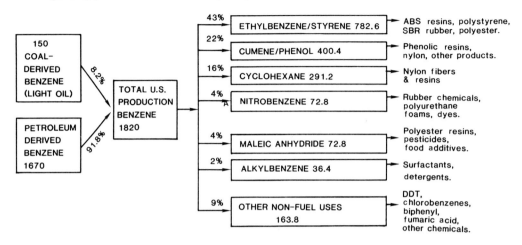

Fig. 3. The commercial uses of nitrobenzene (Cheremisinoff & Morresi, 1979)

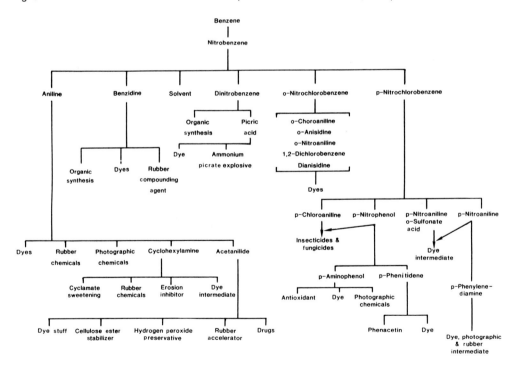

As in the U.S.A., ethylbenzene consumed the largest amounts of benzene in both western Europe and Japan in 1980, followed by cumene in western Europe and cyclohexane in Japan as the second largest consumers. Western Europe accounted for one-third of the non-communist world's total benzene consumption in 1980, compared to 40% for the U.S.A. and 14% for Japan (SRI International, 1983a,b).

In 1979 in western Europe, 4 864 thousand tonnes of recovered benzene were used as follows: ethylbenzene/styrene, 48%; cumene, 20%; cyclohexane, 14%; nitrobenzene/aniline, 7%; detergent alkylate, 4%; maleic anhydride, 3%; chlorobenzenes, 2%; other uses, 2%. The use pattern for recovered benzene in Japan in 1980 was as follows: ethylbenzene/styrene, 51%; cyclohexane, 24%; cumene/phenol, 13%; detergent alkylate, 4%; maleic anhydride, 2%; other uses 6% (IARC, 1982a).

In the past, benzene was widely used as an industrial solvent, but the amounts now employed for this purpose are believed to be relatively small and decreasing, or even abolished, in most Western countries (Holmberg & Lundberg, 1985). Benzene was used in industry (e.g., rubber and tyre manufacturing) (IARC, 1982a,b) as a general-purpose solvent in the 1920s (Davis, 1929), but following reports of toxicity (Hunter, 1939), benzene was supplanted by toluene and other aromatic and aliphatic solvents (Mellan, 1957). However, it is disturbing to realize that in 1968 approximately 50 000 tonnes of benzene were used as a solvent in the U.S.A. (Merian & Zander, 1982). However, it should also be noted that benzene is still extensively used in laboratories as a reagent in sample collection, preparation and extraction, and it has been estimated that there are more than 12 000 laboratories in the U.S.A. alone (Cheremisinoff & Morresi, 1979). It has also been noted recently by Ringen and Addis (1983) that benzene exposure may still occur in industry and is detectable in workroom air in many industrial activities (Holmberg & Lundberg, 1985).

SOURCES OF BENZENE EMISSIONS

The low boiling-point (80.1 °C) and high vapour pressure (100 mm of mercury at 26.1 °C) of benzene cause its rapid evaporation at standard pressures and temperatures. Hypotheses about the stability of benzene in the environment are conflicting. In one view, benzene is basically stable in the atmosphere, hence its contribution to photochemically-induced pollutants may be considered minor (Cheremisinoff & Morresi, 1979). Alternatively, it has been stated that benzene, whether it is emitted directly to air, discharged to water or disposed of on land, will eventually end up in the atmosphere where it is oxidized (Slimak & Delos, 1983–1984).

The degradation of benzene in the environment has recently been reviewed (Cerniglia, 1981; Korte & Klein, 1982; Merian & Zander, 1982). Based on the mobility of benzene and its degradation characteristics, it was concluded by Korte and Klein (1982) that (1) benzene is readily biodegradable; (2) its atmospheric fate is of major importance, with the atmospheric half-life of benzene being less than one day. The pathway for the bacterial oxidation of benzene has been summarized as illustrated in Scheme 1.

Although atmospheric rain washout of benzene to the oceans may be a most probable fate, it rapidly separates from water due to its high vapour pressure. The half-life of benzene in water is about 37 min. Vegetation plays an important role in the absorption of atmospheric benzene (Cheremisinoff & Morresi, 1979).

Scheme 1. The pathway for the bacterial oxidation of benzene (Cerniglia, 1981).

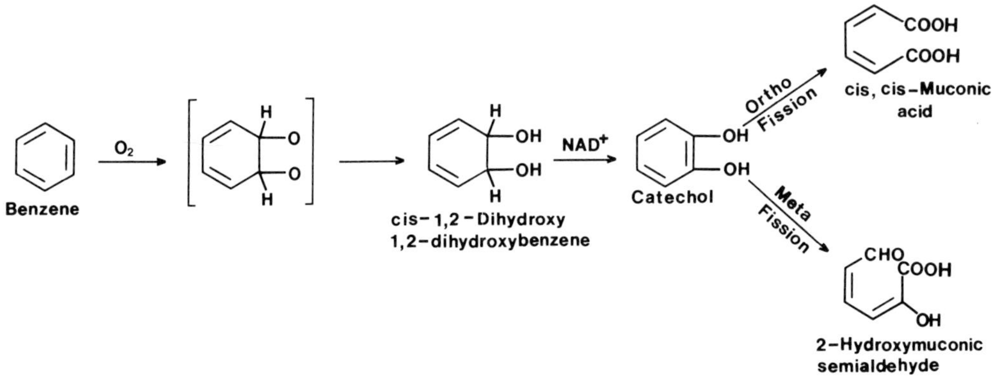

Benzene is found throughout the world with concentrations ranging from 0.3–45 μg/m³ in the ambient atmosphere of even remote regions. The major source of this ambient benzene is believed to be biological (animal and plant matter) rather than industrial (Brief *et al.*, 1980). It has been estimated that, worldwide, about 5 million tonnes of benzene are of natural origin, about 26 million tonnes are produced by refining and cracking oil fractions and 1 million tonnes are produced from coal-tar (Merian & Zander, 1982).

Estimates of annual benzene emissions in the U.S.A. and worldwide vary greatly. For example, fugitive emissions during production, storage, transport and commercial use were estimated by OSHA to be 36 thousand tonnes per year in the U.S.A. in 1976 (OSHA, 1977). This approximates 6–8% of the total produced. While OSHA considers that the fugitive emissions are largely derived from petroleum cracking facilities, a study by Gisser (1978) suggested that the benzene emissions from refineries, olefin plants and alkyl benzene plants were about 40% of earlier estimates of the U.S. Environmental Protection Agency (EPA) (1977). In 1974, the EPA (Howard & Durkin, 1974) estimate of losses from benzene production, transportation and commercial use was an order of magnitude greater than that of OSHA. In the same report, it was estimated that total motor vehicle emissions make up well over half of the benzene released to the environment, with a distribution which probably approximates population density distribution. Release from industrial and commercial sources probably does not exceed 30% of the total. Other sources were considered relatively insignificant. In other reports, it was estimated that 20 000 tonnes of benzene were discharged in 1977 by the U.S. chemical industry from 63% of the identified emission sources. A total of about 40% escapes from storage tanks. On the basis of these figures, it could be calculated that losses at present amount to about 0.17% of the quantities produced (Gisser, 1978; Merian & Zander, 1982).

A summary of emissions of benzene from various sources in the U.S.A. during 1976 is shown in Table 1 (Cheremisinoff & Morresi, 1979). These sources of emissions range from the production of benzene, to its processing into a number of its major derivatives, to its storage and handling and to its usage. As can be noted, all activities associated with benzene give rise to significant emissions. The estimated annual

Table 1. Benzene emissions for 1976 (Cheremisinoff & Morresi, 1979)

No.	Source	U.S. benzene emissions (tonnes/year)
1	Petroleum refineries gasoline production (1976)	1 859
2	Crude oil operations	998

Chemical products derived from benzene (1975)

No.	Source	U.S. benzene emissions (tonnes/year)
3	Nitrobenzene	3 466
4	Aniline	?
5	Styrene	3 046
6	Cumene	227
7	Maleic anhydride	15 782
8	Dichlorobenzene (*o* & *p*)	2 404
9	Monochlorobenzene	
10	Phenol	766
11	Solvent operations	73 014

Storage tanks

No.	Source	U.S. benzene emissions (tonnes/year)
12	Gasoline	771
13	Benzene	272
14	Gasoline distribution (loading and unloading of storage tanks and transfer to service stations)	1 726
15	Benzene distribution	907
16	*Service stations* (loading, car refueling and spillage)	6 585
17	*Car exhausts* (27% uncontrolled, 73% controlled)	168 702
18	*Car evaporative losses*	31 097
	Total	311 622

Table 2. Annual emissions of benzene to air from various sources[a]

Source	Emission (thousand tonnes)
Component of gasoline[b]	40.0–80.0
Production of other chemicals	44.0–56.0
Indirect production of benzene[c]	23.0–79.0
Production of benzene from petroleum	1.8– 7.3
Solvents and miscellaneous sources	1.5
Imports of benzene	0.013

[a] From JRB Associates, Inc. (1980)
[b] Production, storage, transport, vending and combustion
[c] Coke ovens, oil spills, nonferrous metals manufacturing, ore mining, wood processing, coal mining, and textile industry.

Table 3.   Annual benzene emissions to water in the U.S.A. [a]

Source	Emissions (tonnes)
Indirect production of benzene [b]	200–11 000
Solvent and miscellaneous uses	1 450
Production of chemicals other than benzene	1 000
Production of benzene from petroleum	630
Imports of benzene	13

[a] From JRB Associates, Inc. (1980)
[b] Coke ovens, oil spills, nonferrous metal manufacture, ore mining, wood processing, coal mining and textile manufacture

emissions of benzene to air and water from various sources in the U.S.A. is shown in Tables 2 and 3, respectively (IARC, 1982a). An attempt by the U.S. EPA to put pathways for benzene release into better perspective is illustrated in Figure 4, which is based on released amounts for the U.S. 1978 materials balance (Slimak & Delos, 1983–1984). The major emission source involves direct release to the atmosphere and is predominantly due to gasoline combustion, 55%; use of other fuels, 17%; petroleum refining, 9%; gas transport and storage, 8%; benzene use as chemical feedstock, 5%. In contrast, losses of benzene to aquatic and land sources are very much less.

It has been estimated that over 75% of the U.S. population has probably been exposed to benzene, due to its ubiquitous nature (NTP, 1981). In 1976 an estimated 590 thousand tonnes of benzene were released into the atmosphere from 132 million stationary and mobile sources. This includes an estimated 109 thousand tonnes/year from the production, transportation, storage and use of benzene; 450 thousand tonnes/year from the refuelling and operation of motor vehicles and 10 thousand tonnes/year from oil spills.

It was estimated that approximately 7 100 tonnes of benzene from mobile sources were emitted to the ambient air in The Netherlands in 1980, while stationary source emissions contributed an additional 838 tonnes (Guicherit & Schulting, 1985). The main sources of volatile alkanes in The Netherlands are automobile exhaust gas, evaporation losses from gasoline storage and handling, natural gas leaks and petrochemical industries.

On a worldwide basis, benzene losses in the chemical industry probably amount to some 100 000–200 000 tonnes. To this figure must be added losses of the order of 3 million tonnes of benzene during production, transportation and distribution of motor fuel and combustion in gasoline engines (Merian & Zander, 1982).

A significant source of benzene release into the environment is oil spills. The benzene content of crude oil is approximately 0.2%. Tanker washings, accidents, exploration, production, transportation, handling and wastes account for nearly 6 million tonnes of crude oil being discharged into the oceans each year. Of this, nearly 120 000 tonnes are benzene (Cheremisinoff & Morresi, 1979).

Benzene is present in gasoline as a result of its natural occurrence in crude oil and is also a by-product of the catalytic cracking, coking and reforming processes used to

Fig. 4. Pathways for benzene release (Slimak & Delos, 1983–1984)

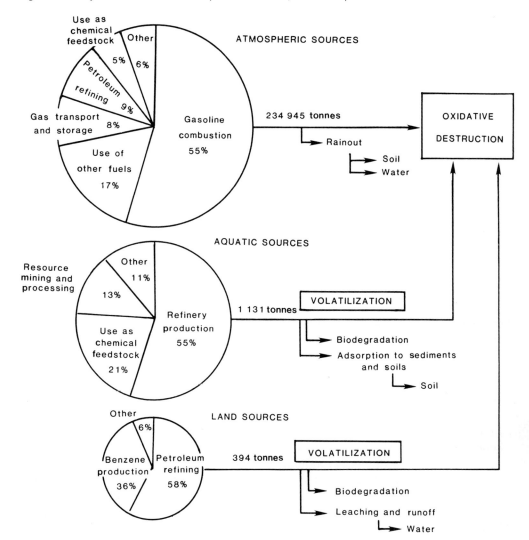

double the yield of gasoline from crude oil (Brief *et al.*, 1980). U.S. gasolines contain an average of 0.8% benzene, while European gasolines contain an average of 5%. Benzene comprises about 2.15% of the total hydrocarbon emissions from a gasoline engine, or approximately 4% of automotive exhaust (U.S. Environmental Protection Agency, 1980).

A further potential source of environmental pollution is the burning of wood, garbage and organic wastes. Since the combustion gases from wood total only about 400 000 tonnes of hydrocarbons per year in the U.S.A., this benzene source is of

Fig. 5. Annual global cycle of benzene (Merian & Zander, 1982)

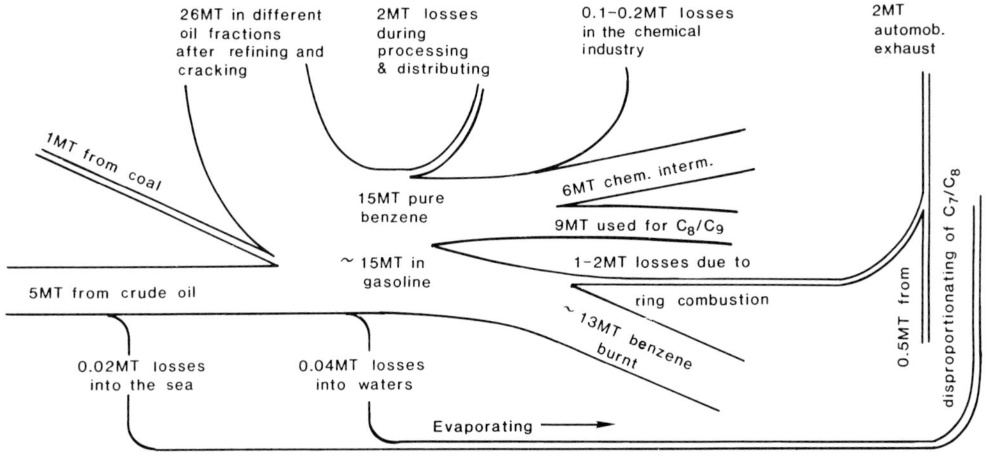

minor significance compared to the 26–30 million tonnes consumed as raw material or in gasoline (Merian & Zander, 1982).

The combustion of various shipboard materials has been reported to form benzene at the following concentrations: wall insulation material, 60 mg/m³ (18.8 ppm), polyvinyl chloride cable jacket, 9 mg/m³ (2.8 ppm) and hydraulic fluid, 800 mg/m³ (250 ppm) (Zinn et al., 1980).

Benzene has been reported to be a thermal degradation product of polyvinyl chloride food-wrapping film when it is cut with a hot wire, giving quantities of benzene ranging from 5–20 ng per cut (Boettner & Ball, 1980).

In addition, benzene has been increasingly reported in abandoned chemical waste dumps and leachates. For example, in the U.S.A., the EPA in mid-1984 had designated 546 sites for its National Priority List. Benzene was among the top five chemicals found (at 94 sites) on this list (Abelson, 1985).

Figure 5 illustrates the global annual cycle of benzene (Merian & Zander, 1982). From this figure it can be concluded that about 15 million tonnes (MT) of benzene are used annually as a base product in the chemical industry, about 13 million tonnes are destroyed through burning and about 4 million tonnes are lost into the environment, mainly into the atmosphere. Assuming the biological and abiotic degradation of benzene to take, on the average, a few days, it can be estimated that there must always be about 100 000 tonnes of benzene in the global environment. It is recognized that this amount must be distributed very irregularly and it is more important to know the local concentration (Merian, 1982).

EXPOSURE LEVELS AND POPULATIONS AT RISK

Industrial exposure

The early uses of benzene, particularly as a solvent, resulted in concentrations in the workplace of about 1 600 mg/m³ (500 ppm), and at times in excess of 3 200 mg/m³

Table 4.   Occupational exposures to benzene in various industries (IARC, 1982a)

Industry	Concentration (mg/m³ air) (ppm)		Year	Reference[a]
	Range	Other		
Rubber coating				
(churn room)	304–832 (95–260)		1935–1937	NIOSH (1974)
(spreader machine)	208–640 (65–200)		1935–1937	NIOSH (1974)
Rubber factory	320[b] (100)	1 600 (500)[c]	1942	EPA (1980)
Rubber coating	83–416 (25–125)		1961	EPA (1980)
	64–80 (20–25)[b, d]	448 (140)[c]	1960–1963	NIOSH (1974)
Rubber raincoat factory	438–698 (137–218)		1977	EPA (1980d)
Printing	32–3 392 (10–1 060)		1939	NIOSH (1974)
Artificial leather,	320–1 600 (100–500)		1936–1939	NIOSH (1974)
rubber goods or				
shoe manufacture				
Leatherette factory	150–1 000 (47–130)		1953–1957	NIOSH (1974)
	80–150 (25–47)[e]		1953–1957	NIOSH (1974)
Shoe factory	1 017–1 504 (318–470)		1956	NIOSH (1974)
	100–500 (31–156)		1960–1963	NIOSH (1974)
	130–140 (41–44)[f]		1964	NIOSH (1974)
	480–2 080 (150–650)		1966–1978	EPA (1980d)
Chemical plant[g]	0.3–1.3 (0.1–0.4)		1979	Evans and Wilcox (1979)
Petroleum refinery	2–103 (0.6–32)[h]		1978	Markel and Elesh (1979)
(quality control lab)				
Waste-water treatment	0.06–1.5 (< 0.02–0.51)		1978	Gorman and Slovin (1980)
plant at petroleum factory	(personal samples)			
	0.06–21.7 (< 0.02–7.22)		1978	Gorman and Slovin (1980)
	(area samples)			
Coal liquefaction plant	0.06 (0.02)		1980	Anon (1980)
Australian Air Force workshop	33–116 (10–35)[b]	4 480 (1 400)[c]	1947	EPA (1980d)
Paint manufacture	trace–362 (trace–78.5)		1963	NIOSH (1974)
Painting of metal products	0.5–10 (0.17–3.1)		1978	McQuilkin (1980)

[a] NIOSH, National Institute for Occupational Safety and Health; EPA, US Environmental Protection Agency
[b] Average
[c] Peak
[d] Following removal of benzene from use in the industry, naphtha solvents containing up to 7.5% benzene were used
[e] Following improved control measures
[f] Following replacement of a technical benzene with toluene in shoe adhesives
[g] Producing hexabromocyclododecane and dialkylaminoethyl chloride hydrochlorides
[h] Maximum measured at benzene distillation operation.

(1 000 ppm). Table 4 shows concentrations of benzene reported in workplace air in various industries since 1935 (IARC, 1982a), Table 5 is a summary of concentrations of benzene in air samples taken near U.S. chemical factories where benzene is used (IARC, 1982a). Although very high levels of exposure to benzene occurred in the past, major improvements in the quality of workplace atmospheres (Table 4) seem generally to have been made in the 1970s (Brief *et al.*, 1980; IARC, 1982a; Holmberg & Lundberg, 1985; Runion & Scott, 1985).

Table 5.   Benzene concentrations in the air near U.S. chemical manufacturing factories (IARC, 1982a)

Source	Concentration		Reference
	(µg/m³)	(ppb)	
Nitrobenzene manufacture	3–11	1–4	Fentiman *et al.* (1979)
Cumene manufacture	25–51	9–19	Fentiman *et al.* (1979)
Maleic anhydride manufacture	2–32	1–10	Fentiman *et al.* (1979)
From pyrolysis gas	6–35	2–13	Fentiman *et al.* (1979)
Detergent alkylate manufacture	2.7–55.4	1–18	Fentiman *et al.* (1979)
Other factories using benzene	1.9–108.8	0.6–34	Suta (1980)

Table 6.   Concentrations of benzene in the US tyre industry, 1973–1977 [a]

Operation	Personal breathing sample		Area sample	
	(mg/m³)	(ppm)	(mg/m³)	(ppm)
Cement mixing	0.6–15.4	0.2–4.8	0–52.8	0–16.5
Extrusion	< 0.3–16.3	< 0.1–5.1	1.3–14.7	0.4–4.6
Tyre building	0.3–7.7	0.1–2.4	0.3–6.4	0.1–2.0
Curing preparation	< 0.3–18.9	< 0.1–5.9	1.3–3.8	0.4–1.2
Inspection and repair	< 0.3–6.1	< 0.1–1.9	0.03–7.0	0.01–2.2
Maintenance	0.6–1.5	0.2–0.5	1.5–4.8	0.5–1.5
Warehouse	–	–	0.03–1.5	0.01–0.5

[a] From Van Ert *et al.* (1980).

Benzene has been reported in many processes associated with the rubber industry (e.g., tyres, tubes, remoulds, retreads, rubber goods, proofed rubber fabrics, adhesives and sealants) (Van Ert *et al.,* 1980; IARC, 1982a,b; Checkoway *et al.,* 1984). Concentrations of benzene found in the air around certain operations in various U.S. rubber tyre factories are shown in Table 6 (Van Ert *et al.,* 1980).

Excessive leukaemia mortality has appeared consistently in epidemiological studies of British and U.S. rubber industry workers, and attempts to identify causative factors have focused on exposure to benzene and other solvents (McMichael *et al.,* 1975; IARC, 1982a,b; Checkoway *et al.,* 1984).

Exposure levels and populations at risk from benzene vary greatly. NIOSH has estimated that some two million workers in the U.S.A. are potentially exposed to benzene in printing, lithography and dry cleaning, and in the manufacture of coke and gas, adhesives, coatings and a variety of chemicals (NIOSH, 1977). Historically, the levels of exposure varied greatly from one process to another, depending on whether they involved open or closed systems. Some industrial exposures are known to have been as high as 320–3 200 mg/m³ on a routine basis (Brief *et al.,* 1980) (see also Table 4, IARC, 1982a). It has recently been suggested by Brief *et al.* (1980) that "industrial establishments in the U.S. with continuous levels over 50 ppm TWA must be very rare". In petroleum refineries during normal operations, there is a low probability ($<5\%$) of benzene levels exceeding a 1-ppm time-weighted average (TWA) and a negligible chance of exceeding 5 ppm. In petroleum plants there is a somewhat higher probability of exceeding 1 ppm, but less than 8% probability of exceeding 5 ppm. This higher potential relative to refineries is related primarily to much higher benzene concentrations in the process streams and products (Brief *et al.*, 1980).

Brief *et al.* (1980) summarized the likely activities wherein workers may be exposed to relatively higher air concentrations of benzene. These include: work in effluent treatment plants (such as API separators); manual tank or stream sampling; laboratory testing of the benzene-containing process materials; maintenance when equipment containing benzene materials is opened or drained without adequate flushing, and loading of ships, barges and tracks with gasoline or benzene-rich streams, particularly if no vapour recovery or remote venting is employed.

Runion and Scott (1985) recently reported an overview of benzene occupational exposure in the U.S.A. for the period 1978–1983. Some 38 000 data points, representing TWA for air samples or persons exposed, were collected from five industries which produce and/or use benzene and from two governmental organizations. Of the reported data, 87% represented exposure levels of 1.0 ppm or less and 98.4% were below 10 ppm. Elevated exposure levels were found in petroleum and chemical operations, including petrochemical and bulk-loading as well as in benzol and by-product plants in the iron and steel industries. Tables 7–12 summarize the percent distribution of exposure to benzene within the various ppm ranges.

The benzene exposure profile for the U.S.A. (Table 7), representing in excess of 38 000 TWA samples, produced an estimated arithmetic mean value of 0.64 ppm and an estimated geometric mean of 0.1 ppm. Eighty-seven percent of all the samples were less than 1.0 ppm, while 11.4% were between 1 and 10 ppm and 1.6% were greater than 10 ppm.

The petroleum industry benzene exposure profile (Table 8) indicated that the petrochemical operations and bulk transfer of benzene and benzene-containing materials offered the highest opportunity for significant exposure. Although benzol plants (Table 9) would appear to offer the iron and steel industry's most significant exposure, the levels were relatively low (2.2 ppm) with an estimated geometric standard deviation of 2.3 ppm. In addition, all of the coke oven data (2 065 employees) were at or below 0.5 ppm. The chemical manufacturing industry benzene exposure profile (Table 10) revealed that barge loading (as also shown by the API data) possessed the most significant exposure, with an estimated geometric mean of 2 ppm and an estimated geometric standard deviation of 1.7 ppm. Table 11, for the rubber industry, suggests that there are no operations where appreciable exposure to benzene exists, most operations involving concentrations less than 0.1 to 0.5 ppm.

Occupational exposure to benzene has also been recently summarized by Berlin (1985) and Holmberg and Lundberg (1985). Table 13 illustrates the results of personal sampling in a number of Swedish workplaces and shows that, although exposure levels about 10 ppm are rather rare, levels between 1 and 5 ppm are rather common for workers handling gasoline or gasoline equipment (Berlin, 1985).

Table 7. U.S. benzene exposure profile (Runion & Scott, 1985)

Data source	No. of samples	% exposed in each range, Exposure range (ppm)						Estimated geometric mean (ppm)	Estimated geometric standard deviation (ppm)	Estimated arithmetic mean (ppm)	Estimated arithmetic standard deviation (ppm)
		< 0.1	0.1–0.5	0.5–1.0	1.0–5.0	5–10	> 10				
American Petroleum Institute	28 561	63.5	25.6	5.1	4.5	0.6	0.7	0.05	6.8	0.29	1.1
National Institute of Occupational Safety and Health	262	62.2	20.2	6.5	8.8	0.8	1.5	0.05	10.4	0.65	3.7
Occupational Safety and Health Administration	189	27.4	28.4	15.2	18.4	5.8	4.8	0.33	8.5	2.87	13.6
National Paint and Coating Association	1 261	81.4	16.1	1.6	0.9	0.0	0.0	0.02	5.0	0.07	0.2
Chemical Manufacturers' Association	2 448		77.1	–	20.6	2.3	0.0	0.39	3.6	0.87	1.6
American Iron and Steel Institute	3 208		77.9	9.6	10.4	1.7	0.4	0.13	6.0	0.61	2.0
Rubber Manufacturers' Association	3 523	52.5	38.3	6.9	2.2	0.1	0.0	0.10	3.3	0.20	0.3
U.S.A. overall	38 317		77.8	9.8	9.3	1.5	1.6	0.10	7.2	0.64	2.5

Table 8. Petroleum industry benzene exposure profile (Runion & Scott, 1985)

Site	No. of samples	% exposed in each range Exposure range (ppm)						Estimated geometric mean (ppm)	Estimated geometric standard deviation (ppm)	Estimated arithmetic mean (ppm)	Estimated arithmetic standard deviation (ppm)
		< 0.1	0.1–0.5	0.5–1.0	1.0–5.0	5–10	> 10				
Other	191	84.4	12.0	1.0	1.6	0.0	1.0	0.01	9.0	0.10	0.5
Retail service stations	1 478	85.6	12.0	1.5	0.7	0.1	0.1	0.02	5.4	0.06	0.2
Exploration/production	3 016	80.0	16.8	1.7	1.2	0.1	0.2	0.03	4.0	0.08	0.2
Pipeline	622	66.9	24.4	3.5	4.7	0.3	0.2	0.05	6.7	0.25	0.9
Trucks, benzene, mixed	1 356	68.4	23.1	5.3	2.9	0.1	0.2	0.05	4.9	0.17	0.4
Refining	14 824	64.6	26.1	4.6	3.8	0.5	0.4	0.05	5.7	0.22	0.7
Rail car, other	19	63.2	26.2	5.3	5.3	0.0	0.0	0.06	5.7	0.26	0.8
Rail car, mixed	674	58.5	28.3	7.6	4.9	0.4	0.3	0.08	5.2	0.28	0.8
Marketing terminal trucks	1 452	57.8	32.8	5.3	3.7	0.3	0.1	0.08	4.1	0.21	0.4
Ship/barge, benzene, mixed	63	61.9	4.8	4.8	19.0	3.2	6.3	0.09	20.0	5.10	49.6
Ship/barge, other	457	44.8	30.9	7.4	12.7	2.2	2.0	0.12	9.2	1.22	6.2
Petrochemical	4 165	44.6	33.2	10.0	9.9	1.3	1.0	0.13	5.5	0.52	1.6
Trucks, benzene	91	12.1	69.2	9.9	2.2	2.2	4.4	0.23	6.1	1.10	3.7
Ship/barge, benzene	90	16.7	17.7	13.3	25.7	8.9	17.7	1.30	9.2	13.2	67.4
Rail car, benzene	63	9.6	7.8	6.3	7.9	7.9	60.5	26.0	38.5	Very large	

Table 9. American iron and steel industry benzene exposure profile (Runion & Scott, 1985)

Site	No. of employees	% exposed in each range Exposure range (ppm)						Estimated geometric mean (ppm)	Estimated geometric standard deviation (ppm)	Estimated arithmetic mean (ppm)	Estimated arithmetic standard deviation (ppm)
		< 0.1	0.1–0.5	0.5–1.0	1.0–5.0	5–10	> 10				
By-product plant	897	41.6	27.8	25.0	4.3	1.3	0.65	3.4	1.35	2.2
Benzol plant	113	6.2	5.3	74.3	13.2	1.0	2.20	2.3	3.11	3.0
Chemical laboratory	133	40.6	40.6	18.8	0.0	0.0	0.56	1.8	0.67	4.2
Coke oven	2 065	100.0	0.0	0.0	0.0	0.0	N.A.	N.A.	N.A.	N.A.

N.A., not available

Table 10. Chemical manufacturing industry benzene exposure profile (Runion & Scott, 1985)

Occupation	No. of employees	% exposed in each range — Exposure range (ppm)						Estimated geometric mean (ppm)	Estimated geometric standard deviation (ppm)	Estimated arithmetic mean (ppm)	Estimated arithmetic standard deviation (ppm)
		<0.1	0.1–0.5	0.5–1.0	1.0–5.0	5–10	>10				
Barge loading	36		8.3	↑	88.9	2.8		2.00	1.7	2.31	1.3
Rail loading	278		87.1	↑	11.9	1.0		0.19	4.2	0.52	1.1
Truck loading	426		90.1	↑	9.4	0.5		0.09	6.0	0.42	1.4
Petrochemical	1 708		73.7	↑	23.4	2.9		0.45	3.6	1.00	1.8

Table 11. Rubber Manufacturers Association benzene exposure profile (Runion & Scott, 1985)

Occupation	No. of samples	% exposed in each range — Exposure range (ppm)						Estimated geometric mean (ppm)	Estimated geometric standard deviation (ppm)	Estimated arithmetic mean (ppm)	Estimated arithmetic standard deviation (ppm)
		<0.1	0.1–0.5	0.5–1.0	1.0–5.0	5–10	>10				
Bead dip operator	64	29.8	64.0	3.1	3.1	0	0	0.14	2.6	0.22	0.3
Cure finisher	96	67.6	24.0	2.1	6.3	0	0	0.04	6.3	0.20	0.7
Calendar operator	33	45.4	42.4	6.1	6.1	0	0	0.12	3.5	0.26	0.4
Spray operator	183	37.7	51.4	9.3	1.6	0	0	0.16	2.4	0.23	0.2
Cement house operator	281	43.0	45.9	9.3	1.8	0	0	0.12	3.0	0.22	0.3
Tyre repair	167	74.2	23.4	2.4	0	0	0	0.04	3.6	0.09	0.2
Casing assembly	139	66.9	26.6	3.6	2.9	0	0	0.05	4.8	0.16	0.4
Tyre builder	1 184	40.5	46.5	10.0	3.0	0	0	0.15	2.8	0.25	0.3
Tuber	433	52.1	35.6	7.4	4.4	0.5	0	0.09	4.3	0.25	0.6
Extruder	43	33.6	58.1	9.3	0	0	0	0.15	2.5	0.23	0.2
Miscellaneous	897	69.0	27.4	3.3	0.3	0	0	0.05	3.5	0.11	0.2
Banbury operator	3	100.0	0	0	0	0	0	N.A.	N.A.	N.A.	N.A.

N.A., not available

Table 12.   U.S. Agency profile of benzene exposures (Runion & Scott, 1985)

Data source (activity)	No. of samples	% exposed in each range Exposure range (ppm)						Estimated geometric mean (ppm)	Estimated geometric standard deviation (ppm)	Estimated arithmetic mean (ppm)	Estimated arithmetic standard deviation (ppm)
		< 0.1	0.1–0.5	0.5–1.0	1.0–5.0	5–10	> 10				
Occupational Safety and Health Administration (Refining)	66	9.1	40.9	21.2	19.7	3.0	6.1	0.50	6.0	9.33	30.5
National Institute of Occupational Safety and Health (Refining)	74	39.1	29.7	14.9	13.5	1.4	1.4	0.18	6.1	0.87	2.9
National Institute of Occupational Safety and Health (Petrochemical)	20	30.0	40.0	5.0	10.0	0.0	15.0	0.21	25.7	10.51	98.6

Table 13. Occupational exposure to benzene in Sweden measured by personal sampling (Berlin, 1985)

Occupation	Sampling time (min)	Benzene concentration (ppm–mean) (range in parentheses)
Tank lorry drivers	45	0.4 (4.13–0.01)
Loading	45	4.0 (45.5–0.03)
Unloading	45	0.33 (2.9–0.01)
Driving	45	0.026 (0.11–< 0.005)
Petrol station attendants	45	0.054 (0.31–0.02)
Coast tanker crew	45	6.56 (22.8–0.33)
Coke work	9–25	2.72 (12.0–0.16)
Rock depots for oil	17	< 1 [a]
Automobile servicemen	10	0.052 (0.053–0.005)
Lumberjacks	8–10	0.29 (0.92–0.02)
Chemical laboratory	10	0.44 (2.0–0.04)
Manual cleaning of petrol tanks	4–8	195 [b]
Petrol pump servicemen	6–10	0.41 (0.64–0.23)

[a] Stationary measurement 2–12 ppm
[b] Stationary measurement 1 m above the tank opening

Table 14. Exposure measurements during gasoline loading of tankers [a]

Concentration (mg/m³)	Winter period		Summer period	
	No. of samples	Percentage of samples	No. of samples	Percentage of samples
0–2	41	62	23	38
2–6	11	17	12	20
6–10	4	6	6	10
10–16 TWA [b]	2	3	4	6.5
16–30 STEL [b]	3	4.5	6	10
30–50	2	3	4	6.5
> 50	3	4.5	5	9
Total	66	100	60	100

[a] As quoted from (Gjörlof et al. 1982)
[b] The Swedish Occupational Standard Values (1981) TWA for 8-h exposure is 16 mg/m³ (5 ppm) and the short-term exposure limit (STEL), defined as a time-weighted average for 15 min, is 30 mg/m³ (10 ppm).

Measurements of levels of exposure to benzene during gasoline loading of tankers (Table 14) show that few lie above the Swedish occupational standard values for benzene (8-h TWA of 5 ppm (16 mg/m³) with a 15 min TWA of 10 ppm (30 mg/m³)). Deck personnel were occasionally exposed to up to 350 mg/m³ in the late phase of gasoline loading of ships (Bachs, 1979).

Table 15. National occupational exposure limits for benzene[a]

Country	Year	Concentration		Interpretation[b]	Status
		mg/m³	ppm		
Australia	1978	30	10	TWA[c]	Guideline
Belgium	1978	30	10	TWA[c]	Regulation
Czechoslovakia	1976	50	–	TWA	Regulation
		80	–	Ceiling (10 min)	
Denmark	1981	30	10	TWA	Regulation
Federal Republic					Technical
of Germany	1983	26	8		guideline
Finland	1975	32	10	TWA[c]	Regulation
Hungary	1974	20	–	TWA[d]	Regulation
Italy	1978	30	10	TWA[c]	Guideline
Japan	1980	32	10	Ceiling	Guideline
The Netherlands[e]	1978	30	10	TWA[c]	Guideline
Poland	1976	30	–	Ceiling[c]	Regulation
Romania	1975	50	–	Maximum[c]	Regulation
Sweden	1978	15	5	TWA[c]	Guideline
		30	10	Maximum (15 min)	
Switzerland	1978	6.5	2	TWA[c]	Regulation
USA[a]					
OSHA	1980	–	10	TWA	Regulation
		–	25	Ceiling	
		–	50	Peak[f]	
ACGIH	1981	30	10	TWA	Guideline
		75	25	STEL	
NIOSH	1980	3.2	1	Ceiling (60 min)	Guideline
USSR	1980	5	–	Ceiling[c]	Regulation
Yugoslavia	1971	50	15	Ceiling[c]	Regulation

[a]From American Conference of Governmental Industrial Hygienists (ACGIH) (1981); International Labour Office (1980); National Institute for Occupational Safety and Health (NIOSH) (1980); US Occupational Safety and Health Administration (OSHA) (1980); Holmberg and Lundberg (1985)
[b]TWA, time-weighted average; STEL, short-term exposure limit
[c]Skin irritant notation added
[d]May be exceeded 5 times per shift as long as average does not exceed value
[e]Proposal: 1 ppm (TWA) from 1983
[f]Peak limit above ceiling − 10 min

Seventeen countries have been reported to limit occupational exposure to benzene by regulation or recommended guideline. Table 15 lists the national occupational exposure limits for benzene (IARC, 1982a; Holmberg & Lundberg, 1985). The 8-h TWA occupational standard value for benzene is 5 or 10 ppm in most countries. Many countries have also listed benzene as a carcinogen. In the Federal Republic of Germany there are no occupational standard values for carcinogens such as benzene, but there are "technical guidelines" which specify 26 mg/m³ (8 ppm) for benzene (Holmberg & Lundberg, 1985). In the USSR, the maximum allowable concentration (MAC) of benzene in the air of the working zone is 5 mg/m³, with the working zone defined as the space up to 2 m above the level of the site occupied by the workers.

It should be noted that the present OSHA standard for benzene in the U.S.A. (originally adopted in 1971) is an 8-h TWA of 10 ppm, with a ceiling limit of 25 ppm and a maximum peak concentration of 50 ppm for a 10-min period. In 1978, OSHA promulgated a new permanent standard (OSHA, 1978) for occupational exposure to benzene, based on evidence that there is a causal connection between benzene exposure and leukaemia. This standard limited exposure to 1 ppm of benzene in air (8-h TWA), the level then estimated to be the lowest feasible. The standard included a ceiling limit of 5 ppm for any 15-min period during an 8-h day. This standard was vacated by the U.S. Court of Appeals in 1978, principally due to the failure of OSHA to clarify and evaluate the benefits of changing the permissible exposure level for benzene from 10 ppm to 1 ppm. This judgement was confirmed by the U.S. Supreme Court in 1980 (Brief *et al.*, 1980). In early December 1985, OSHA once again proposed a permissible exposure limit of 1 ppm TWA and an action level of 5 ppm (Anon., 1985c). The four principal industrial sectors covered by the standard are: petrochemicals, petroleum refining, coke and coal chemicals and tyre manufacturers. The Agency estimates that some 270 000 workers are exposed to benzene and that, at the current 10 ppm exposure level, benzene represents a risk of 44 to 156 excess deaths per 1 000 employees. The proposed 1 ppm level is expected to reduce this risk by about 90%, with the result that an estimated 822 lives would be saved over a working lifetime.

Very much less is known with certainty concerning environmental or community exposure to benzene (Brief *et al.*, 1980).

In a survey of 12 states of the U.S.A., Suta (1980) estimated that 300 000 people were exposed to benzene in air from coke-oven operations. In a survey of 22 states, it was estimated that about 6 million people were exposed to $0.3–3.0\,\mu g/m^3$ (0.1–1.0 ppb) benzene from chemical factories, about 1 million to $3.0–13.0\,\mu g/m^3$ (1.1–4.0 ppb), about 200 000 people to $13.0–32.0\,\mu g/m^3$ (4.1–10.0 ppb) and about 80 000 people to more than $32.0\,\mu g/m^3$ (10.0 ppb) (Suta, 1980). The National Toxicology Program (1981) estimated that 800 000 persons in the U.S.A. may be exposed to benzene from coke-oven emissions at levels greater than $0.32\,mg/m^3$, and 5 million persons from petroleum refinery emissions at levels of $0.32–3.2\,mg/m^3$. During chemical manufacturing, anywhere from 80 000 to 6 million persons may be exposed to benzene concentrations ranging from $0.32–32\,\mu g/m^3$.

Benzene measurements near U.S. refineries and chemical plants handling benzene or benzene-containing streams ranged from $1–400\,\mu g/m^3$ in areas inside these facilities, $0.1–480\,\mu g/m^3$ in the vicinity of chemical plants and $1.6–830\,\mu g/m^3$ in the vicinity of refineries (Brief *et al.*, 1980).

In western Europe, community air close to industrial establishments has been reported to have a concentration of benzene about one-thirtieth of the concentration present in factory air (Brief *et al.*, 1980).

General sources of exposure to benzene

In the general population, the respiratory route is the major source of human exposure to benzene and much of this exposure is by way of gasoline vapours (Howard & Durkin, 1974). Exposure of the general public occurs at concentrations at least 2 to 3 orders of magnitude lower than have been recorded for industrial situations (Van Raalte, 1982).

As noted earlier, benzene comprises about 2.15% of total hydrocarbon emissions from a gasoline engine, or about 4% of automotive exhaust (U.S. Environmental Protection Agency, 1980). The most polluting fuels in terms of benzene levels are leaded gasoline and gasohol (50–115 mg/km), in contrast to diesel (10–20 mg/km), while unleaded gasoline (catalyst equipped) engines emit only 1–15 mg benzene/km (Egeback, 1982; Holmberg & Ahlborg, 1983; Holmberg & Lundberg, 1985). Higher ambient air levels of benzene are found near major roadways and metropolitan areas and are reported to correlate with traffic levels (Fentiman et al., 1979; Thorburn & Colenutt, 1979; Brief et al., 1980; Suyama et al., 1980; Jonsson & Berg, 1980; IARC, 1982a). Motor vehicles contribute benzene to the community air from incompletely combusted exhaust emissions, from dealkylation of benzene homologues in the fuel and from direct evaporation from fuel tanks (Brief et al., 1980). The EPA estimated that the contribution of benzene to the environment from motor vehicles will drop from 82 to 46% of the total industrial emissions, which were estimated in 1976 to exceed 246 thousand tonnes by 1985 (Brief et al., 1980).

Suta (1980) estimated that 37 million people in the U.S.A. are exposed to benzene in the air from self-service gasoline stations. Ambient air benzene concentrations in gasoline service stations in the U.S.A. have been reported to be in the range 1–10 mg/m^3 in one study and 0–5.4 mg/m^3 in another, as well as in the range 0.08–0.8 mg/m^3 (Ollison, 1977; Brief et al., 1980). Large variations of levels were found, anywhere from 4.5–32 mg/m^3 to a few exposures at 64–96 mg/m^3, as well as up to 320–800 mg/m^3. These variations were due to the type of bulk terminal, the ambient temperature, whether top or bottom loading was employed and the presence or absence of a vapour recovery system (Brief et al., 1980).

Servicemen working at adjustment and trimming of gasoline pumps at gasoline service stations may be exposed to 0.5–20 mg benzene/m^3, with the highest exposure occurring at pump shops (Moberg et al., 1981). Although low average levels of benzene occur in large automobile garages, in smaller garages the exposure can be expected to be much higher.

Information concerning the levels of benzene in the atmosphere is limited. Ambient monitoring data suggest that levels of benzene range from 3 to 320 µg/m^3 (IARC, 1982a; NTP, 1983a).

Rural background concentrations of benzene have been reported to range from 0.3–54 µg/m^3; these levels are related to biological sources, ambient benzene concentrations tending to increase after forest fires and oil seeps (Brief et al., 1980).

The general urban atmosphere reportedly contains 0.05 mg benzene/m^3 of air. Assuming a daily inhalation of 24 m^3 of air and a benzene retention of 50%, human beings would absorb 0.6 mg of benzene/day (National Research Council, 1980).

Data concerning indoor concentrations of benzene (as well as other aromatic hydrocarbons) are extremely sparse. Average indoor benzene concentrations below 20 µg/m^3 have been measured in one limited study with sampling periods from one to several days. The mean value for simultaneous sampling of outdoor air next to the dwellings investigated has been found to be about 30 µg/m^3 (Seifert & Abraham, 1982, 1983).

Benzene is slightly soluble in water (0.8 mg/L at 20 °C) and has been detected in lake, river and well water, raw and finished drinking-water, and in effluents from oil and coal processing, chemical factories, raw sewage and sewage treatment plants (Shackelford & Keith, 1976; Hushon *et al.,* 1980; IARC, 1982a). Benzene has been identified in some samples of drinking-water at levels of 0.1 to 0.3 µg/L, with the highest concentration reported to be 20 µg/L, and in subsurface water at concentrations up to 32 mg/m^3 (NTP, 1981). Assuming an intake of 2 L/day and a level of 1 µg/L in U.S. drinking-water, the dose of benzene to humans would be 2 µg/day (National Research Council, 1980).

Benzene is reported to occur in fruits, fish, vegetables, nuts, dairy products, beverages, eggs, cooked chicken and heat-treated or canned beef (Chang & Peterson, 1977; U.S. Environmental Protection Agency, 1980; IARC, 1982a). Various levels of benzene have been reported in cigarette smoke (150–204 mg/m^3, Lauwerys, 1979). Inhaled benzene from this source may approach 10 µg/cigarette (Brief *et al.,* 1980). Berlin *et al.* (1977) reported that the smoke from one cigarette contains 60–80 µg of benzene. In another report, it was suggested that the average cigarette gives rise to about 31 µg benzene, so that daily consumption of 10 cigarettes results in an uptake of about 310 µg; this is equivalent to the quantity of benzene inhaled over a 24-h period when the air contains 7.5 µg/m^3 benzene at a respiratory-minute volume of 28.6 L (for light work). Under resting conditions (respiratory-minute volume = 8 L), the benzene concentration in the inhaled air would have to be about 27 µg/m^3 in order that 310 µg benzene be inhaled in 24 h (Kluge, 1980).

In May 1981, the U.S. Consumer Products Safety Commission (CPSC) withdrew its proposed ban on benzene in consumer products, except for gasoline and laboratory reagents that contain benzene as an intentional ingredient or as a contaminant at 0.1% or greater by volume. This decision was based on CPSC findings that benzene is no longer used as an intentional ingredient in consumer products and that the contaminant levels remaining were unlikely to result in significant consumer exposure to benzene vapour. It was suggested that, since the intentional use of benzene in consumer products has essentially been eliminated, between 400 000 and 800 000 persons in the U.S.A. would no longer be exposed (NTP, 1981). However, a labelling regulation established in 1962 for products containing more than 5% benzene and a 1977 safety packaging requirement for paint solvents and thinners containing 10% or more of petroleum distillates, such as benzene, remains in effect (NTP, 1983a).

It has been estimated that the average U.S. urban dweller may receive about 850 µg benzene daily from food and air and that the dietary intake of benzene may be as high as 250 µg/day (National Research Council, 1980; NTP, 1983a). The estimated quantity of 250 µg/day is equivalent to a concentration of benzene which would be inhaled and absorbed over a 24-h period if the atmospheric benzene level were 12.2 µg/m^3, based on a respiratory-minute volume of 28.6 L during light work, with a 50% retention of benzene. Under resting conditions (respiratory-minute volume = 8 L), the benzene concentration of the inhaled air would have to be about 43 µg/m^3 in order that 250 µg benzene be absorbed in 24 h (Kluge, 1980). Benzene levels of 24–60 µg/m^3 have been found in the breath of some individuals without specific exposure to benzene, suggesting that the source may be the diet (National Research

Council, 1980; IARC, 1982a). The intake of benzene based on an inhalation volume of 10 m³ will be 32 μg/day for each 1 ppb in the air (Brief *et al.,* 1980).

A recent, important five-year study by the U.S. EPA has revealed that people can be exposed to far greater concentrations of common toxic organic chemicals (e.g., benzene, xylenes, halogenated alkanes) *indoors* than they are outdoors, even in cities where plants manufacture or use these chemicals. Using personal and stationary outdoor air monitors, median indoor levels were found to be five times greater than median outdoor levels for the major 11 volatile organic chemicals. Benzene was found to be 30 to 50% higher in the air of homes of smokers than in the homes of non-smokers (Wallace *et al.,* 1984; Ember, 1985).

There is an additional aspect of exposure to benzene (i.e., solvent abuse) that has recently been disclosed. The scope and consequences of such exposure cannot be critically determined at this time. For example, benzene sniffing is said to be widespread among the youth of some isolated Pacific islands. Of 14 schizophrenics under the age of 35 so far questioned, nine had sniffed benzene at some time (Daniels & Fazakerley, 1983).

REFERENCES

Abelson, P.H. (1985) Chemicals from waste dumps. *Science, 229,* 335

Aksoy, M. (1985) Malignancies due to occupational exposure to benzene. *Am. J. Ind. Med., 5,* 395–402

American Conference of Government Industrial Hygienists (1981) *Threshold Limit Values for Chemical Substances and Physical Agents in the Workroom Environment with Intended Changes for 1981,* Cincinnati, OH, p. 10

Anon. (1980) Low levels of suspect carcinogens found in coal liquefaction facilities. *Occup. Saf. Health Rep., 9,* 1163–1164

Anon. (1985a) Key chemicals – benzene. *Chem. Eng. News,* May 25, p. 26

Anon. (1985b) Facts and figures for the chemical industry. *Chem. Eng. News,* June 10, pp. 53–55

Anon. (1985c) Benzene, formaldehyde: workplace exposure limits proposed. *Chem. Eng. News,* Dec. 9, p. 4

Arp, E.W., Wolf, P.H. & Checkoway, H. (1983) Lymphocytic leukemia and exposures to benzene and other solvents in the rubber industry. *J. Occup. Med., 25,* 598–602

Bachs, A. (1979) *Exposure to Benzene and Alkylbenzenes During Loading of Petrol* Goteborg, Inst. Teknisk Kemi, Chalmers Tekniska Hogskola

Berlin, M. (1985) Low level benzene exposure in Sweden: effect on blood elements and body burden of benzene. *Am. J. Ind. Med., 7,* 365–373

Berlin, M. & Tunek, A. (1984) Benzene. In: Aitio, A., Riihimaki, U. & Vainio, H., eds, *Biological Monitoring and Surveillance of Workers Exposed to Chemicals,* New York, Hemisphere, pp. 23–34

Berlin, M., Fredga, K., Gullberg, B., Holm, S., Knutsson, P., Reitalu, J. & Tunek, A. (1977) *Biological Monitoring and Chromosome Changes at Exposure to Benzene,*

Report to Swedish Labour Protection Board, No. 771018, Lund, Institutes of Hygiene and Genetics, University of Lund

Berlin, M., Gage, J.C., Gullberg, B., Holm, S., Knudsen, P., Eng, C. & Tunek, A. (1980) Breath concentration as an index of the health risk from benzene: studies on the accumulation and clearance of inhaled benzene. *Scand. J. Work Environ. Health, 6,* 104–111

Boettner, E.A. & Ball, G.L. (1980) Thermal degradation products from PVC film in food wrapping operations. *Am. Ind. Hyg. Assoc. J., 41,* 513–522

Brief, R.S., Lynch, J., Bernath, T. & Scala, R.A. (1980) Benzene in the workplace. *Am. Ind. Hyg. Assoc. J., 41,* 616–623

Cerniglia, C.E. (1981) Aromatic hydrocarbons: metabolism by bacteria, fungi and algae. In: Hodgson, E., Bend, J.R. & Philpot, R.M., eds, *Reviews in Biochemical Toxicology,* Vol. 3, Amsterdam, Elsevier/North Holland, pp. 321–361

Chang, S.S. & Peterson, R.J. (1977) Symposium: the basis of quality in muscle food. Recent developments in the flavor of meat. *J. Food Sci., 42,* 298–305

Checkoway, H., Wilcosky, T., Wolf, P. & Tyroler, H. (1984) An evaluation of the associations of leukemia and rubber industry solvent exposures. *Am. J. Ind. Med., 5,* 239–249

Cheremisinoff, P.N. & Morresi, A.C. (1979) *Benzene — Basic and Hazardous Properties,* New York, Marcel Dekker

Daniels, A.M. & Fazakerley,R.C. (1983) Solvent abuse in the Central Pacific. *Lancet, 1,* 75

Davis, P. (1929) Toxic substances in the rubber industry, Part 2: Benzol. *Rubber Age, 13,* 367–368

Dean, B.J. (1985) Recent findings on the genetic toxicology of benzene, toluene, xylenes and phenols. *Mutat. Res., 154,* 153–181

DGMK (1980) *Evaluation of Benzene Toxicity in Man and Animals,* Research Rept. No. 174–6, Hamburg, Deutsche Gesellschaft für Mineralölwissenschaft und Kohlechemie eV., June

Egeback, K.E., ed. (1982) *Chemical and Biological Characterization of Vehicle Exhausts Emissions When Using Different Engine/Fuel Combinations,* Stockholm, National Swedish Environment Protection Board

Ember, L. (1985) Toxic chemical levels higher indoors than out. *Chem. Eng. News,* June 24, pp. 22–23

Fentiman, A.F., Neher, M.B., Kinzer, G.W., Sticksel, P.R., Coutant, R.W., Jungclaus, G.A., Edit, N.A., McNulty, J. & Townley, C.W. (1979) *Environmental Monitoring Benzene* (PB-295 641), Prepared for the U.S. Environmental Protection Agency by Battelle Columbus Laboratories, Springfield, VA, National Technical Information Service, pp. 9–15, 26–110

Fishbein, L. (1984) An overview of environmental and toxicological aspects of aromatic hydrocarbons. I. Benzene. *Sci. Total Environ., 40,* 189–218

Fishbein, L. (1985a) An overview of environmental and toxicological aspects of aromatic hydrocarbons. II. Toluene. *Sci. Total Environ., 42,* 267–288

Fishbein, L. (1985b) An overview of environmental and toxicological aspects of aromatic hydrocarbons. III. Xylene. *Sci. Total Environ., 43,* 165–183

Fishbein, L. (1985c) An overview of environmental and toxicological aspects of aromatic hydrocarbons. IV. Ethylbenzene. *Sci. Total Environ., 44,* 169–287

Gisser, P. (1978) *Benzene Emission Control Costs in Selected Segments of the Chemical Industry,* Foster D. Snell, Inc., Florham Park, NY, June 12 (National Technical Information Service. Report PB 283781)

Gjörloff, K., Skardin, B. & Svedung, I. (1982) *Occupational Conditions During Loading of Petrochemicals on Tankers,* IVL Report B653, Frysta, Institutet for Vatten och Luftvardsforskning

Goldstein, B.D., Snyder, C.A., Snyder, R. & Wolman, S.R. (1978) *Assessment of Health Effects of Benzene Germane to Low-level Exposure,* Washington DC, U.S. Environmental Protection Agency, September, 112, pp. 89–117

Guicherit, R. & Schulting, F.L. (1985) The occurrence of organic chemicals in the atmosphere of The Netherlands. *Sci. Total Environ., 43,* 193–219

Holmberg, B. & Ahlborg, U. (1983) Mutagenicity and carcinogenicity of car exhausts and cool combustion emissions. *Environ. Health Perspect., 47,* 1–30

Holmberg, B. & Lundberg, P. (1985) Benzene standards, occurrence, and exposure. *Am. J. Ind. Med., 7,* 375–383

Howard, P.H. & Durkin, P.R. (1974) *Sources of Contamination, Ambient Levels and Fate of Benzene in the Environment,* EPA 560/5-75-005, Washington DC, US Environmental Protection Agency

Hunter, F.T. (1939) Chronic exposure to benzene (benzol). II. The clinical effects. *J. Ind. Hyg., 21,* 331–354

Hushon, J., Clerman, R., Small, R., Good, S., Taylor, A. & Thoman, D. (1980) *An Assessment of Potentially Carcinogenic Energy Related Contaminants in Water,* Prepared for U.S. Dept. of Energy and National Cancer Institute, McLean, VA, Mitre Corporation, p. 68

IAES/SECOTOX (1980) *Benzene — Interpretation Data and Evaluation of Current Knowledge,* International Academy of Environmental Safety and Society of Ecotoxicology and Environmental Safety Workshop, Vienna, June 10–11

IARC (1979) *IARC Monographs on the Evaluation of the Carcinogenic Risk of Chemicals to Humans,* Vol. 19, *Some Monomers, Plastics and Synthetic Elastomers and Acrolein,* Lyon, International Agency for Research on Cancer, pp. 231–274

IARC (1982a) *Benzene.* In: *IARC Monograph on the Evaluation of the Carcinogenic Risk of Chemicals to Humans,* Vol. 29, *Some Industrial Chemicals and Dyestuffs,* Lyon, International Agency for Research on Cancer, pp. 93–148

IARC (1982b) *IARC Monographs on the Evaluation of the Carcinogenic Risk of Chemicals to Humans,* Vol. 28, *The Rubber Industry,* Lyon, International Agency for Research on Cancer, pp. 195, 332

ILO (1971a) *Convention 136 concerning protection against hazards of poisoning arising from benzene, adopted by the Conference at its 56th session,* International Labour Conference, Geneva, June

ILO (1971b) *Recommendation 144 concerning protection against hazards of poisoning arising from benzene, adopted by the Conference at its 56th session,* International Labour Conference, Geneva, June

Infante, P.F. & White, M.C. (1983) Benzene: epidemiologic observations of leukemia by cell type and adverse health effects associated with low level exposure. *Environ. Health Perspect., 52,* 75–82

Infante, P.F. & White, M.C. (1985) Projections of leukemia risk associated with occupational exposure to benzene. *Am. J. Ind. Med., 7,* 403–414

International Labour Office (1980) *Occupational Exposure Limits for Airborne Toxic Substances,* 2nd (rev.) Ed. *(Occupational Safety and Health Series No. 37)*, Geneva, pp. 48–49, 271–290

Jonsson, A. & Berg, S. (1980) Determination of 1,2-dibromoethane, 1,2-dichloroethanol and benzene in ambient air using porous polymer traps and gas chromatographic-mass spectrometric analysis with selected ion monitoring. *J. Chromatogr., 190,* 97–100

JRB Associates, Inc. (1980) *Materials Balance for Benzene, Level I-Preliminary* (EPA-560/13-80-014), Prepared for the U.S. Environmental Protection Agency, McLean, VA, p. xiii

Kluge, A. (1980) Benzene in the environment. *Regul. Toxicol. Pharmacol., 1,* 244–263

Korte, F. & Klein, W. (1982) Degradation of benzene in the environment. *Ecotoxicol. Environ. Saf., 6,* 311–327

Lauwerys, R.R. (1979) *Industrial Health and Safety, Human Biological Monitoring of Industrial Chemicals. 1. Benzene,* CEC Report EUR 6570/11979, Luxembourg, Commission of the European Communities

Maltoni, C., Conti, B. & Cotti, G. (1983) Benzene: a multipotential carcinogen. Results of long term bioassays performed at the Bologna Institute of Oncology. *Am. J. Ind. Med., 4,* 589–630

Maltoni, C., Conti, B., Cotti, G. & Belpoggi, F. (1985) Experimental studies on benzene carcinogenicity at the Bologna Institute of Oncology: current results and ongoing research. *Am. J. Ind. Med., 7,* 414–446

McMichael, A.J., Spirtas, R., Kupper, L.L. & Gamble, J.F. (1975) Solvent exposure and leukemia among rubber workers: an epidemiologic study. *J. Occup. Med., 17,* 234–239

Mehlman, M.A., ed. (1983) *Carcinogenicity and Toxicity of Benzene,* Princeton, NJ, Princeton Scientific Publ., pp. 1–15

Mehlman, M.A., Schreiner, C.A. & Mackerer, C.R. (1980) Current status of benzene teratology: a brief review. *J. Environ. Pathol. Toxicol., 4,* 123–131

Mellan, I. (1957) *Handbook of Solvents,* Vol. I, *Pure Hydrocarbons,* New York, Reinhold

Merian, E. (1982) The environmental chemistry of volatile hydrocarbons. *Toxicol. Environ. Chem., 5,* 167–175

Merian, E. & Zander, M. (1982) Volatile aromatics. In: Hutzinger, O., ed., *Handbook of Environmental Chemistry,* Vol. 3, Part B, *Anthropogenic Compounds,* Berlin (West), Springer-Verlag, pp. 117–161

Moberg, B., Norvlinder, R. & Ramnas, O. (1981) *Exposure to Benzene and Alkylbenzenes during Adjustment and Trimming of Gasoline Pumps,* Goteborg, Inst. Teknisk Kemi, Chalmers Tekniska Hogskola

National Research Council (1980) *Drinking Water and Health,* Vol. 3, Washington DC, National Academy of Sciences Press, pp. 80–86, 261–262

NIOSH (1977) *Revised Recommendation for an Occupational Exposure Standard for Benzene,* National Institute for Occupational Safety and Health, Cincinnati, OH, US Dept. of Health, Education and Welfare

NIOSH (1980) *Summary of NIOSH Recommendations for Occupational Health Standards,* Rockville, MD, National Institute for Occupational Safety and Health

NTP (1981) Benzene, In: *2nd Annual Report on Carcinogens – Report NTP81-43,* National Toxicology Program, US Dept. of Health and Human Services, December, pp. 49–52

NTP (1983a) *3rd Annual Report on Carcinogens – Summary 1983, Report No. 82-330,* National Toxicology Program, NIEHS, Research Triangle Park, NC, pp. 28–29

NTP (1983b) *Technical Report on the Toxicology and Carcinogenesis Studies of Benzene in F344/N Rats and B6C3F1 Mice, NTP Report, 83-072,* National Toxicology Program, NIEHS, Research Triangle Park, NC

Occupational Safety and Health Administration (1980) Benzene. *US Code Fed. Regul.,* Title 29, Parts 1910.19, 1910.1000, 1910.1028

Ollison, W.M. (1977) *Human Exposure to Atmospheric Benzene. A Review.* Washington DC, American Petroleum Institute

OSHA (1977) Occupational exposure to benzene. Occupational Safety and Health Administration, *Fed. Regist., 42,* 27452–27478, May 27

OSHA (1978) Occupational exposure to benzene. Occupational Safety and Health Administration, *Fed. Regist.,* 4510–26, June 27

Purcell, W.P. (1978) Benzene. In: Kirk, R.E. & Othmer, D.F., eds, *Encyclopedia of Chemical Technology,* 3rd ed., Vol. 3, New York, John Wiley and Sons, pp. 744–771

Ringen, K. & Addis, P. (1983) Protecting workers from benzene exposure. In: Mehlman, M.A., ed., *Carcinogenicity and Toxicity of Benzene,* Princeton, NJ, Princeton Scientific Publ., pp. 77–89

Rinsky, R.A., Young, R.J. & Smith, A.B. (1981) Leukemia in benzene workers. *Am. J. Ind. Med., 2,* 217–245

Runion, H.E. & Scott, L.M. (1985) Benzene exposure in the United States, 1978–1983: an overview. *Am. J. Ind. Med., 7,* 385–393

Seifert, B. & Abraham, H.J. (1982) Indoor air concentrations of benzene and some other aromatic hydrocarbons. *Ecotoxicol. Environ. Saf., 6,* 190–192

Seifert, B. & Abraham, H.J. (1983) Use of passive samplers for the determination of gaseous organic substances in indoor air at low concentration levels. *Int. J. Anal. Environ. Chem., 13,* 237–253

Shackelford, W.M. & Keith, L.H. (1976) *Frequency of Organic Compounds Identified in Water,* EPA-600/4-76-062, Athens, GA, US Environmental Protection Agency, pp. 37, 63–65

Slimak, M. & Delos, C. (1983–1984) Environmental pathways of exposure to 129 priority pollutants. *J. Toxicol. Clin. Toxicol., 21,* 39–63

Snyder, R. & Kocsis, J.J. (1975) Current concepts of chronic benzene toxicity. *CRC Crit. Rev. Toxicol., 3,* 265

SRI International (1983a) *Directory of Chemical Producers,* Menlo Park, CA, pp. 452–454

SRI International (1983b) *CEH Report Abstract Benzene Chem. Industries Div. Newsletter,* Menlo Park, CA, January–February, pp. 5–6

Suta, B.E. (1980) *Definition of Population-at-risk to Environmental Toxic Pollutant Exposures,* Vol. II, Appendix C, *Human Population Exposures to Atmospheric Benzene,* Prepared for U.S. Environmental Protection Agency, Washington DC, pp. 22, 34, 55, 63

Suyama, Y., Katabiri, Y. & Saiki, Y. (1980) Photochemical pollution. Measurements of aromatic hydrocarbons near intersections and non-methane hydrocarbons on highways. *Kanogawa-Ken Kogai Senta Nempa, 11,* 25 (*Chem. Abstr. 93,* 172772q)

Thorburn, S. & Colenutt, B.A. (1979) A gas chromatographic comparison of volatile organic compounds in urban and rural atmospheres. *Int. J. Environ. Stud., 13,* 265–271

Tobin, H.H. (1985) *World Aromatic Market Trends,* SRI Chem. Industries Div. Newsletter, Menlo Park, CA, SRI International, April, pp. 2–3

U.S. Environmental Protection Agency (1977) *Atmospheric Benzene Emissions.* EPA Publication No. EPA-400/3-72029, Washington DC, October

U.S. Environmental Protection Agency (1978) *Assessment of Health Effects of Benzene Germane to Low Level Exposure.* EPA Rept. 600/1-78-061, Office of Health and Ecological Effects, Washington DC, p. 20

U.S. Environmental Protection Agency (1980) *Ambient Water Quality Criteria for Benzene* (EPA-440/5-80-018) Washington DC, pp. C1–C8, C16–C35, C67–C100

U.S. International Trade Commission (1981) *Preliminary Report on U.S. Production of Selected Synthetic Organic Chemicals (Including Synthetic Plastics and Resin Materials) Preliminary Totals, 1980 (SOC Series C/P81-1),* Washington DC, pp. 1, 4, 5

Van Ert, M.D., Arp, E.W., Harris, R.L., Symons, M.J. & Williams, T.M. (1980) Worker exposure to chemical agents in the manufacture of rubber tires: solvent vapor studies. *Am. Ind. Hyg. Assoc. J., 41,* 212–219

Van Raalte, H.G.S. (1982) A critical look at hazards from benzene in workplace and community air. *Regul. Toxicol. Pharmacol., 2,* 67–76

Van Raalte, H.G.S. & Grasso, P. (1982) Hematological, myelotoxic, clastogenic carcinogenic and leukemogenic effects of benzene. *Regul. Toxicol. Pharmacol., 2,* 153–176

Wallace, L.A., Pellizzari, E., Hartwell, T., Rosenzweig, M., Erickson, M., Sparacino, C. & Zelon, H. (1984) Personal exposure to volatile organic compounds. I. Direct measurements in breathing zone air, drinking water, food, and exhaled breath. *Environ. Res., 35,* 293–319

Watanabe, T., Endo, A., Kato, Y., Shima, S., Watanabe, T. & Ikeda, M. (1980) Cytogenetics and cytokinetics of cultured lymphocytes from benzene-exposed workers. *Int. Arch. Occup. Environ. Health, 46,* 31–41

Webber, D. (1985) C & EN's top 50 chemical products. *Chem. Eng. News,* May 6, pp. 12–13

Zinn, B.T., Browner, R.F., Powell, E.A., Pasternak, M. & Gardner, R.O. (1980) *The Smoke Hazards Resulting from the Burning of Shipboard Materials Used by the US Navy* (NRL Rept. 8414). Prepared for the US Naval Research Laboratory, Georgia Institute of Technology, Atlanta, GA

CHAPTER 5

TOLUENE: USES, OCCURRENCE AND EXPOSURE

L. Fishbein[1]

Department of Health and Human Services
Food and Drug Administration
National Center for Toxicological Research
Jefferson, AR 72079, USA

INTRODUCTION

Toluene is an agent of major chemical, environmental and occupational significance. It is produced in enormous quantities and is extensively employed in a broad spectrum of applications, primarily as a solvent (for which its use is increasing as a "safe" replacement for benzene), as a component in gasoline, and in the production of benzene and a host of other chemicals (e.g., benzoic acid, nitrotoluenes, tolyl diisocyanates, dyes, pharmaceuticals, food additives, plastics, etc.). Toluene is also present in many consumer products, including household aerosols, paints, varnishes, adhesives and glues. In addition, it has been widely abused by "glue sniffers". Hence, there is a broad potential for exposure involving both industrial workers and the general public (e.g., *via* vehicle exhausts and consumer products).

Although there is general agreement that toluene does not have the haematotoxic properties of benzene and that the narcotic and neurotoxic properties of toluene represent the major health hazards in humans, note should be made of the recent studies of Maltoni *et al.* (1983), in which the tumorigenicity of toluene in experimental animals was reported, and of the conflicting reports on the clastogenic properties of toluene both in man and experimental animals. It should also be noted that commercial toluene contains varying amounts of benzene and that toluene is frequently employed in industry with benzene and alkyl benzenes (e.g., xylenes, ethylbenzene).

As in the case of benzene, the importance of toluene with regard to its production, use, occurrence, dispersion and human toxicity has spawned an extensive literature (McMichael *et al.,* 1975; ILO, 1977; Dean, 1978; Cohr & Stokholm, 1979; Criteria Group for Occupational Standards, 1981; WHO, 1981; Benignus, 1981a,b; Merian,

[1]Present address: ENVIRON Corporation, 1000 Potomac Street NW, Washington DC 20007, USA

1982; Merian & Zander, 1982; NAS, 1982; Maltoni *et al.,* 1983; Lauwerys, 1983; Dean, 1985; Fishbein, 1985).

PRODUCTION AND USE

Toluene is produced in large quantities, primarily in the U.S.A., western Europe and Japan. U.S. production of all grades of toluene in 1981 was 2.92 million tonnes (887 million gallons), ranking 23rd in importance among the chemical products (Anon., 1982). U.S. production of toluene in 1979 and 1980 was 3.13 million tonnes (950 million gallons) and 2.90 million tonnes (883 million gallons), respectively, which ranked 22nd and 23rd among the chemical products for this period (Storck, 1981). In 1983 and 1984, production of toluene was 2.57 and 2.39 million tonnes, respectively 22nd and 27th in importance for this period (Anon., 1985). Production of toluene in 1984 was estimated to have been as follows (in millions of kilograms): France, 39; Italy, 312; Federal Republic of Germany, 358; Japan, 356 (Anon., 1985). World production of toluene is estimated at more than 10 million tonnes (approximately one-third the amount of benzene produced) and the European Economic Community consumed approximately 1.0 million tonnes of toluene in 1980 (Merian & Zander, 1982).

Toluene is produced as an aromatic mixture with benzene and mixed xylenes, primarily from catalytic reformate from refineries and secondarily from petroleum-derived pyrolysis gasoline as a by-product of olefin manufacture during the cracking of hydrocarbons. (Catalytic reforming involves the dehydrogenation of selected petroleum fractions rich in naphthalenes to yield an aromatic mixture consisting of toluene, benzene and mixed xylenes. Toluene is isolated by distillation, followed by washing with sulfuric acid and redistillation) (Cier, 1969; Ring, 1979; Ring & Gunn, 1979). Small amounts of toluene as an aromatic mixture are also obtained from coal-derived coke-oven light oil and as a by-product from the manufacture of styrene (Cier, 1969; Clement Associates, 1977; SRI, 1979).

There are currently 201 locations in the U.S.A. where toluene is produced as an aromatic mixture from catalytic reformate, nine locations where it is produced as an aromatic mixture from pyrolysis gasoline manufacture and six others where toluene is derived from coal (SRI, 1979).

Benzene is a common contaminant of toluene. While highly purified toluene (reagent grade and nitration grade) contains less than 0.01% benzene, industrial grade and cruder grade toluenes (90–120 °C boiling range) can contain significant quantities of benzene (e.g., as much as 25%), and probably other hydrocarbons as well (Clement Associates, 1977). For example, samples of commercial toluene (toluol) in the U.S.A. were stated to contain 2–10% of benzene in the 1940s (Wilson, 1943), and levels of 15% and 10% of benzene and xylene, respectively, were reported in samples of commercial toluene in the Federal Republic of Germany in the 1950s (Humperdinck, 1954).

It should be noted that commercial toluene, like benzene, can also contain a spectrum of polycyclic aromatic hydrocarbons (e.g., pyrene, fluoranthene and benzo-[*ghi*]perylene (Lijinsky & Raha, 1961).

Table 1. Toluene production and consumption in 1978 (U.S.A.)[a]

A. Production

Source	Isolated toluene (10^6 kg)	Toluene in BTX (10^6 kg)	Total toluene produced (10^6 kg)
Catalytic reformate	3 629	25 798	29 427
Pyrolysis gasoline	376	331	708
Coal derived	66	14	79
Styrene by-product	100	45	145
Total	4 171	26 188	30 359

B. End use consumption

End use	Isolated toluene used (%)	Toluene used (10^6 kg/yr)
Gasoline as BTX		26 189
Gasoline isolated (back blended)	35.1	1 465
Benzene dealkylation	40.2	1 675
Paints and coating solvent	6.3	263
Adhesives, inks, pharmaceutical solvent	3.2	132
Toluene diisocyanate	4.8	200
Xylenes (disproportionation)	2.3	98
Benzoic acid	1.6	65
Benzyl chloride	0.8	36
Vinyl toluene	0.6	25
Benzaldehyde	0.2	8
p-Cresol	0.1	6
Miscellaneous others	0.6	24
Net export	4.2	174
Total	100.0	30 360

[a] Ring (1979) and Ring & Gunn (1979).

In 1980, over 85% of the toluene recovered and consumed in the world was accounted for by the U.S.A., western Europe and Japan. It should be noted that the three regions differ significantly in sources of supply and in the relative importance of chemical and solvent markets. While over 90% of recovered toluene in 1981 was derived from catalytic reformate in the U.S.A., in Japan and western Europe most toluene is recovered from pyrolysis gasoline (SRI, 1982). These differences occur because U.S. refineries are heavily committed to the production of gasoline, while refineries in western Europe and Japan concentrate more heavily on distillate fuel oils. In all three regions, coke-oven light oil provides less than 10% of the toluene supply.

A summary of the production and consumption of isolated toluene and toluene as an aromatic mixture in 1978 in the U.S.A. is shown in Table 1 (Ring, 1979; Ring & Gunn, 1979). As indicated, all the toluene produced as an aromatic mixture and not

Fig. 1. Uses of toluene in the USA (Cier, 1969)

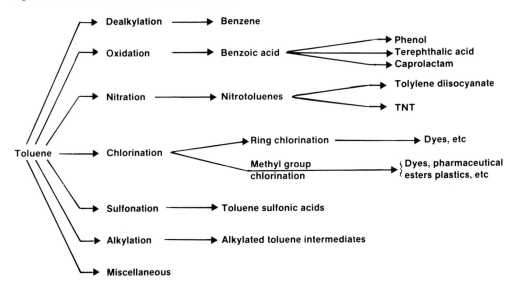

isolated (26 188 million kg) was blended into gasoline. The remaining isolated toluene (4 171 million kg) has a large variety of end uses; these are shown in Figure 1 (Cier, 1969) as well as in Table 1. The single largest end use of toluene is in the manufacture of benzene *via* dealkylation, which represents 40.2% of isolated toluene production. The second largest use of isolated toluene is back-blending into gasoline, which consumed an estimated 1 465 million kg isolated toluene, or 35.1% of 1978 production. An estimated 9.5% of isolated toluene is used in solvent applications. The major use of toluene as a solvent is in paints and coating formulations which consumed an estimated 263 million kg, while 132 million kg toluene were used in adhesives, inks, pharmaceuticals and other products requiring a solvent carrier (SRI, 1979). In addition to the end uses listed in Table 1, significant amounts of toluene are also employed in the production of explosives (TNT), and in the manufacture of saccharin and detergents (toluene sulfonates).

Because of its strong solvent power, toluene is a preferred solvent in many applications, including coatings, adhesives, inks, pharmaceuticals and chemical processing. Solvent applications accounted for 40% or more of the non-fuel demand for recovered toluene in Japan and western Europe in 1980. In the U.S.A., solvent uses for toluene in 1981 were second only to its use in the production of benzene *via* hydrodealkylation and accounted for about 26% of non-fuel consumption (SRI, 1982). As noted earlier, benzene is the most important of the 20 significant derivatives of toluene in the U.S.A., followed by dinitrotoluene (for toluene diisocyanate, TDI), benzoic acid and benzyl chloride. In western Europe, phenol is the most important chemical derivative of recovered toluene, followed by TDI and caprolactam, whereas Japan uses toluene primarily to produce benzene and cresol (SRI, 1982).

Table 2. Global losses of toluene into the environment[a]

Emissions	Amount (millions of tonnes)
Losses into the sea	0.5
Losses from refineries into the air	2.5
Evaporation of gasoline	0.05
Automobile exhaust	2.0
Solvent losses	1.0
Losses from the chemical industry	0.1
Total	6.2

[a] Merian (1982).

Toluene is also widely distributed in a large number of consumer products. An average content of 12.2% toluene was found in 1 393 products surveyed. The categories with the largest number of toluene-containing products were household aerosols, paints, varnishes, shellac, rust preservatives, etc., adhesives and adhesive products containing glue, paint and varnish thinners, flame-retardant chemicals and solvent-based cleaning and sanitizing agents (Clement Associates, 1977; CPSC, 1977).

SOURCES OF EMISSIONS

Estimates of the total annual emissions of toluene to the environment cover a broad range of values. For example, it has been estimated that about 6 million tonnes of toluene are lost into the global environment, mainly into the atmosphere (Merian, 1982; Merian & Zander, 1982). Approximately 1–1.5 million tonnes of toluene are lost from its use as a solvent. Toluene emissions associated with the production, transportation and processing of petroleum are estimated to be of the order of 3–4 million tonnes, and some 2 million tonnes are emitted as a component of automobile exhaust gases. These figures include toluene emissions which are produced through dealkylation of higher volatile aromatics (NAS, 1976), in combustion processes or through the burning of wood and garbage (Bradowsky et al., 1976; NAS, 1976; Merian & Zander, 1982). Compared with these emissions, those occurring during transportation and distribution of gasoline (estimated worldwide at about 50 000 tonnes) and in the chemical industry (about 50 000–100 000 tonnes) are considered to be relatively modest (Merian & Zander, 1982). The total annual load of toluene lost into the sea as part of petroleum fractions is estimated to be about 500 000 tonnes. Table 2 summarizes the global losses of toluene into the environment (Merian, 1982).

The U.S. Environmental Protection Agency (1977a; Clement Associates, 1977) estimated the total annual emissions of toluene in the U.S.A. to be about 450 000 tonnes, with 99.3% of this amount going to the atmosphere and 0.7% to waste water. Another estimate of total emissions in the U.S.A. in 1978 amounted to approximately 1.0 million tonnes (Table 3). The most significant emissions arose from losses of toluene due to its use as a solvent and from automobile exhaust and evaporation of

Table 3.   Total 1978 toluene emissions (U.S.A.)[a]

Source	Toluene emissions (kg/yr)
Toluene production – catalytic reformate	2 942 700
Toluene production – pyrolysis gasoline	636 900
Toluene production – coal-derived	99 230
Toluene production – styrene by-product	110 300
Paint and coatings solvent	262 634 000
Adhesives, inks, pharmaceutical solvent	112 039 000
Benzene production	335 030
Toluene diisocyanate production	255 500
Benzoic acid production	98 000
Benzyl chloride production	35 800
Vinyl toluene production	25 000
Benzaldehyde production	12 200
p-Cresol production	12 700
Xylene disproportionation production	19 600
Other/miscellaneous uses	9 140
Gasoline – marketing evaporative loss	17 460 000
Gasoline – automobile evaporative loss	16 060 000
Gasoline – automobile exhaust emissions	589 747 000
Coke ovens	11 648 000
Total	1 014 180 100

[a] SRI (1979)

gasoline. Since gasoline consumes approximately 90% of all toluene produced, it is the largest source of toluene emission. Toluene emissions were estimated to have been 17 460 tonnes from gasoline marketing activities, using an emission factor of 0.002148 kg hydrocarbon lost per kilogram gasoline consumed and assuming toluene is 1.26% by weight of the hydrocarbon emission. Toluene emissions were estimated to have been 16 057 tonnes from automobile gasoline evaporation, using an emission factor of 0.83 g/mile (0.52 g/km) hydrocarbon evaporated loss; average mileage was assumed to be 14.7 mile/gal (16.0 L/100 km). Toluene emissions in automobile exhaust were estimated to have been 589 747 tonnes using an emission factor of 3.2 g/mile (2.0 g/km) of hydrocarbons in the exhaust, 14.7 mile/gal mileage and assuming toluene constituted 12% by weight of the exhaust emission.

In Japan, toluene is extensively used as a solvent in paint and printing inks, and annual emissions of 254 000 tonnes (Kankocho, 1976) to 610 000 tonnes (Tsuritani, 1974) are estimated from this application alone (Merian & Zander, 1982).

In the absence of reactive impurities, the major reaction for volatile alkylated aromatic hydrocarbons in the environment involves oxidation of the side chains (Merian & Zander, 1982). Toluene, xylenes and other alkyl benzenes are autooxidized in the atmosphere by oxygen at roughly the same rate as ethylene, especially in the presence of catalysing impurities in the air (NAS, 1976).

During the combustion process in gasoline engines, benzene, toluene, acetylene, acrolein and aromatic aldehydes are formed from volatile aromatic compounds by

Table 4. Occupational exposure limits for toluene[a]

Country	Limits (mg/m³)	Remarks
Australia	375	
Belgium	375	
Bulgaria	50	
Czechoslovakia	200	Average
	1 000	Ceiling
Finland	750	
German Democratic Republic	200	
	800	Short-term
Germany, Federal Republic of	750	
Hungary	50	
Italy	300	
Japan	375	
Netherlands	375[b]	
Poland	100	
Romania	300	Average
	400	Ceiling
Sweden	375	
Switzerland	380	
USA[c]	750	Ceiling
USSR	50	Time-weighted average
Yugoslavia	200	

[a]International Labour Office (1977)
[b]Absorption through intact skin (mucosae) possible
[c]Occupational Safety and Health Administration

cracking and disproportionation, and also by oxidation. When automobile exhaust gases are exposed to ultraviolet light in the presence of nitric oxides, 30% of the benzene, 68% of the toluene and 84% of the xylene decompose within 6 h (Shinoyama, 1975). Aromatic compounds with side chains, and aldehydes formed from them, contribute towards the formation of photochemical smog (NAS, 1976; Merian & Zander, 1982).

EXPOSURE LEVELS AND POPULATIONS AT RISK

Estimates of exposure to toluene vary greatly. NIOSH has variously estimated that 100 000 workers (Weaver, 1974) or 4 million workers (NIOSH, 1976) are potentially exposed to toluene. Most exposures have occurred in relation to its use as a solvent, vapour inhalation being the mode of entry of major concern. Skin contact and ingestion of toluene are of far less significance (Weaver, 1974; WHO, 1981; Lauwerys, 1983). Table 4 lists the national occupational exposure limits for toluene (ILO, 1977).

Since data have been available primarily since the early 1970s, it is difficult to state whether (and where) environmental pollution by many of the major volatile aromatic compounds is decreasing, is more or less constant or is increasing (Merian & Zander, 1982). Merian and Zander (1982) state that "unfortunately, nothing is known to what extent volatile aromatics are present in the gas phase in air, and as true solutions in water and to what extent they are adsorbed to aerosols or to suspended particulate matter".

While it is known that workers and segments of the general public are exposed to toluene from chemical manufacturing processes, coke ovens, petroleum refineries, solvent operations, the storage and distribution of gasoline, urban automobile emissions, urban gasoline service stations and using self-service gasoline, as well as consumer products containing toluene, data concerning the extent of this exposure is extremely meagre (especially compared to what is known of exposure to benzene) (Merian & Zander, 1982).

In urban atmospheres, the composition of aromatic pollutants is generally considered to be similar to that of gasoline, suggesting the latter as the source (Merian & Zander, 1982; NAS, 1976; Pellizzari & Sawicki, 1977; Mendenhall, 1978). Since gasoline consumes 91% of all toluene produced, it is the largest source of toluene emissions (SRI, 1979).

In urban areas with a heavy flow of traffic, air contains some 0.6 mg/m^3 aliphatic compounds, plus about 0.15–0.2 mg/m^3 aromatic compounds, including about 0.08 mg/m^3 toluene, about 0.04 mg/m^3 xylenes and about 0.04 mg/m^3 higher benzenes (Merian & Zander, 1982).

Table 5 shows some emission values for volatile aromatic compounds. Since locations and sampling times, as well as sampling and analytical methods applied, differ widely, the data in this table can be compared only to a limited extent.

It was estimated that approximately 20 000 tonnes of toluene from mobile sources were emitted in the ambient air in The Netherlands in 1980, while stationary source emissions contributed an additional 6 278 tonnes (Guicherit & Schulting, 1985).

In addition to the chemical and petroleum industries, other significant sources of toluene emissions are found in printing and certain plastics processing operations (Merian & Zander, 1982). Another source of pollution is the smoke from forest fires, which can contain substantial amounts of volatile aromatic compounds, e.g., 97–891 mg/m^3 toluene, 25–320 mg/m^3 benzene and 116–684 mg/m^3 xylenes (Merian & Zander, 1982; NAS, 1976).

Surface waters generally contain relatively small quantities of volatile aromatic hydrocarbons. Although to date approximately 65 different, non-halogenated, benzenoid hydrocarbons have been identified in surface and drinking-waters (Garrison, 1976; Merian & Zander, 1982) and very much more is known concerning the presence of chlorinated derivatives of these compounds, data concerning the presence of toluene in water are relatively meagre (Merian & Zander, 1982; US Environmental Protection Agency, 1977b, c). Low levels of toluene, generally ranging from 1–5 µg/L, have been found in a number of American surface, tap and drinking-waters, although levels up to 12 µg/L have been reported in the drinking-water and tap water of New Orleans, Louisiana (US Environmental Protection Agency, 1977b,c; Merian & Zander, 1982).

Toluene (as well as other aromatic hydrocarbons such as benzene, xylenes and ethyl benzene) has been increasingly reported in indoor environments and, on occasion, at levels exceeding those in outdoor air (Seifert & Abraham, 1982; De Bortolie et al., 1984). For example, the concentrations of toluene, benzene and m-/p-xylene have

Table 5.   Emission values (mg/m³) for volatile aromatic compounds [a]

City	Benzene	Toluene	Xylenes	Higher alkyl benzenes
Los Angeles 1966/67 average values	0.05–0.10	0.11–0.17	0.10–0.12	0.10
Los Angeles 1966/67 maximum values	0.18	0.42	0.38	0.36
Los Angeles 1967/71 average values		0.10–0.12	0.08–0.12	0.10
Azusa, CA 1967/71 average values		0.04–0.06	0.03–0.06	0.05
Zurich, average values of				
8 locations, 1972	0.04	0.06	0.02	
Zurich, maximum values				
Milchbuck 1972	0.08	0.15	0.05	
New York, New Jersey		0.15	0.15	
Sheffield, London	0.4	0.9	0.7	
Sendai, Shiogama, Tagajo 1974	0.06–0.08	0.02	0.06–0.39	0.02–0.07
Dallas, Los Angeles, St Louis,				
Chicago 1976	0.003–0.014			
Columbus, Ohio 1978	0.004–0.030			
Newbury Park, CA 1978	0.005–0.020	0.01–0.04		
Newark industrial site, NJ	300	and traces of chlorobenzene		
Bound Brooke industrial site, NJ	9	and 20 mg chlorobenzene/m³		
Torrance industrial site, CA	13.6	and 20.7 mg chlorobenzene/m³		
Other industrial sites NY & NJ	2–3	and traces of chlorobenzene		
The Hague 1975	0.03	0.07	0.07	0.06
Paris 1974			0.003–0.01	0.007–0.025
Houston 1974	0.004–0.05	0.001–0.04	0.04–0.07	
Pretoria, Johannesburg, Durban				
1975/76	0.007–0.02	0.03–0.05	0.02–0.03	0.03–0.04
Frankfurt 1980	0.005–0.14	0.005–0.21	0.003–0.15	
Berlin (West) 1978	0.002–0.015			

[a] Merian & Zander (1982)

been determined inside and outside homes. With sampling periods from one to several days, average indoor toluene concentrations of 60 µg/m³ were measured, using passive sampling and gas chromatography. The mean value for simultaneous sampling of outdoor air next to the dwellings investigated was about 35 µg/m³ (Seifert & Abraham, 1982).

A recent WHO (1985) study has reported that the ambient air concentrations of toluene range from background levels of 0.1 µg/m³ to 20 mg/m³ while indoor concentrations in non-industrial buildings range from 17 µg/m³ to 700 µg/m³ (mean values).

In a recently reported U.S. Environmental Protection Agency Total Exposure Assessment Methodology (TEAM) study assessing personal exposure to volatile organic compounds in selected home environments, toluene was frequently found in air and breath samples (Wallace et al., 1984).

It should be further noted that toluene, as well as benzene, has been reported as an indoor pollutant, derived primarily from tobacco smoke, with toluene levels in public places ranging from 40–4 600 μg/m^3. Benzene levels ranged from 20–317 μg/m^3 (Hoffmann *et al.*, 1983).

REFERENCES

Anon. (1982) C & EN's top 50 chemical products. *Chem. Eng. News,* June 14, p. 33

Anon. (1985) Facts and figures for the chemical industry. *Chem. Eng. News,* June 10, pp. 25–55

Benignus, V.A. (1981a) Health effects of toluene – a review. *Neurotoxicology,* **2,** 567–568

Benignus, V.A. (1981b) Neurobehavioral effects of toluene – a review. *Neurobehav. Toxicol. Teratol.,* **3,** 407–415

Bradowsky, T.P., Wilson, N.B. & Scott, W.J. (1976) Chromatographic analysis of gaseous products from pyrolysis. *Anal. Chem.,* **48,** 1812

Cier, H.E. (1969) Toluene. In: Standen A., ed., *Kirk-Othmer Encyclopedia of Chemical Technology,* Vol. 20, 2nd ed., New York, Interscience/Wiley, pp. 56

Clement Associates (1977) Toluene. In: *Information Dossiers on Substances Designated by TSCA Interagency Testing Committee* (October, 1977). Contract #NSF-C-ENV-77-15417, Washington DC, December, pp. 65–70

Cohr, K.H. & Stokholm, J. (1979) Toluene: a toxicologic review. *Scand. J. Work Environ. Health.,* **5,** 71–90

CPSC (1977) *Chemical Consumer Hazard Information System,* Washington DC, Consumer Product Safety Commission

Criteria Group for Occupational Standards (1981) Scientific basis for Swedish occupational standards, toluene. *Arb. Hälsa,* **21,** 40–45

Dean, B.J. (1978) Genetic toxicology of benzene, toluene, xylenes and phenols. *Mutat. Res.,* **47,** 75–97

Dean, B.J. (1985) Recent findings on the genetic toxicology of benzene, toluene, xylenes, and phenols. *Mutat. Res.,* **154,** 153–181

DeBortoli, M., Knoppel, H., Pecchio, E., Peil, A., Rogora, L., Schauenburg, H., Schlitt, H. & Vissers, H. (1984) Integrating "real life" measurements of organic pollution in indoor and outdoor air of homes in northern Italy. In: Berglund, B., Linduall, T. & Sundell, J., eds, *Indoor Air,* Vol. 4, *Chemical Characterization and Personal Exposure,* Stockholm, Swedish Council for Building Research, pp. 21–26

Fishbein, L. (1985) An overview of environmental and toxicological aspects of aromatic hydrocarbons, II. Toluene. *Sci. Total Environ.,* **42,** 267–288

Garrison, A.W. (1976) *Consultants Rept. Technical Paper No. 9 to the WHO Internal Reference Center for Community Water Supply,* December

Guicherit, R. & Schulting, F.L. (1985) The occurrence of organic chemicals in the environment of The Netherlands. *Sci. Total Environ.,* **43,** 193–219

Hoffmann, D., Haley, N.J., Brunnemann, K.D., Adams, J.D. & Wynder, E.L. (1983) *Cigarette Sidestream Smoke: Formation, Analysis, and Model Studies on the Uptake by Non-smokers.* Presented at the U.S.-Japan Meeting on New Etiology of Lung Cancer in Honolulu, Hawaii, March 21–23

Humperdinck, K. (1954) Besondere Form der Knochenmarkschädigung bei einem Tiefdrucker. *Berufsgenossensch,* p. 89

ILO (1977) *Occupational Exposure Limits for Airborne Toxic Substances, (Occupational Safety and Health Series, No. 37),* Geneva, International Labour Office

Kankocho, K. (1976) *Report Commission Control of Hydrocarbon Sources* (*Air Pollution Abstract* 100154), Tokyo Sept.

Lauwerys, R.R. (1983) *Industrial Chemical Exposure Guidelines for Biological Monitoring,* Davis, CA, Biomedical Publications

Lijinsky, W. & Raha, L.R. (1961) Polycyclic hydrocarbons in commercial solvents. *Toxicol. Appl. Pharmacol., 3,* 469

Maltoni, C., Conti, B. & Cotti, G. (1983) Benzene: a multipotential carcinogen. Results of long-term bioassays performed at the Bologna Institute of Oncology. *Am. J. Ind. Med., 4,* 589–630

McMichael, A.J., Spirtas, R., Kupper, L.L. & Gamble, J.F. (1975) Solvent exposure and leukemia among rubber workers: an epidemiologic study. *J. Occup. Med., 17,* 234–239

Mendenhall, D.D. (1978) *Organic Characterization of Aerosols and Vapor Phase Compounds in Urban Atmospheres,* EPA Report No. 600/3-78-031, Washington DC, US Environmental Protection Agency

Merian, E. (1982) The environmental chemistry of volatile hydrocarbons. *Toxicol. Environ. Chem., 5,* 167–175

Merian, E. & Zander, M. (1982) Volatile aromatics. In: Hutzinger, G., ed., *Handbook of Environmental Chemistry,* Vol. 3, Part B, *Anthropogenic Compounds,* Berlin (West), Springer-Verlag, pp. 117–161

NAS (1976) *Vapor Phase Organic Pollutants,* Washington DC, National Academy of Sciences

NAS (1982) *Alkylbenzenes,* Washington DC, National Academy of Sciences

NIOSH (1976) *National Occupational Hazards Survey (NOHS),* Cincinnati, OH, National Institute for Occupational Safety and Health

Pellizzari, E.D. & Sawicki, E. (1977) *The Measurement of Carcinogenic Vapors in Ambient Atmospheres,* EPA Report No. 600, Washington DC, US Environmental Protection Agency

Ring, K. (1979) Toluene. In: *Chemical Economics Handbook,* Menlo Park, CA, SRI, July, p. 300.7200A-300.7202L

Ring, K. & Gunn, T.C. (1979) BTX aromatics supply. In: *Chemical Economics Handbook,* Menlo Park, CA, SRI, February, pp. 300.6500A-300.6502F

Seifert, B. & Abraham, H.J. (1982) Indoor air concentrations of benzene and some other aromatic hydrocarbons. *Ecotoxicol. Environ. Saf., 6,* 190–192

Shinoyama, E. (1975) Progress in automotive exhaust gas measurement industries. *J. Jpn Soc. Air Pollut., 10,* 264

SRI (1979) *Human Exposure to Atmospheric Concentrations of Selected Chemicals.* Vol. I, Research Triangle Park, NC, U.S. Environmental Protection Agency, Office of Air Quality Planning and Standards

SRI (1982) *Chem. Ind. Div. Newsletter,* July–August, pp. 5–7

Storck, W.J. (1981) C & EN's top 50 chemical products, *Chem. Eng. News,* May 4, p. 37

Tsuritani, K. (1974) *Labor Health and Pollution Control. Air Pollution Abstracts,* (069282)

US Environmental Protection Agency (1977a) *A Study of Industrial Data on Candidate Chemicals for Testing,* Washington DC, August

US Environmental Protection Agency (1977b) *Survey of Two Municipal Wastewater Treatment Plants,* Cincinnati, OH, Wastewater Research Division

US Environmental Protection Agency (1977c) *Information System. Monitoring to Detect Previously Unrecognized Pollutants in Surface Water,* EPA Report No. 560/6-77-0157, Washington DC

Wallace, L.A., Pellizzari, E., Hartwell, T., Rosenzwell, M., Erickson, M., Sparacino, C. & Zelon, H. (1984) Personal exposure to volatile organic compounds. I. Direct measurement in breathing zone air, drinking water, food, and exhaled breath. *Environ. Res., 35,* 293–319

Weaver, N.K. (1974) Commentary. *J. Occup. Med., 16,* 109–111

WHO (1985) *Working Group on Air Quality Guidelines for Certain Organic Air Pollutants, Prague, April 22–26,* Geneva, pp. 1–3

WHO (1981) *Recommended Health Based Limits in Occupational Exposure to Selected Organic Solvents (WHO Technical Reports Series No. 664),* Geneva, pp. 7–24

Wilson, R.H. (1943) Toluene poisoning. *J. Am. Med. Assoc., 123,* 1106–1108

CHAPTER 6

XYLENES: USES, OCCURRENCE AND EXPOSURE

L. Fishbein[1]

Department of Health and Human Services
Food and Drug Administration
National Center for Toxicological Research
Jefferson, AR 72079, USA

INTRODUCTION

Xylene (dimethylbenzene) exists in three isomeric forms: *ortho-, meta-* and *para-xylene* (1,2-dimethyl-, 1,3-dimethyl- and 1,4-dimethylbenzene). The commercial product, which is commonly known as "xylol", is a mixture of all three isomers, with *m*-xylene predominating (usually 60–70%). It should also be noted that the term "mixed xylenes" is frequently used for the xylenes *plus* ethylbenzene (Cier, 1970). [The technical product contains approximately 40% *m*-xylene and 20% each of ethylbenzene, *o*-xylene and *p*-xylene. Small quantities of toluene and C_9 aromatic fractions may also be present (SRI, 1975)]. Xylene is produced in very large quantities and is extensively employed in a broad spectrum of applications, primarily as a solvent (increasingly as a "safe" replacement for benzene), and in gasoline as part of the BTX component (benzene-toluene-xylene). There is a broad potential for exposure, both of industrial workers (production and use of the xylenes) and the general public (*via* vehicle exhausts, consumer products, etc.).

Salient aspects of xylene production, use, dispersion, exposure and toxicology have been extensively reviewed (Cier, 1969; NIOSH, 1975; ILO, 1977; Åstrand, 1975; Åstrand *et al.,* 1978; Nordic Expert Group, 1979; SRI, 1979, 1980; WHO, 1979; Riihimäki & Savolainen, 1980; Criteria Group for Occupational Standards, 1981; Merian, 1982; Merian & Zander, 1982; NAS, 1982; Henschler, 1983; Lauwerys, 1983; DGMK, 1984; Dean, 1985; Fishbein, 1985; Jori *et al.,* 1986).

---

[1]Present address: ENVIRON Corporation, 1000 Potomac Street NW, Washington DC 20007, USA.

Table 1.   General composition of commercial xylenes
from petroleum and coal-tar

Constituent	Petroleum product (%)	Coal-tar product (%)
o-Xylene	20	10–15
m-Xylene	44	45–70
p-Toluene	20	23
Ethylbenzene	15	6–10

PRODUCTION AND USE

Until the early 1940s, virtually all of the aromatic solvents, e.g., benzene, toluene, xylene and solvent naphtha, which is a mixture of solvents (primarily xylene), were produced from coal. Xylene from petroleum was first produced in the U.S.A. in 1944 (U.S. Tariff Commission, 1946; Arp *et al.,* 1983).

Most of the xylene isomers now produced occur together as mixed xylenes in an aromatic mixture (BTX) containing benzene and toluene. The majority of mixed xylenes are currently produced in the U.S.A. by catalytic reforming of petroleum (Cier, 1970; Ransley, 1970; Clement Associates, 1977; SRI, 1979). They are also obtained from pyrolysis gasoline as a by-product of olefin manufacture during the cracking of hydrocarbons. Small amounts of mixed xylenes (as BTX) are also obtained from coal-derived coke-oven light oil and from the disproportionation of toluene (Ring, 1979; Ring & Gunn, 1979; SRI, 1979).

The differences in the composition of commercial xylenes produced from petroleum and from coal-tar are indicated in Table 1. Commercial xylene may also contain small amounts of toluene, ethylbenzene, trimethylbenzene (pseudocumene), phenol, thiophene, pyridine and non-aromatic hydrocarbons and has frequently been contaminated with benzene (NIOSH, 1975; Clement Associates, 1977; WHO, 1981).

Approximately 3 880 thousand tonnes of mixed xylenes were isolated in the U.S.A. in 1978, from a total of 35 369 thousand tonnes of mixed xylenes produced as BTX. The non-isolated mixed xylenes (BTX) are blended into gasoline, while the isolated mixed xylenes are used primarily for the production of the individual isomers and for solvent applications (Ransley, 1970; Ring, 1979; Ring & Gunn, 1979).

Mixed xylenes occur naturally in only small quantities in petroleum stocks, necessitating their production by the reforming of selected naphtha streams which are rich in naphthalenes (alicyclics). Catalytic reforming involves the hydrogenation of naphtha fractions that are unsatisfactory for use as gasolines. The aromatic fractions, consisting primarily of benzene, toluene and mixed xylenes, are isolated by the reformate and by a combination of extraction and distillation (Cier, 1970; SRI, 1979). The total mixed xylene produced from catalytic reformate in 1978 is estimated to have been 34 889 thousand tonnes, of which 3 625 thousand were isolated for chemical use (Ring, 1979; Ring & Gunn, 1979). The second largest source of mixed xylenes is from pyrolysis gasoline, which yielded an estimated 375 thousand tonnes of mixed xylene

Table 2.   Mixed xylenes production in the U.S.A. (1978)[a, b]

Source	Isolated mixed xylenes	Non-isolated mixed xylenes	Total mixed xylenes
Catalytic reformate	3 625	31 264	34 889
Pyrolysis gasoline	195	180	375
Toluene disproportionation	48	42	90
Coal-derived	13	2	15
Total	3 881	31 488	35 369

[a] Ring (1979); Ring & Gunn (1979)
[b] In thousand tonnes/year

as BTX, from which an estimated 195 thousand tonnes were isolated for chemical use (SRI, 1979).

New sources of xylenes from petroleum reforming operations are provided by the Toyo Rayon and Atlantic-Richfield processes, which involve the disproportionation of toluene or the transalkylation of toluene with trimethylbenzenes. The products are principally benzene and xylenes. If the transalkylation feed stocks are limited to toluene and polymethylbenzenes (no benzene derivatives), the product xylenes from these operations will contain no ethylbenzene (Cier, 1970). In 1978, the disproportionation of toluene produced an estimated 90 thousand tonnes of mixed xylenes of which 48 thousand tonnes were separated for chemical use. In addition, 15 thousand tonnes of mixed xylenes were produced from coal-derived BTX, with an estimated 13 thousand tonnes separated for chemical use. Table 2 summarizes isolated and non-isolated mixed xylenes production by source in the U.S.A. for 1978 (Ring, 1979; Ring & Gunn, 1979; SRI, 1979). In the U.S.A. there are currently 201 locations where mixed xylenes are produced from catalytic reformate, nine locations where they are produced as BTX from pyrolysis gasoline manufacture, three devoted to coal-derived mixed xylenes production and two where mixed xylenes are produced from toluene disproportionation.

In 1982 and 1983, respectively, U.S. production of xylenes amounted to 2.26 and 2.53 million tonnes, ranking respectively 27th and 24th in importance among the chemicals produced during those years (Webber, 1984). The production of mixed xylenes in 1984 rose to 2.78 million tonnes, ranking 22nd among the chemicals produced (Anon., 1985a). The production of p-xylene in 1983 and 1984 was 1.86 and 1.94 million tonnes, respectively, ranking 29th (Anon., 1985b). It was projected that the output of p-xylene would increase slightly in 1985 to 2.0 million tonnes, with the final figure depending on the availability of mixed xylenes, on the export markets for p-xylene (as well as for o-xylene) and on the size of imports of apparel made from polyester fibres. (The production capacity for p-xylene was expected to reach 2.6 million tonnes in 1985; Anon., 1985a). The production of o-xylene for 1983 and 1984 was 354 and 316 thousand tonnes, respectively.

The production of mixed xylenes in the Federal Republic of Germany in 1979 amounted to 223 thousand tonnes (compared to 1 626 thousand tonnes xylenes produced in the U.S.A. in that period). For western Europe, production of xylenes in 1980 was expected to be about three times that in 1970 (Ullman, 1974; Merian & Zander, 1982). The production of xylenes in 1984 was estimated to have been as follows (in thousands of tonnes): France, 85; Italy, 395 and the Federal Republic of Germany, 455 (Anon., 1985a).

World production of *p*-xylene in 1983 was 3.9 million tonnes, of which the U.S.A. accounted for 48%; western Europe, 23% and Japan, 16%. The U.S.A. and western Europe exported 324 thousand and 327 thousand tonnes of *p*-xylene, respectively, in this period (Bromberger & Kridyl, 1985).

World production of *o*-xylene in 1983 was 1.3 million tonnes, of which western Europe produced 30% and the U.S.A. 18%. Eastern Europe was the other large producer. Western Europe and the U.S.A. exported 191 thousand and 66 thousand tonnes of *o*-xylene in this period (Bromberger & Kridyl, 1985).

Table 3 shows the end-use distribution of mixed xylenes and individual xylene isomers in the U.S.A. in 1978 (Klapproth, 1978; Ring, 1979; Ring & Gunn, 1979; SRI,

Table 3. End-use distribution of mixed xylenes and xylene isomers (1978)[a]

	Use	
	10^6 kg/yr	%
Mixed xylene as BTX (not isolated)	31 488	
Gasoline	31 488	100.0
Isolated mixed xylene	3 880	
p-Xylene isomer	1 863	48.0
o-Xylene isomer	497	12.2
m-Xylene isomer	40	1.0
Ethyl benzene	100	2.6
Gasoline backblending	979	25.2
Paint and coating solvent	225	5.8
Adhesives solvent	35	0.9
Chemical manufacturing solvent	35	0.9
Agricultural solvent	30	0.8
Other miscellaneous solvents	25	0.7
Net export	75	1.9
o-Xylene	474	
Phthalic anhydride	304	64.1
Gasoline backblending	10	2.0
Exports	161	33.9
p-Xylene	1 863	
Terephthalic acid	649	34.8
Dimethyl terephthalate	925	49.7
Net exports	281	15.1
Gasoline backblending	8	0.4
m-Xylene	40	
Isophthalic acid	40[b]	100.0

[a] Klapproth (1978), Ring (1979), Ring & Gunn (1979), SRI (1979)
[b] Difference between production and use supplied by imports

1979). All mixed xylenes produced as BTX and not isolated (31 488 thousand tonnes) are blended into gasoline. The remaining isolated mixed xylenes (3 881 thousand tonnes) are used in a variety of solvent applications, as well as to produce the individual isomers of xylene.

Xylenes are used *inter alia* as solvents, particularly in the paint and printing ink industries, e.g., 183 000 tonnes per year in the U.S.A. (NAS, 1976) and 91 000 tonnes per year (Merian & Zander, 1982). In eastern Europe it is also used for numerous applications in the shoe industry (Merian & Zander, 1982).

The single largest end-use of mixed xylene is in the production of the *p*-xylene isomer, which consumed an estimated 1.86 million tonnes in the U.S.A. in 1978 (SRI, 1979). Production of *p*-xylene was about 1.63 million tonnes in 1980, down about 16% from 1979 (Anon., 1980), and 1.72 million tonnes in 1981 (Anon., 1981). The production of *p*-xylene in the U.S.A. in 1982 and 1983 was 1.46 and 1.86 million tonnes, respectively, ranking 31st and 29th, respectively, among the chemicals produced during those years (Webber, 1984). In 1981, the major derivatives produced from *p*-xylene were dimethylterephthalate (55%) and terephthalic acid (45%), the major end uses (almost 100%) being polyester fibre, film and fabricated items, mostly bottles (Anon., 1981).

During 1983–1988, U.S. consumption of mixed xylenes for *p*-xylene production is expected to increase annually at about 1.4%. Domestic consumption of *p*-xylene for polyester fibres will grow at an annual rate of about 1.1%, while consumption for film and bottle resins will increase annually at 6.8% and 6.5%, respectively (Bomberger & Kridyl, 1985).

In 1984, the synthesis of dimethylterephthalate and terephthalic acid again consumed 55% and 45%, respectively, of the production of *p*-xylene. In that year, the major end uses were polyester fibres, 80%; blow-moulded items (mostly bottles), 10%; and films, 5% (Anon., 1985b).

The production of *o*-xylene in the U.S.A. in 1978 consumed 450 thousand tonnes of mixed xylenes, with phthalic anhydride the predominant outlet as an intermediate for plasticizers used in vinyl plastics (SRI, 1980). The production of *m*-xylene in 1978 consumed 40 thousand tonnes of mixed xylenes (Table 3).

U.S. consumption of mixed xylenes for *o*-xylene production for the period 1983 to 1988 is expected to decline annually at a rate of 3.4%. While the market for phthalic anhydride is increasing, more *o*-xylene is being imported and more anhydride is being produced from naphthalene.

U.S. *m*-xylene consumption for isophthalic acid production is expected to grow at 8.9% per year between 1983 and 1988. Isophthalic acid is used in the production of unsaturated polyester resins.

U.S. production of ethylbenzene from mixed xylenes streams is expected to drop from 91 thousand tonnes per year in 1983 to about 45 thousand tonnes in 1988. This projected drop is due primarily to the high energy cost of separation, making synthesis a more practical production method (Bomberger & Kridyl, 1985).

SOURCES OF EMISSION

Sources of emissions of mixed xylenes arise during its production (principally from catalytic reformating) and end use. Process emissions originate from the reactor, distillation, and crystallization vents. Storage emissions represent the loss from both working and final product storage, as well as loading and handling losses, while fugitive emissions are those which result from plant equipment leaks (SRI, 1979). Estimates of the extent of emissions of the xylenes vary greatly. Total emissions of mixed xylenes from catalytic reformate production in the U.S.A. in 1978 were estimated to have been approximately 4 000 tonnes. Individual isomer emissions from the mixed xylenes were 16.7% p-xylene, 20.5% o-xylene, 35.7% m-xylene, 2.9% toluene, 23.7% ethylbenzene and 0.5% others. Individual emission estimates from catalytic reformating production of p-xylene, o-xylene and m-xylene were approximately 680 tonnes, 860 tonnes and 1 500 tonnes, respectively, during this period (SRI, 1979).

The mixed xylene emissions from pyrolysis gasoline, toluene disproportionation and coal-derived production sources were 150 tonnes, 18 tonnes and 18.7 tonnes, respectively, in the U.S.A. in 1978 (SRI, 1979). The emissions due to production of the individual isomers of xylene in the U.S.A. in 1978 were estimated to have been approximately 1 180 tonnes, 2 950 tonnes and 79.8 tonnes for o-xylene, p-xylene and m-xylene, respectively (SRI, 1979). Clement Associates (1977) estimated that approximately 408 000 tonnes of xylenes are released to the environment each year.

Guicherit and Schulting (1985) estimated that approximately 51 tonnes and 2 070 tonnes of o-xylene and m-/p-xylene, respectively, were emitted in the ambient air in The Netherlands in 1980 from stationary sources, while mobile source emissions for o-xylene and m-/p-xylene combined totalled 13 200 tonnes.

Globally, the xylene introduced into the environment was estimated by Merian and Zander (1982) to be made up of some 0.5 million tonnes from solvent losses, about 2 million tonnes from losses during the production, transportation and processing of petroleum and some 0.5 to 1 million tonnes as a component of automobile exhaust gases. Compared with these emissions, the losses during transportation and distribution of gasoline (estimated worldwide at 10 000 tonnes) and the losses in the chemical industry (estimated at less than 50 000 tonnes) are considered to be relatively low. It should also be noted that emission is low because the vapour pressure of the C_8 aromatics is lower than that of benzene and toluene (Merian & Zander, 1982).

Table 4 summarizes the global losses of benzene, toluene, xylenes and other C_8 and C_9 aromatics and higher alkylated benzols and naphthalenes into the environment (Merian, 1982).

The concentrations of toluene and xylenes in streets are higher than those of benzene, probably because gasoline contains much higher amounts. For example, xylene levels of 0.05 to 0.15 mg/m^3 and toluene levels of 0.05 to 0.2 mg/m^3 have been reported in the atmosphere of some streets, and some surface waters have been found to contain 3 µg/L xylenes, about 1–2 µg/L ethylbenzene and 2 µg/L toluene (US Environmental Protection Agency, 1977a,b; Merian & Zander, 1982).

Table 4. Global losses of volatile aromatics into the environment[a, b]

Loss	Benzene	Toluene	Xylenes and other C_8 and C_9's	Higher alkylated benzols and naphthalenes
Losses into the sea	0.07	0.5	0.6	0.1
Losses of refineries into the air	2	2.5	1.5	2
Evaporation of gasoline	0.1	0.05	0.02	
Automobile exhaust	2	2	0.5	0.5
Diesel exhaust				0.2
Solvent losses		1	0.5	
Losses in the chemical industry	0.1	0.1	0.05	0.01
Total	4.3	6.2	3.2	2.8

[a] Merian & Zander (1982)
[b] Million tonnes

CHEMICAL AND PHOTOCHEMICAL REACTIONS

The major reaction for volatile alkylated aromatic hydrocarbons in the environment (in the absence of reactive impurities) involves oxidation of the sidechains (Merian & Zander, 1982). Xylenes, like toluene and other alkylbenzenes, are autoxidized in the atmosphere by oxygen at roughly the same rate as ethylene, especially in the presence of catalysing air impurities (NAS, 1976).

The photochemical reactivity of alkylbenzenes is enhanced by nitric oxide or solid particles on whose surfaces catalytic reactions occur (Korte & Boedefeld, 1978). When automobile exhaust gases are exposed to ultraviolet light in the presence of nitric oxides, 30% of the benzene, 68% of the toluene and 84% of the xylene decompose within 6 h (Shinoyama, 1975).

The reactivity of xylenes to oxidation has been suggested to be low, with estimated half-lives of 2 200 years to peroxy radical and 100 years to ozone. The half-life for reactions of xylenes with hydroxyl radical was reported to be 3 days (Brown, 1975). Products of microbial degradation of xylenes in soil are reported to include *alpha*-hydroxy-*p*-toluic acid, *p*-methylbenzyl alcohol, benzyl alcohol, *m*- and *p*-toluic acids and 4-methylcatechol (Davis, 1968; Omori & Yamada, 1970; Brown, 1975). Since xylenols, benzoic acids, phenols, etc., are hydrophilic decomposition products of volatile aromatic compounds, they are easily subject to microbial biodegradation (Merian & Zander, 1982).

EXPOSURE LEVELS AND POPULATION AT RISK

Compared to benzene and toluene, very much less is known of the populations at risk and the levels of exposure to mixed xylenes or the individual isomers of xylene. As noted earlier, mixed xylenes are produced in large amounts in an aromatic mixture (BTX), are extensively employed as solvents and are present in gasoline and a broad range of consumer products (mostly in household aerosols and paints, varnishes,

Table 5. Occupational exposure limits for xylenes [a]

Country	Xylene [b]	Remarks
Australia	435	
Belgium	435 [c]	
Bulgaria	50	
Czechoslovakia	200	Average
	1 000	Ceiling
Finland	435 [c]	
German Democratic Republic	600	Short-term
Germany, Federal Republic of	870	
Hungary	50	
Italy	400	
Japan	670 (435 [c]) [d]	
Netherlands	435	
Poland	100	
Romania	300 [c]	Average
	400	Ceiling
Sweden	435 [c]	
Switzerland	435 [c]	
USA [e]	435	Time-weighted average
USSR	50	
Yugoslavia	50	Ceiling

[a] ILO (1977)
[b] All values expressed in mg/m^3
[c] Absorption through intact skin (mucosae) possible
[d] Recommended by the Japan Association of Industrial Health in 1980
[e] Occupational Safety and Health Administration

shellac and rust preventatives, etc.). Although the individual isomers are employed in extensive amounts for the synthesis of a relatively small number of chemicals (e.g., phthalic acid, isophthalic acid, terephthalic acid and dimethylterephthalate), these derivatives are very extensively employed for the further production of phthalate esters as plasticizers for vinyl plastics and, in the case of terephthalic acid, for polyester resins and fibres such as Davron, Mylar and Terylene.

The population exposed belongs mainly to the industrial workforce, which can be exposed to airborne mixed xylenes during their production and end use, and wide application as an industrial solvent. Exposure of the general public can arise from automobile exhausts and the many consumer products containing xylenes.

In the NIOSH survey of occupational exposure, xylene (mixed isomers) was ranked 13th out of approximately 7 000 agents, with an estimated 4 million workers in the U.S.A. believed to be exposed to it (NIOSH, 1976). It has been estimated that approximately 408 thousand tonnes of xylenes are released to the environment each year (US Environmental Protection Agency, 1977b). It has also been estimated that 2 000 workers in the U.S.A. are exposed to *m*-xylene, 3 000 to *o*-xylene and 3 000 to *p*-xylene (NIOSH, 1976; Clement Associates, 1977). Table 5 lists national occupational exposure limits for xylene (ILO, 1977). Potential exposure of a segment of the general population may also arise from the presence of mixed xylenes in a wide variety of consumer products, including such household items as degreasing cleaners, insecticides, lacquers, paint removers and pesticides (Gleason *et al.,* 1969; CPSC, 1977). The 1 095 products surveyed by the Consumer Products Safety Commission (CPSC, 1977) contained an average of 9.5% mixed xylenes. The largest number of mixed xylene-containing products was found in the household aerosols and paints, varnishes, shellac and rust preventatives categories. Exposure of the general population can also result from the approximately 408 thousand tonnes of mixed xylenes which are reported to be released into the environment annually (Clement Associates, 1977; SRI, 1979).

Indoor air concentrations of aromatic hydrocarbons, such as benzene, toluene and the isomeric xylenes, have often been found at levels which exceed those outdoors (Seifert & Abraham, 1982, 1983; Seifert *et al.,* 1983; Wallace *et al.,* 1984; Berglund *et al.,* 1987). Benzene, the isomeric xylenes and ethylbenzene (as well as six chlorinated alkanes and alkenes) were consistently present in personal air and breath samples at higher concentrations than in outdoor samples in a recent survey of 355 urban residents in two cities in New Jersey, U.S.A. (Wallace *et al.,* 1984).

The isomeric xylenes are among the 11 most often measured chemicals indoors in U.S. Environmental Protection Agency surveys and have been detected by the National Aeronautics and Space Administration in nearly 800 of the 10 000 materials tested which are used in space shuttles; marking pens released the highest levels of xylene (Ember, 1985).

Data concerning environmental levels of the xylenes are scant. In urban atmospheres, the relative amounts of aromatic pollutants are similar to those in gasoline (Merian & Zander, 1982).

The aromatic compounds in a premium unleaded gasoline can include the following (percentages by weight): benzene, 1.9; toluene, 13.6; ethylbenzene, 2.7; *p*-xylene, 4.2; *m*-xylene, 12.2; and *o*-xylene, 5.2 (Korte & Boedefeld, 1978).

In urban areas with a heavy flow of traffic, air can contain about 0.15–0.2 mg aromatic compounds/m^3, including about 0.04 mg xylene/m^3, about 0.08 mg toluene/m^3 and about 0.04 mg benzene/m^3, in addition to some 0.6 mg aliphatic compounds/m^3 (Merian & Zander, 1982). Individual isomers of xylene have been reported in air (0.07–0.27 mg/m^3 for the *m* isomer and less for the others) (Brown, 1975). In a study of exposure by inhalation in an urban population in the Chicago, IL, area (54 selected normal, healthy volunteers; categories according to race, sex and age) in the presence of endogenous effluents, Krotoszynski *et al.* (1979) reported *o*-, *m*- and *p*-xylene mean levels of 1.0, 0.324 and 3.1 ng/L, respectively.

Levels of 116–684 mg xylenes/m^3 have been reported in the smoke from forest fires (NAS, 1976; Merian & Zander, 1982). Generally low levels of xylenes (e.g., 3 µg/L) have been reported in surface waters (Merian & Zander, 1982).

REFERENCES

Anon. (1980) Key chemicals – p-xylene. *Chem. Eng. News,* November, p. 24
Anon. (1981) Key chemicals – p-xylene. *Chem. Eng. News,* November 30, p. 18

Anon. (1985a) Facts and figures for the chemical industry. *Chem. Eng. News,* June 10, p. 15

Anon. (1985b) Key chemicals: *p*-xylene. *Chem. Eng. News,* March 25, p. 27

Arp, E.W., Jr, Wolf, P.H. & Checkoway, H. (1983) Lymphocytic leukemia and exposures to benzene and other solvents in the rubber industry. *J. Occup. Med., 25,* 598–602

Åstrand, I. (1975) Uptake of solvents in the blood and tissues of man. A review. *Scand. J. Work Environ. Health, 1,* 199–218

Åstrand, I., Engström, J. & Ovrum, P. (1978) Exposure to xylene and ethylbenzene. I. Uptake, distribution and elimination in man. *Scand. J. Work Environ. Health, 4,* 185–194

Berglund, B., Berglund U., Lindhall, T. & Sundell, J., eds (1987) *Indoor Air,* Vols. 1–5, Stockholm, Swedish Council for Building Research

Bomberger, D.C. & Kridyl, A.G. (1985) *CEH Report Abstract Mixed Xylenes,* Menlo Park, CA, SRI International, *SRI Chem. Ind. Newsletter,* May–June, p. 5

Brown, S.L. (1975) *Research Program on Hazard Priority Ranking of Manufactured Chemicals, Phase II-Final Report to National Science Foundation,* Menlo Park, CA, SRI

Cier, H.E. (1970) Xylenes and ethylbenzene. In: Standen, H., ed., *Kirk-Othmer Encyclopedia of Chemical Technology,* Vol. 22, 2nd Ed., New York, Interscience/ Wiley, pp. 467–507

Clement Associates (1977) *Xylenes.* In: *Information Dossiers on Substances Designated by TSCA Interagency Testing Committee* (October, 1977), Contract NSF-C-ENV-77-15417, Washington DC, December

CPSC (1977) *Chemical Consumer Hazard Information System,* Washington DC, Consumer Product Safety Commission

Criteria Group for Occupational Standards (1981) Scientific basis for Swedish occupational standards. *Arb. Hälsa, 21,* 46–58

Davis, R.S (1968) Catabolism of *p*-xylene by *Pseudomonas. Can. J. Microbiol., 14,* 1005–1009

Dean, B.J. (1985) Recent findings on the genetic toxicology of benzene, toluene, xylenes and phenols. *Mutat. Res., 154,* 153–181

DGMK (1984) Deutsche Gesellschaft für Mineralölwissenschaft und Kohlechemie eV, *Wirkung von Xylol auf Mensch und Tier,* Hamburg, pp. 174–178

Ember, L. (1985) Toxic chemical levels higher indoors than out. *Chem. Eng. News,* June 24, pp. 20, 21

Fishbein, L. (1985) An overview of environmental and toxicological aspects of aromatic hydrocarbons. III. Xylene. *Sci. Total Environ., 43,* 165–183

Gleason, M.N., Gosselin, R.E., Hodge, H.C. & Smith, R.P. (1969) *Clinical Toxicology of Commercial Products: Acute Poisoning,* 3rd Ed., Baltimore, Williams and Wilkins, pp. 227–230

Guicherit, R. & Schulting, F.L. (1985) The occurrence of organic chemicals in the atmosphere of The Netherlands. *Sci. Total Environ., 43,* 193–219

Henschler, D., ed. (1983) *Gesundheitsschädliche Arbeitsstoffe. Toxikologisch. arbeitmedizinische Begründung von Marktwerten,* Weinheim, Verlag Chemie

ILO (1977) *Occupational Exposure Limits for Airborne Toxic Substances (Occupational Safety and Health Series No. 37),* Geneva International Labour Office

Jori, A., Calamari, D., Di Domenico, A., Galli, C.L., Galli, E., Marinovich, M. & Silano, V. (1986) Ecotoxicological profile of xylenes. *Ecotoxicol. Environ. Saf., 11,* 44–80

Klapproth, E.M. (1978) Xylene isomers. In: *Chemical Economics Handbook,* Menlo Park, CA, SRI, December, pp. 30.7400A-300.7404M

Korte, F. & Boedefeld, E. (1978) Ecotoxicological review of global impact of petroleum industry and its products. *Ecotoxicol. Environ. Saf., 2,* 55–62

Krotoszynski, B.K., Bruneau, G.M. & O'Neill, H.J. (1979) Measurement of chemical inhalation exposure in urban population in the presence of endogenous effluents. *J. Anal. Toxicol., 3,* 225–234

Lauwerys, R. (1983) *Industrial Chemical Exposure Guidelines for Biological Monitoring,* Davis, CA, Biomedical Publications

Merian, E. (1982) The environmental chemistry of volatile hydrocarbons. *Toxicol. Environ. Chem., 5,* 167–175

Merian, E. & Zander, M. (1982) Volatile aromatics. In: Hutzinger, G., ed., *Handbook of Environmental Chemistry,* Vol. 3, Part B, *Anthropogenic Compounds,* Berlin (West), Springer-Verlag, pp. 117–161

NAS (1976) *Vapor-phase Organic Pollutants,* Washington DC, National Academy of Sciences

NAS (1982) *Alkylbenzenes,* Washington DC, National Academy of Sciences

NIOSH (1975) *Criteria for a Recommended Standard Occupational Exposure to Xylene,* Washington DC, National Institute for Occupational Safety and Health

NIOSH (1976) *National Occupational Hazards Survey (NOHS),* Cincinnati, OH, National Institute for Occupational Safety and Health

Nordic Expert Group (1979) Xylene. *Arb. Hälsa, 35,* 21–24

Omori, T. & Yamada, K. (1970) Utilization of hydrocarbons by microorganisms. XVII. Metabolism of xylene and related compounds. *Agric. Biol. Chem., 34,* 664–669

Ransley, D.L. (1970) BTX Processing. In: Grayson, M. & Eckroth, D., eds, *Kirk-Othmer Encyclopedia of Chemical Technology,* Vol. 4, 3rd Ed., New York, Wiley and Sons, pp. 264–277

Riihimäki, V. & Savolainen, K. (1980) Human exposure to m-xylene – kinetics and acute effects on the central nervous system. *Ann. Occup. Hyg., 23,* 411–422

Ring, K. (1979) Mixed xylenes. In: *Chemical Economics Handbook.* Menlo Park, CA, SRI, February, pp. 300.7300A-300.7301D

Ring, K. & Gunn, T.C. (1979) BTX aromatics supply. In: *Chemical Economics Handbook,* Menlo Park, CA, SRI, February, p. 300.6500A-300.6502F

Seifert, B. & Abraham, H.J. (1982) Indoor air concentrations of benzene and some other aromatic hydrocarbons. *Ecotoxicol. Environ. Saf., 6,* 190–192

Seifert, B. & Abraham, H.J. (1983) Use of possible samplers for the determination of gaseous organic substances in indoor air at low concentration levels. *Int. J. Environ. Anal. Chem., 13,* 237–253

Seifert, B., Ullrich, D. & Schmahl, H.J. (1983) Occurrence of carcinogenic organic substances in kitchen air. In: *Proceedings VI World Congress on Air Quality, Paris, May 16–20,* Paris, SEPIC, pp. 75–79

Shinoyama, E. (1975) Progress in automotive exhaust gas measurement industries. *J. Jpn Soc. Air Pollut., 10,* 264–268

SRI (1975) *Chemical Economics Handbook,* Menlo Park, CA, Chemical Information Services, December, pp. 699.5022I-U

SRI (1979) *Human Exposure to Atmospheric Concentrations of Selected Chemicals,* Vol. I, Office of Air Quality Planning and Standards, Research Triangle Park, NC, U.S. Environmental Protection Agency, pp. A-29-4 to A-29-72

SRI International (1980) *Directory of Chemical Producers in the U.S.,* Menlo Park, CA

Ullman, T. (1974) *Ullman's Encyclopädie der Technischen Chemie,* Vol. 8, 4th Ed., Weinheim, Verlag-Chemie

US Environmental Protection Agency (1977a) *Information System EPA-RS-73-277. Monitoring to Detect Previously Unrecognized Pollutants in Surface Water (EPA Report No. 560/6-77-0157)* Washington DC

US Environmental Protection Agency (1977b) *A Study of Industrial Data on Candidate Chemicals for Testing,* Washington DC, November 1976, August 1977

U.S. Tariff Commission (1946) *Synthetic Organic Chemicals, US Production and Sales, 1944 (Report No. 155),* Washington DC

Wallace, L., Pellizzari, E.D., Hartwell, T.D., Zelon, H., Sparacino, C. & Whitmore, R. (1984) Analyses of exhaled breath of 355 urban residents for volatile organic compounds. In: Berglund, B., Berglund, U., Lindhall, T. & Sundell, J., eds, *3rd Indoor Air Symposium, August 20–24,* Stockholm, Swedish Council for Building Research, pp. 15–20

Webber, D. (1984) Top 50 chemical products. *Chem. Eng. News,* May 7, pp. 8–10

WHO (1979) *Internationally Recommended Health Based Occupational Exposure Limits of Selected Organic Solvents,* Geneva, World Health Organization

WHO (1981) Xylene. In: *Recommended Health Based Limits in Occupational Exposure to Selected Organic Solvents (WHO Technical Reports Series No. 664),* Geneva, World Health Organization, pp. 25–38

SAMPLING, SAMPLING STRATEGY AND ANALYSIS OVERVIEWS

CHAPTER 7

PAST AND PRESENT EXPOSURE DETERMINATION TECHNIQUES FOR BENZENE, TOLUENE AND XYLENE

L. Fishbein[1]

Department of Health and Human Sciences,
Food and Drug Administration,
National Center for Toxicological Research,
Jefferson, AR 72079, USA

I.K. O'Neill & A. Tossavainen

International Agency for Research on Cancer,
Lyon, France

INTRODUCTION

The aromatic hydrocarbons (primarily benzene, toluene, the xylenes, ethylbenzene and styrene) are among the most important volatile aromatic compounds of commercial and environmental significance (IARC, 1979, 1982a,b; Merian, 1982; Merian & Zander, 1982; Fishbein, 1984, 1985a,b,c). Although hygienists, until recently, have been concerned primarily with exposure to benzene, and to a lesser extent toluene and xylene, in the workplace, it is increasingly recognized that large segments of the general public can also be exposed to these agents as a result of the broad spectrum of activities in which they are generated, processed, dispersed and used (Fishbein, 1984, 1985a,b,c). However, it should be noted that although there have been many case reports, case series and epidemiological studies associating exposure to benzene with leukaemia in humans, very few of them have provided quantitative information concerning the relative risk under specified conditions of exposure, and conflicting reports have appeared concerning the models used to extrapolate risk (Chapter 1, this volume; NAS, 1976; Berlin *et al.,* 1980; Brief *et al.,* 1980; OSHA, 1981; Rinsky *et al.,* 1981; Van Raalte, 1982; Van Raalte & Grasso, 1982; White *et al.,* 1982; Maltoni *et al.,* 1983; Chandler, 1984; Checkoway *et al.,* 1984; Irvine, 1984; Van Raalte *et al.,* 1984; Infante & White, 1985; Runion & Scott, 1985)

---

[1] Present address: ENVIRON Corporation, 100 Potomac Street NW, Washington DC, USA

as well as aspects of occupational exposure to mixed solvents (e.g., those encountered in the rubber industry, see McMichael *et al.,* 1975; Wolf *et al.,* 1981; IARC, 1982b; Arp *et al.,* 1983; Checkoway *et al.,* 1984).

The few large-scale epidemiological studies involving exposure to benzene, toluene and xylene, either individually or in admixture, have generally provided little unambigous information about the levels and duration of exposure (McMichael *et al.,* 1975; Ott *et al.,* 1978; IARC, 1982b; Checkoway *et al.,* 1984). It is generally conceded that exposure levels in factories where benzene and/or mixed solvents were employed were not well documented and that there were no previous exposure data for a number of plants where leukaemia deaths have occurred as a result of exposure to solvents.

One such study reported that the peak concentration of benzene in the working environment of Turkish shoe-workers ranged from 210 to 650 ppm (Aksoy, 1977). In another study, it was stated only that benzene levels in air near rotogravure machines in some Italian factories were 200 to 400 ppm with peaks up to 1 500 ppm and were 25 to 6 000 ppm near shoe-workers handling glue, but were 'mostly' around 200 to 500 ppm (Vigliani, 1976). It is rather difficult to judge the representativeness of these few measurements with respect to the entire cohorts for which the leukaemia incidence rates were calculated. In recreating the exposure conditions of the workers included in the epidemiological studies, attempts have been made to describe the range of average individual exposures, both by level and by duration (White *et al.,* 1982). Inevitably, however, the exposure indices are model-dependent and, in most cases, the lack of biological knowledge does not allow one to evaluate their appropriateness. For example, no unambiguous method is available for combining data on cumulative doses with short-term exposure levels.

It is also suggested that the actual exposures pertaining to the benzene-initiated leukaemia cases during the etiologically meaningful period in the 1940s and 1950s are largely unknown (Infante *et al.,* 1977; Van Raalte *et al.,* 1984). Berlin *et al.* (1980) have stated that the limited knowledge available concerning the occupational dose-response relationship for benzene is derived from the clinical examination of men working in environments periodically subjected to air analysis. Such measurements are not very satisfactory for assessing the cumulative exposure to a volatile liquid which may produce relatively high transient concentrations in air.

It is important to note that benzene has been produced commercially from coal-tar since 1849, from coal gas since 1876 and from petroleum since 1941. Petroleum is currently the major global source of benzene production (Chapter 4; Purcell, 1978; IARC, 1982a; Fishbein, 1984). In order to improve the assessment of potential risk from exposure to aromatic toxicants, both prospectively and retrospectively, it is necessary to obtain more accurate knowledge of the sources and levels to which humans are exposed *via* all significant environmental routes.

Industrial hygiene measurements made for labour inspection and monitoring purposes may provide some knowledge of current exposure levels in the workplace. During 1978–83, benzene data from more than 60 US companies were collected and reviewed (Runion & Scott, 1985). About 38 000 personal samples of four or more hours' duration gave an arithmetic mean of 0.64 ppm; 87% of all samples contained less than 1 ppm and 11.4% more than 10 ppm. Elevated levels were reported from benzene production and the petrochemical and rubber industries, as well as from bulk loading and shipping operations. In the early 1980s, the Finnish Institute of Occupational Health visited about 600 workplaces annually and more than 10 000 air samples were taken (Kokko, 1982). Of these, about 1 000 were analysed for benzene, toluene or xylene content. Next to carbon monoxide, toluene and xylene were the most common compounds measured in the surveys. Less than 5% of the samples exceeded the current exposure limits (10 ppm benzene, 200 ppm toluene, 100 ppm xylene). Most of the high-exposure situations were related to manual or other open use of organic solvents, e.g., in spray painting, degreasing and cleaning work. Similar results were reported by the Danish National Institute of Occupational Health; in 1983–84 about 4 000 determinations of toluene and xylene were made and the exposure limits were exceeded in 1.7% and 2.5% of the samples, respectively (Arbeijdstilsynet, 1985). The geometric mean concentration of benzene in 50 255 workplaces in China was 5.75 ppm, and 1.3% of the samples exceeded 312.5 ppm. More than 500 000 workers were exposed to benzene in painting, printing, shoe-making and chemical industries (Yin et al., 1987).

Benzene comprises about 2% of the total hydrocarbon emission from a gasoline engine. In a Swedish study, urban atmospheres were reported to contain 5 to 500 g/mg^3, associated with automobile use, (Holmberg & Lundberg, 1985). The correlation between benzene and toluene concentrations and the toluene:benzene ratio, which normally approximates 2.4:1, can be used as indicators of traffic-induced air pollution (Tsani-Bazaca et al., 1982).

The purpose of this chapter is primarily to review the exposure measurements reported and the technical facilities employed prior to 1970. With few exceptions, exposure measurements reported before that time for groups of workers subjected to epidemiological studies were scarce or very limited. In order to avoid repeating inadequate exposure measurements and better to appreciate the advantages of the sampling and analytical methods detailed in this volume, earlier exposure measurements and methods are contrasted with presently available techniques.

MEASUREMENT OF EXPOSURE TO BENZENE

The literature dealing with the analysis of benzene in industrial gases, organic solvents, air (ambient and industrial), water and biological tissues is particularly voluminous and reveals the almost continuous need for enhanced selectivity and sensitivity. Many of these procedures have had a long history of use for a variety of purposes, including toxicological investigations (Snyder, 1977; IARC, 1982a). The air concentrations to be measured may vary by a factor of 10^6, from ambient levels of micrograms/m^3 in rural areas to high occupational exposures of thousands of milligrams/m^3. Before personal samplers were widely available, area samplers were used extensively by industrial hygienists in assessing exposure, and thus early measurements do not accurately reflect real exposures, particularly of individuals closely involved in the use of these volatile substances.

With regard to human exposure, there are several unique problems which greatly complicate the evaluation of 'safe' levels of exposure to benzene. When occupationally exposed groups are studied in detail, pancytopenia is far more frequently observed than is leukaemia (Snyder & Kocsis, 1975; Laskin & Goldstein, 1977; IARC, 1982a,b). As noted earlier, there is a paucity of unambiguous information (especially in the earlier literature) concerning the relationship between leukaemia and levels of occupational exposure to benzene. Many of the procedures that were employed before the advent of gas chromatography (GC) in the late 1950s (e.g., gravimetric, visible and ultraviolet (UV) spectrophotometric, infra-red and gas interferometry) involved procedures that were both cumbersome and somewhat non-selective and insensitive by today's standards (Snyder, 1977). Nearly all the early methods of analysis suffered from interference, so that the presence of other airborne substances must be considered in examining early exposure data. Some have questioned the sensitivity and reliability of benzene measurements in the 1940s indicating levels ranging from zero to 10–15 ppm (Tabershaw & Lamm, 1977). Additionally, it is recognized that, because of limited sampling, the estimation of exposure intensities and cumulative doses may be conservative for individuals occupationally exposed to benzene prior to 1960 (Ott et al., 1978).

Industrial or work-room air

Because benzene is one of the most toxic of the common organic solvents, its determination in work-room air has long been an important industrial hygiene procedure (Elkins et al., 1962; Snyder, 1977). The earliest major studies of exposure to benzene, reported in 1926 and 1928, were made by adsorption of the vapour on activated charcoal, followed by gravimetric determination (Greenberg, 1926; Posner, 1928). This technique suffered from interference from other vapours. The procedures of Smyth (1929, 1931) involved bubbling air containing benzene through a concentrated sulfuric acid/nitric acid mixture and reducing the resultant dinitrobenzene to diaminobenzene, which was then titrated with ferric alum. The method was reported to be satisfactory for concentrations as low as 30 ppm (Smyth, 1931), but is not specific for benzene. Schrenk et al. (1935) determined the dinitrobenzene colorimetrically after addition of methylethyl ketone and strong alkali. Modifications of this procedure were employed by Dolin (1943) and Fabre et al. (1950). The procedure of Dolin (1943) permitted the determination of benzene in the presence of toluene, xylene and other substances and was reported to be sensitive to 0.27 ppm in 10-mL samples of air. Benzene concentrations of 18 mg/m^3 or more (5.6 ppm) could be determined with an error of less than 1% in a sample of 100 mL of air. The reaction with concentrated sulfuric acid and formaldehyde (Dietrich, 1932) yields a brown precipitate in the presence of benzene. When air is drawn through a tube containing this mixture on a solid support, the length of the resulting brown section can be used as a measure of benzene concentration (Hubbard & Silverman, 1950; Elkins et al., 1962; Krynska, 1971). The procedure was also used in the UK in 1939 for determining benzene (DSIR, 1939). Hubbard and Silverman (1950) adapted this reaction to a direct-reading indicator tube. The most simple direct-reading instrument is the colorimetric tube, usually used with a hand pump, a wide variety of which are available. These colorimetric tubes were generally found to function optimally in the 20 to 160 ppm range and were accurate to within ± 50% at the 95%

confidence level. However, while colorimetric tubes are inexpensive, simple and convenient to use, their inherent limitations and potential errors should be recognized (AIHA, 1976). Present-day manufacturers include Mine Safety Appliances (Model No. 93074), Scott-Draeger (Model No. CH-248) and Unico-Kitagawa. Indicator tubes have been widely employed in the USA, the Federal Republic of Germany and Japan for the determination of benzene vapour concentrations (Auergesellschaft, 1955; Kobayaschi, 1952; Küh, 1957). Benzene colorimetric tubes have been employed with available ranges from 0.15 to 150 mg/m^3, sensitive to other aromatic compounds and somewhat sensitive to hydrocarbons (WHO, 1982). An indicator tube method based on the colour rection between benzene vapours and 0.2 mm silica gel treated with a 5% solution of cerium sulfate (forming sulfuric acid) has been reported by Kol'kovsky (1969). The method is sensitive to 5 mg/m^3 (1.5 ppm), with an accuracy of $\pm$ 15% for low concentrations of benzene and of $\pm$ 5% for high concentrations. Although the procedure is applicable for the determination of benzene in the presence of hydrocarbons and carbon monoxide, it is not applicable in the presence of toluene and xylene vapours.

Quantitative determinations of benzene in air samples have been achieved by direct gas-phase UV spectrophotometry and by absorption measurements in benzene solutions prepared by bubbling air through non-UV-absorbing solvents. However, both of these procedures involve samples with a small number of UV-absorbing components and identification of any interfering compounds (Snyder, 1977). Air contaminated with benzene (Bouillot & Berton, 1951) or with benzene and toluene (Cole, 1942) has been monitored by gas-phase UV spectrophotometric analyses at several wavelengths, with a detection limit of approximately 10 ppm. UV gas analysers have been developed to monitor benzene specifically in industrial atmospheres with the same sensitivity (Konosu & Mashiko, 1965; Konosu et al., 1972).

Although gas-phase analysis requires a minimum of sample preparation, it also requires special instrumentation (e.g., sample cuvettes of sufficient size to hold the large cells required for trace gas analysis) not available in most commercial laboratory spectrophotometers. Hence, the procedure has been modified by bubbling the air sample through a liquid solvent. Sensitivity may thus be enhanced by increasing the volume of air passing through the solvent and/or by reducing its flow rate. The solvent (methanol or ethanol) is cooled with dry ice/acetone to increase the extraction efficiency (Laurian, 1938). This procedure has permitted the determination of benzene in air in the presence of other hydrocarbons with a limit of detection of 5 ppm (Alekseeva et al., 1969). A variation of this technique utilizing silica gel to adsorb the benzene, which is then eluted with ethanol and analysed, has been reported (Ovrum, 1956).

Maffett et al. (1956) reported a rapid method for the determination of pure benzene in air (less than 35 ppm) which involved the collection of benzene at a rate of 1.2–1.5 L/min in a sampling tube containing silica gel. The amount of benzene retained was determined spectrophotometrically by measuring the absorbance in iso-octane at 254.5 nm.

Infra-red detection of benzene in air has been reported using direct gas-phase analysis (Steger & Kahl, 1969; Kreuzer et al., 1972). One of the techniques utilizes infra-red absorption from CO and CO_2 laser beams and permits the detection of 3 ppb (Kreuzer *et al.*, 1972).

Sampling benzene in air containing other hydrocarbons to measure occupational exposure or environmental conditions is generally acknowledged to be best achieved by drawing a known volume of air through a tube containing a solid absorbent (e.g., activated charcoal, Porapak Q, Tenax GC), using a low-flow-rate sampling pump (Brief *et al.*, 1980). When charcoal is used as the absorbent, the benzene is subsequently desorbed using a solvent such as carbon disulfide, then determined by GC on 50/80 Porapak, Type Q, using flame-ionization detection (NIOSH 1974, 1977a,b; Brief *et al.*, 1980).

The NIOSH charcoal tube technique, P & CAM 127 (NIOSH, 1977b) was recently evaluated and found suitable, under certain conditions, for the simultaneous quantitative determination of seven solvents (i.e., toluene, benzene, xylene, dichloromethane, acetone, 1,1,1-trichloroethane, hexane) at and below their respective 8-h threshold limit value (TLV) and time-weighted average (TWA) (Otson *et al.*, 1983). The analyses were performed using a gas chromatograph equipped with a flame-ionization detector. Detection limits for all components were less than 0.05 mg/mL (0.3 L injections). Analytical precision (coefficient of variation) of better than 5% was obtained for triplicate 2-L air samples at 22 C and 95% relative humidity, with each compound at or below its 1980 8-h TLV-TWA.

The NIOSH standard method number S-311 (NIOSH, 1977b) for the determination of benzene in air employs a tube (7 cm × 4 mm i.d.) filled with 20/40 mesh activated coconut charcoal separated into two sections (100 mg and 50 mg) and uses carbon disulfide desorption. The air flow rate through the tube can vary from 50 to 200 mL/min, but is held constant during the sampling period. Typically, a total volume of about 2 L is sampled. The NIOSH S-311 method has been validated over the range of 13–52 ppm and found to work for levels of 1 to 10 ppm as well. The sensitivity of the method is presumed to be 1 ppm if one liter of air is sampled. The accuracy should be at least ± 25% at a confidence level of 95%, and the total coefficient of variation found by NIOSH for the range 13–52 ppm was 5.9%. Results from collaborative testing revealed that personal sampling pumps operating at approximately 1 L/min for 10 min collected a quantity of benzene that upon analysis yielded a coefficient of variation of 11.6% (NIOSH, 1974, 1977a) for a mean concentration of 22.8 ppm. Results from collaborative testing indicated that sampling at 1 L/min for 2 h will collect a sufficient quantity of benzene from an airborne concentration of 1 ppm to allow analysis with a coefficient of variation which is considered acceptable (NIOSH, 1974, 1977a). According to NIOSH (1977a), 1 ppm represents the lowest level at which a reliable estimate of occupational exposure to benzene can be determined at this time.

However, it should be noted that thermal (rather than solvent) desorption of the vapour into the gas chromatograph permits the sensitivity of the above procedure to be enhanced by a factor of 100 (Brief *et al.*, 1980). Two detailed methods which are suitable for measuring benzene in air from around 1 ppb upwards and can be used for monitoring personal exposure or fixed locations were recently described (Baxter *et al.*, 1980). Both methods are designed to use modern, small, low-flow-rate sampling pumps, with small sample tubes using adsorbents which are relatively unaffected by atmospheric moisture. The first is a new method based on sampling tubes which enable the whole sample to be heat-desorbed directly into an isothermal gas chromatograph, giving greatly enhanced sensitivity and eliminating sample preparation, as well as the problems of solvent interference on the chromatogram.

Interest in sampling organic vapours with a passive sampling device in place of the pump/solid sorbent tube method has been growing rapidly (Bailey & Hollingdale-Smith, 1977; Evans *et al.*, 1977; Tompkins & Goldsmith, 1977; Bamberger *et al.*, 1978; Brief *et al.*, 1980; Lautenberger *et al.*, 1980; Sefton *et al.*, 1982). The passive dosimeters in general are based on permeation-controlled, diffusion-controlled and permeation/diffusion-controlled mass transport mechanisms across a membrane to a charcoal absorbent bed (Brief *et al.*, 1980; Lautenberger *et al.*, 1980). After exposure, the activated carbon is removed from the device and analysed by GC. In comparative testing, the above passive monitor was demonstrated to possess an overall accuracy at least equivalent to that of the charcoal tube method in determining ambient concentrations of several organic compounds, including benzene, over the range 0.5–1 100 ppm. Both field and laboratory tests were conducted, and parameters such as temperature, relative humidity, air movement, sampling rates, desorption efficiencies, sampling range bias and precision were all examined (Lautenberger *et al.*, 1980). The passive dosimeters were found to be less sensitive to benzene in a mixture, but are useful for monitoring environments which have been carefully evaluated with charcoal tubes. Passive dosimeters are more effectively applied to 8-h average samples than to 15+ min (ceiling) samples (Brief *et al.*, 1980).

Passive dosimeters with instant readout capability have recently been devised by combining the principles of gas indicator tubes and membrane control of mass transfer. The membrane controls the diffusion of the gas or vapour to the reagent-impregnated support, where it reacts to produce a stain. Results with both benzene and hydrogen-sulfide monitors demonstrated that TWA concentrations of ambient gas or vapour could be measured accurately and precisely by following the movement of the coloured stain in the specific, calibrated indicator tube. The 95% confidence interval for measurements at the TLV (80 ppm-h) is $\pm$ 15% for benzene and $\pm$ 20% for hydrogen sulfide—well within NIOSH limits of acceptability (Sefton *et al.*, 1982). The specificity of the dosimeter is limited by the specificity of the colour-change chemistry. Since there is no requirement for follow-up analysis by GC, spectrophotometry or other method, monitoring of worker exposure is claimed to be much simpler and less expensive than by currently available techniques.

Area sampling was used extensively prior to the availability of personal samplers. Modern area samplers employ (1) flame-ionization detection, sometimes preceded by GC separation, (2) photo-ionization, using intense UV light, and (3) infra-red absorption at a wavelength of 3.3 m or at 15.2 m with a CO_2 optical filter. Area monitors are available in portable, semi-portable and fixed installations (Cheremisinoff & Morresi, 1979; Brief *et al.*, 1980).

Ambient air

As noted earlier, exposure of the general public to benzene occurs at concentrations that can be at least two or three orders of magnitude lower than those recorded for industrial situations. The greatest single contribution to the concentration of benzene in community air in the USA, western Europe and Japan comes from the manufacture, transport, storage and use of motor gasoline (Chapter 4; Howard & Durkin, 1974; Laskin & Goldstein, 1977; Brief *et al.*, 1980; IARC, 1982a; Van Raalte, 1982; Fishbein, 1984). However, the formation of benzene by combustion processes also contributes notably for those exposed indoors to side-stream cigarette smoke (Wallace *et al.*, 1987). Almost all methods used for the analysis of organic pollutants in air involve a preconcentration step, commonly using charcoal (White *et al.*, 1970; Burghardt & Jeltes, 1975; Louw *et al.*, 1977; NIOSH, 1977b; Seifert & Abraham, 1982a,b) to adsorb volatile organic compounds, followed by elution with carbon disulfide. The eluate can then be analysed by GC, using flame-ionization detection or mass spectrometry (Cooper *et al.*, 1971). The disadvantage of carbon disulfide is that it cannot be used with electron-capture or photoionization detectors. Freeze-concentration of samples before analysis has also been employed (Stephens, 1973; Siegel *et al.*, 1974). These preconcentration steps are usually necessary because of the limited sensitivity of flame-ionization detection.

More recently, commercially available polymers (Holzer *et al.*, 1977; Louw *et al.*, 1977; Brown & Purnell, 1979), especially Tenax GC, Porapak/N and some modified charcoals (Raymond & Guichon, 1974; Patzelova *et al.*, 1978), are increasingly being used for concentrating pollutants in air. Although Tenax GC is not affected by the presence of water, its trapping efficiency is drastically reduced in the presence of carbon dioxide (Piecewicz *et al.*, 1979).

An automated GC technique has been developed to monitor benzene and alkylbenzene concentrations in ambient air, enabling the measurement of sub-parts-per-billion concentrations in air without using preconcentration or trapping techniques (Hester & Meyer, 1979). Benzene, substituted arenes and various volatile halo-organic compounds in air have been analysed with detection limits of 1 to 5 g/m^3, *via* initial trapping on Porapak N at ambient temperatures, followed by GC (Van Tassel *et al.*, 1981). The application of Tenax collection and high-resolution GC/mass spectrometric/computer analysis for the determination of organic vapour emissions near industrial and chemical disposal sites was recently described by Pellizzari (1982).

A variety of volatile hydrocarbons may be emitted from motor vehicle exhausts, depending on fuel composition. These are principally benzene, toluene and derivatives thereof, as well as 1,2-dibromoethane and 1,2-dichloroethane. It has been shown that correlations between the hydrocarbon concentrations in ambient air may be useful to identify their sources. The correlation between benzene and toluene and the establishment of the toluene:benzene ratio as an indicator of traffic-induced air pollution is now widely acknowledged (Pilar & Graydon, 1973; Tsani-Bazaca *et al.*, 1982). Variations in this ratio, which is normally about 2.4:1, observed in certain countries may be due to differences in fuel composition (Jonsson & Berg, 1978; Tsani-Bazaca *et al.*, 1982). A correlation between benzene and 1,2-dibromoethane concentrations has also been cited as a possible guide to identifying motor vehicle-related air pollution (Jonsson & Berg, 1978; Tsani-Bazaca *et al.*, 1982). Variation between countries is evident, with ratios of approximately 161:1 for Sweden and approximately 100:1 for the UK, this difference being due to the higher benzene and lower 1,2-dibromoethane content of petrol in Sweden following progressive reduction of the alkyl lead content (Tsani-Bazaca *et al.*, 1982). A sensitive and precise method was described for the determination of trace components in air, with a detection limit by serial mass spectrometry which is better by two or three orders of magnitude than for earlier GC-mass spectrometric methods (Fujii *et al.*, 1979).

The sampling techniques described earlier for the measurement of occupational exposure to benzene are generally employed for monitoring benzene levels in community (ambient) environments. For ambient air monitoring, the sizes of the sampling tubes are usually increased to contain up to 600 mg of absorbent (charcoal, Tenax) and the sampling times are as long as 8 h (Brief *et al.*, 1980). The samples are desorbed and analysed as already described.

It is increasingly recognized that indoor air quality must be more rigorously evaluted for the presence of contaminants which can arise from smoking, the use of consumer products, emanations from building materials, burning processes, etc. Indoor air concentrations of benzene and some other aromatic hydrocarbons were determined (Seifert & Abraham, 1982a,b) by means of a passive sampler with a charcoal pad of known surface area (Gas Badge, National Mine Service Co.; Bamberger *et al.*, 1978) followed by extraction and analysis by GC. A more extensive investigation has been carried out by Wallace and Pellizzari and their co-workers (Wallace *et al.*, 1982), who report a strong association between active-passive smoking and benzene exposure (Wallace *et al.*, 1987). The authors report[1] that cigarette smoke is the predominant source of exposure to benzene in the general environment.

EXPOSURE MEASUREMENT FOR TOLUENE

As noted previously, earlicr studies of the toxicology of toluene were complicated by the frequent contamination of toluene with benzene (Chapter 5; Casarett & Doull, 1975; Cohr & Stokholm, 1979; Fishbein, 1985a). In addition, many occupational situations involve exposure to solvent mixtures (benzene, xylenes, ethyl benzene, chlorinated hydrocarbons, etc.). It can also be anticipated that the maximum allowable concentrations of many solvents (e.g., benzene, halogenated hydrocarbons and perhaps toluene and xylene) in the workplace will be lowered; hence sensitive procedures will be required for their determination in work environments and for biological monitoring.

Industrial or work-room air

Determination of the levels of exposure to solvent vapours in the industrial atmosphere has long been a difficult problem, with sample collection and concentration being the most troublesome aspects of the assessment of solvent vapour hazards (Rushing, 1958; White *et al.*, 1970).

The earliest procedures for the determination of toluene in air were based on modifications of the colorimetric procedures mentioned above, which were originally

---

[1] Wallace, L.A., private communication.

developed for the determination of benzene (Hubbard & Silverman, 1950; Kol'kovsky, 1967).

A later procedure of Blake and Rose (1960) used a formaldehyde solution (5% formalin in orthophosphoric/sulfuric acid mixture) for the colorimetric determination of toluene in air. This early procedure for determining toluene was checked by comparison with a method in which toluene was nitrated and dinitrotoluene was determined colorimetrically with butanone (Jacobs, 1941).

A number of specialized collection/concentration techniques developed primarily in the late 1950s and early 1960s have been reported. The usual methods involve absorption in solvents (Mansur et al., 1959; Levadie & Harwood, 1960; Urone & Smith, 1961), or adsorption on coated or non-coated adsorbents or activated charcoal (West et al., 1958; Altshuller et al., 1962; Cropper & Kaminsky, 1963; Otterson & Guy, 1964; Whitman & Johnston, 1964; Novak et al., 1965; Faust & Hermann, 1966; Reid & Halpin, 1968; White et al., 1970; Kupel & White, 1971). Adsorbed analytes were subsequently desorbed in the laboratory by heat (West et al., 1958; Altshuller et al., 1962) or a suitable solvent (Otterson & Guy, 1964; Whitman & Johnston, 1964; Faust & Hermann, 1966) and determined by GC (Mansur et al., 1959; Williams, 1965; Faust & Hermann, 1966; Reid & Halpin, 1968). Among the numerous analytical procedures reported for the determination of toluene, GC offers the greatest specificity and sensitivity. The colorimetric methods, as well as the direct spectrophotometric methods, are subject to interferences from a broad spectrum of compounds, and the removal of these interferences is in many cases incomplete and tedious (Yant et al., 1936; NIOSH, 1973).

White et al. (1970) described a convenient method for the determination of solvent vapours (including toluene, xylenes, benzene, chloroform, carbon tetrachloride and perchloroethylene) in atmospheric samples. A glass tube (5 cm × 4 mm i.d.) packed with activated charcoal was used to take an integrated 10-L sample. The activated charcoal was desorbed with 1 mL carbon disulfide and an aliquot (5 μL) was analysed by flame-ionization GC. NIOSH (1973, 1977b) described a compliance method giving sampling and analytical procedures for the determination of toluene in air, based on a modification of the method described by White et al. (1970) and Kupel and White (1971). The NIOSH charcoal tube technique, P & CAM 127 (NIOSH, 1977b) was recently evaluated and found suitable, under certain conditions, for the simultaneous quantitative determination of seven solvents (toluene, benzene, xylene, dichloromethane, acetone, 1,1,1-trichloroethane, hexane) at and below their respective 8-h TLV-TWA (Otson et al., 1983). Air sampling with activated charcoal tubes and subsequent desorption and analysis is probably the procedure most widely used by industrial hygienists for monitoring vapour-phase organic pollutants (Bencsath et al., 1978; Dharmarajan & Smith, 1981). Indeed, more than 50% of the methods listed in the five volumes of the NIOSH Manual of Analytical Methods (e.g., NIOSH, 1977b) are based on this technique.

Between 1960 and the mid 1970s, a number of basic studies were published concerning the calibration and evaluation of gas detecting tubes (Ash & Lynch, 1971; Roper, 1971). All pertained to short-term detector tubes with sample times less than 5 min. It was found that the behaviour of nearly all tubes was influenced by the pressure (Saltzman, 1962; Leichnitz, 1977). The tubes were sometimes sensitive to the flow rate (Kusnetz *et al.,* 1960; Saltzman, 1962), and the stain was generally not affected by humidity or temperature. More recently, tubes designed for long-term sampling have become available. It has been suggested by Jentzsch and Fraser (1981) that the precision and accuracy of modern long-term detector tubes may encourage industrial hygienists to use these devices for monitoring personnel for toluene exposure, as they appear to meet the accuracy requirement of the Joint Committee of the American Conference of Governmental Industrial Hygienists and the American Industrial Hygienists Association, e.g., 'readings are produced that are within ± 25% of the time concentration at multiples of 1, 2 and 5 times the test standard for the contaminant, and within ± 35% of the true value at one-half the test standard. The test standard is usually the TLV' (AIHA, 1976). It should be noted that the same reactions are used for the indicating layers of the toluene and the benzene tubes, so that if benzene and toluene are present in unknown amounts, these tubes cannot be used to measure the concentration. Unfortunately, some of the older exposure measurements did not eliminate this interference problem. The accuracy and precision of the indicator tube may be achieved only with a single, known contaminant, unless the description of the tube includes the relative deviations and limitations due to interfering substances.

Several other methods for toluene have become available since 1970: (a) passive dosimeters (see p. 129), which possess multiple advantages, including lighter weight, compactness and simplicity when compared to sampling methods using pumps (Hill & Fraser, 1980); (b) portable infra-red gas analysers (e.g., Miran-1A and other similar models), which are now extensively used for either instantaneous measurement or continuous monitoring of a large variety of air contaminants (Samimi, 1983); and (c) UV spectrometry, which has also been employed for the determination of benzene and xylene in admixture with toluene (Yuan & Ma, 1981).

EXPOSURE MEASUREMENTS FOR XYLENES

As noted above, any consideration of the analysis of xylenes, particularly in the industrial workplace and general environment, must take into consideration concomitant exposure to other aromatic hydrocarbons, primarily benzene, toluene and ethylbenzene (Chapters 4, 5 and 6; Fishbein, 1984, 1985a,b,c).

The earlier methods employed for the determination of xylene were similar to those used for toluene and benzene in air. Methods of collection included the use of plastic bags (Smith & Pierce, 1970), absorption in scrubbers by nitrating solutions (Baernstein, 1943) and organic solvents (Maffett *et al.,* 1956; Dambrauskas & Cook, 1963) and adsorption on silica gel (Whitman & Johnston, 1964) or activated charcoal (Reid & Halpin, 1968; White *et al.,* 1970; Kupel & White, 1971).

The earliest procedures for the determination of xylenes in air, like those for toluene, were based on modifications of colorimetric procedures originally developed for the determination of benzene (Hubbard & Silverman, 1950; Kol'kovsky, 1967). The techniques were useful during this period for field measurements of airborne aromatic hydrocarbons at levels generally greater than 25 ppm (Hubbard & Silverman, 1950; Kol'kovsky, 1967).

A number of specialized collection-concentration techniques developed primarily in the 1960s have been reported. These were discussed for toluene on p. 132. The resulting samples were subsequently analysed by GC, with flame-ionization detection (West *et al.,* 1958; Mansur *et al.,* 1959; Levadie & Harwood, 1960; Otterson & Guy, 1964; Williams, 1965; Faust & Hermann, 1966; Reid & Halpin, 1968). The earlier GC procedures permitted the determination of aromatic hydrocarbons in the range 1–50 ppm in 20-L air samples (West *et al.,* 1958) and at somewhat higher levels in 5-mL samples (Cropper & Kaminsky, 1963).

Reid and Halpin (1968) employed a simple activated charcoal tube (13 cm × 6 mm i.d.) for collecting air samples and a desorption procedure using carbon disulfide to effect the determination of a number of the commonly encountered aromatic hydrocarbons (benzene, toluene, xylene, as well as a variety of halogenated hydrocarbons). More recently (NIOSH, 1974, 1977b), this has been adopted as a standard procedure. The lower limit of detection was found to be less than 12 μg/sample. In a collaborative test, the coefficient of variation in the range 60–200 ppm was 9.5%, and rose to 13% at approximately 5 ppm (NIOSH, 1974). Although charcoal tubes are employed for the detection of xylene vapours in occupational environments (NIOSH, 1975), the development of more sophisticated detection tubes and personal passive dosimeters for the detection of xylene vapours, either alone or in admixture with other aromatic hydrocarbons, is rather scant. Mueller and Miller (1979) have criticized the utility of the charcoal tube method for the determination of airborne organic vapour mixtures (including xylene isomers found in xylol and toluene) in factory environments.

BIOLOGICAL MONITORING

It has been increasingly observed that measurements of airborne pollutant concentrations do not provide an entirely satisfactory measurement of exposure and of the physiological effects of exposure (Brief *et al.,* 1980; Gompertz, 1980; Grunder & Moffitt, 1982). The biological effects of organic solvents are more directly related to the amount absorbed than to the concentration in the working atmosphere. It follows that a better estimate of individual risk can be obtained by measuring uptake rather than exposure. It is recognized that there are great variations in worker uptake, depending on respiratory fitness, excercise and the amount stored in adipose tissue. Additionally, clearance and metabolism of the solvent may vary from one individual to another, being affected by genetic and environmental conditions (Gompertz, 1980). A WHO Expert Committee (WHO, 1973) observed that 'using man as a biological monitor may or may not give a better estimate of magnitude of exposure than direct measurement of environmental concentration, depending on how well the measured internal concentration reflects the magnitude of the effective dose to critical organs or sites within the body'.

The most frequent and significant route by which humans are exposed to toxic solvents is by inhalation, although it is recognized that toxic effects in humans have often been attributed to combined exposure through respiration and skin contact (e.g., rotogravure workers wash ink from their hands in open vats of benzene; Hunter, 1978; IARC, 1982a,b).

Biological monitoring for benzene (analytical methods 4, 5, 6)

Historically, levels of phenylsulfate (ratio of inorganic: organic sulfates) and phenol in a normalized urine sample were used to monitor levels of exposure to benzene. Since the biological half-life of benzene metabolites is usually short (< 12 h), it should be noted that the time of biological material sampling in relation to exposure is critical. This is discussed in Chapter 12.

One recommended biological method for the determination of urine levels following benzene exposure is that described by NIOSH (1977b). Urine samples are treated with perchloric acid at 95 °C to hydrolyse the phenol conjugates, phenylsulfate and phenylglucuronide. The total phenol is then extracted with diisopropyl ether and the concentration determined by GC, using flame-ionization detection and a 1.5 m × 5 mm column, packed with polyethylene glycol adipate on universal 'B' support and operated at 200 °C.

Brief *et al.* (1980) have cautioned that, because of the rather small differences in phenol levels following exposure to benzene, care should be exercised that other sources of urinary phenol do not alter these levels. The following factors can influence the level of phenol in urine: intake of salicylates, dermal application of phenol-containing preparations, gastrointestinal disorders favouring bacterial degradation of tyrosine and phenylalanine and intake of ethanol (Fishbeck *et al.,* 1975). In view of these possibilities, it was suggested by Brief *et al.* (1980) that phenol monitoring would be of minimal value as an index of exposure to benzene at levels of 10 ppm or less. (According to Truhaut and Murray (1978), a concentration of phenol in urine of more than 25 mg/L indicates some exposure to benzene.) Similarly, the ratio of inorganic: organic sulfates would appear to be an insensitive tool at these levels of exposure.

A more promising biological test of exposure may be the determination of benzene in breath (exhaled air) (Brief *et al.,* 1980). A benzene level of 0.12 ppm was proposed as a limit for exposure to 10 ppm for 8 h (measurement made 16 h after exposure) (Lauwerys, 1976, 1979; Sherwood, 1976). It was cautioned that confounding factors such as cigarette smoke should be taken into account in this determination.

When inhaled, benzene may induce a variety of blood dyscrasias, such as leukopenia, leukocytosis, thrombocytopenia and anaemia. A detailed study of benzene toxicity may thus require measurement of the benzene concentration in blood relative to the inhaled concentration. Several procedures for determining benzene in blood have been reported. These require either large quantities of blood or incubation of small blood samples for extended periods (Gerarde & Guertin, 1959; Sato, 1971; Withey & Martin, 1974). The more recent and most useful methods are based on the analysis of an extract by GC (Snyder & Kocsis, 1975; Snyder *et al.,* 1977; Ghimenti *et al.,* 1978) or head-space GC (Withey & Martin, 1974; Sato *et al.,* 1975).

Sato (1971) showed that it was possible, by means of a GC equilibration method using 1 mL of blood, to separate and detect benzene at 0.02 g/mL, toluene at 0.04 g/mL and *m*-xylene at 0.1 mg/mL. Sato and Fujiwara (1972) reported an average concentration of approximately 0.08 g benzene/mL of blood 30 min after three human subjects inhaled benzene at 25 ppm for 2 h. The results seem to indicate that a linear relationship exists between inhaled levels of benzene and the amounts found in blood. Sato *et al.* (1975) described a GC determination of toluene and benzene from a small sample of blood, e.g., 0.02 or 0.1 mL. The procedure involves equilibration of the sample in a sealed 2-mL hypodermic syringe at 37 °C for about 30 min. After establishing equilibrium, 1 mL of the overlying air is analysed by GC.

Biological monitoring for toluene (analytical methods 4, 5, 7, 8, 9)

Numerous GC procedures have been employed for the determination of toluene in inhaled and exhaled air, as well as in arterial and venous blood. The rationale for the use of breath is based on the fact that volatile substances capable of crossing the alveolar-capillary membrane will partition between the bloodstream and alveolar air. Hence the concentration of a substance in breath will be related to the concentration in blood (Wilson & Ottley, 1981). For example, Åstrand *et al.* (1972) have shown that the content of solvent in alveolar air samples collected during exposure is related to the intensity of exposure. At rest, the mean value for alveolar air concentration found during exposure to 100 ppm of toluene is 18.1 ppm (SE = 1.41 ppm; n = 15). The corresponding value for an exposure to approximately 200 ppm at rest was 37.5 ppm. The correlation between environmental exposure to toluene and its alveolar concentration measured in workers during the work shift seems to agree with these estimates (Brugnone *et al.*, 1976; Lauwerys, 1983). However, it should be noted that Åstrand *et al.* (1972) were of the opinion that 'neither alveolar air samples (nor venous blood samples) taken at given intervals after the *conclusion* of a period of exposure provide sufficiently accurate information on the average amount of solvent in inspired air at a working place or on the magnitude of an individual's uptake'.

The conventional test for monitoring uptake of toluene is based on the excretion of hippuric acid in the urine. Earlier studies (Ogata *et al.*, 1969, 1970; Veulemans & Masschelein, 1979) reported that about 70% of the toluene absorbed in humans is expected to be excreted in the urine as hippuric acid. Hippuric acid is a conjugation product of benzoic acid and is a normal constituent of urine, originating mainly from food containing benzoic acid or benzoates. In non-occupationally exposed workers, the concentration of hippuric acid in spot urine samples rarely exceeds 1.5 g/g creatinine (Buchet & Lauwerys, 1973).

Early procedures for the determination of hippuric acid were reviewed by Ellman *et al.* (1961). These methods, which are tedious and do not always produce quantitative results, are not employed today. A variety of more acceptable procedures includes colorimetry (Gaffney *et al.*, 1954; Pagnotto & Lieberman, 1967; Ikeda & Ohtsuji, 1969; Ogata *et al.*, 1969, 1970; Mikulski *et al.*, 1972), UV spectrophotometry (Elliott, 1957; Rieder, 1957) and fluorimetry (Ellman *et al.*, 1961; Elliott & Walker, 1964; Elster *et al.*, 1978). Improved specificity has been achieved in some of the above methods by preliminary sample treatment with ion-exchange resin (Elliott, 1957), paper chromatography (Gaffney *et al.*, 1954; Ikeda & Ohtsuji, 1969; Ogata *et al.*, 1969) or alcohol/ether extraction (Pagnotto & Lieberman, 1967). More recent determinations of hippuric acid in urine are based on GC (Buchet & Lauwerys, 1973; Engstrøm *et al.*, 1976; Apostoli *et al.*, 1982).

Colorimetric procedures are used most frequently for the determination of total hippuric acid (together with methyl hippurates, if present) and require small samples of urine (1 mL or less). These methods stem from studies of El Masri *et al.* (1956) and Umberger and Fiorese (1963) and exist in several versions. In the procedure of Umberger and Fiorese (1963), hippuric acid dissolved in pyridine produces a red-orange colour upon the addition of benzene sulfonyl chloride. The colour has a stable absorbance at 380 nm and is sensitive to microgram quantities of hippuric acid.

The method used by Pagnotto and Lieberman (1967), based on UV spectrophotometry (230 nm) of a urine extract in an isopropanol-ether mixture, is not specific for hippuric acid, since it also measures methyl hippuric acid and uric acids at the same wavelength. Using this procedure, Pagnotto and Lieberman (1967) reported average hippuric acid values to be 0.8 g/L for unexposed subjects and 7.0 g/L for workers exposed to 200 ppm toluene.

Improved and more specific methods for the quantitative determination of hippuric and *m*- and *p*-methyl hippuric acids in urine were described by Ogata *et al.* (1969). The acids were extracted from urine with ether/ethanol, which was dried with silica gel or with ethyl acetate. After removal of the solvent by evaporation, coloured azolactones were formed by reaction with *p*-dimethylaminobenzaldehyde in acetic anhydride, or benzene sulfonyl chloride in pyridine, and the absorbances were measured. The sensitivities were about 4 µg/mL of urine using the *p*-dimethylaminobenzaldehyde reagent and 20 µg/mL using benzene sulfonyl chloride. Both methods are characterized by good recovery (94–100%). Separation of hippuric acid and methyl hippuric acids was achieved by paper and thin-layer chromatography before estimation. This improved method is particularly advantageous for monitoring workers exposed to mixed vapours of toluene and *m*- or *p*-xylene, since it provides for the separation of the respective xylene metabolites.

It is widely acknowledged that the excretion rate of hippuric acid at the end of the exposure period is much more closely related to the time-weighted toluene load than concentration alone (Veulemans & Masschelein, 1979; Lauwerys, 1983). On a group basis, a time-weighted average exposure to 100 ppm corresponds to a hippuric acid excretion rate of 4 mg/min, according to Veulemans and Masschelein (1979). However, it is recognized that for practical reasons the collection of a timed urine sample is frequently impossible.

Utidjian and Weaver (1974) suggest that the measurement of urinary hippuric acid is probably more valuable as qualitative evidence of toluene exposure than as a precise index of the level of exposure, since there is a wide interpersonal variation in hippuric acid excretion. More recent methods of hippuric acid analysis are discussed in Chapter 12, as well as methods involving other metabolites of toluene.

Biological monitoring for xylene (analytical methods 4, 5, 10, 11)

The biological monitoring of xylene in exposed individuals has been reviewed elsewhere (Piotrowski, 1977; WHO, 1981; Lauwerys, 1983). The biological tests which have been considered for evaluating exposure to xylene are methylhippuric acid in urine, xylene in blood and xylene in expired air (WHO, 1981; Lauwerys, 1983). It is generally acknowledged that the evaluation of exposure by analysis of xylene in exhaled air or in blood is not currently considered adequate for routine monitoring purposes.

Methylhippuric acids provide the best test of exposure, since they are not normally present in urine (Buchet & Lauwerys, 1973) and are the metabolic products of almost all the retained xylene (Flek & Sedivec, 1975). This is discussed in more detail in Chapter 12.

Earlier procedures for the determination of hippuric and methylhippuric acids in urine relied primarily on spectrophotometric techniques (Gaffney *et al.*, 1954; Pagnotto & Lieberman, 1967; Ogata *et al.*, 1969). The colorimetric technique cannot be used for the simultaneous determination of hippuric acids in urine without a preliminary chromatographic separation on paper or silica gel. The molar extinctions of azolactones obtained from hippuric acid and *m*- and *p*-methylhippuric acids are similar and amount to 1.5×10^4 and 1.4×10^4, respectively. Hence, it is generally acknowledged that colorimetric and direct UV spectrophotometric methods have a rather low specificity and sensitivity and are subject to interference from a wide variety of compounds. Removal of this interference is tedious and in many cases incomplete (Slob, 1973; Caperos & Fernandez, 1977; Poggi *et al.*, 1982).

The gas chromatographic procedures of Van Roosmalen and Drummond (1978) and Caperos and Fernandez (1977) permit the simultaneous determination of the major urinary metabolites of toluene, xylenes and styrene. The limit of detection for methylhippuric acid using the procedure of Van Roosmalen and Drummond (1978) was 4 mg/L. A detection limit of 5 mg/L was obtained for hippuric acid and *o*-, *m*-, and *p*-methylhippuric acids using the procedure of Caperos and Fernandez (1977). With larger urine samples, a considerably higher sensitivity could be achieved.

REFERENCES

Aksoy, M. (1977) Leukaemia in workers due to occupational exposure to benzene. *New Istanbul Contrib. Clin. Sci., 12,* 3–14

Alekseeva, M.V., Krylova, N.A. & Khrustaleva, V.A. (1969) Spectrophotometric determination of benzene, isopropylbenzene and alpha-methyl-styrol in the air. *Air Pollut. Trans.,* Vol. 1 *(DHEW D–4064, AP 56)*

Altshuller, A.P., Bellar, T.A. & Clemons, C.A. (1962) Concentration of hydrocarbons on silica gel prior to gas chromatographic analysis. *Am. Ind. Hyg. Assoc. J., 23,* 164

AIHA (1976) *Direct Reading Colorimetric Indicator Tubes Manual,* Akron, OH, American Industrial Hygiene Association

Apostoli, P., Burgnone, F., Perbellini, L., Cocheo, V., Bellomo, M.L. & Silvestri, R. (1982) Biomonitoring of occupational toluene exposure. *Int. Arch. Occup. Environ. Health, 50,* 153–168

Arbeijdstilsynet (1985) *Data Base for Workplace Measurements* [in Danish], Copenhagen, Danish National Institute of Occupational Health

Arp, E.W., Wolf, P.H. & Checkoway, H. (1983) Lymphocytic leukemia and exposures to benzene and other solvents in the rubber industry. *J. Occup. Med., 25,* 598–602

Ash, R.M. & Lynch, J.R. (1971) The evaluation of gas detector tube systems: benzene. *Am. Ind. Hyg. Assoc. J., 32,* 410

Åstrand, I., Ehrner-Samuel, H., Kilbom, A. & Ovrum, P. (1972) Toluene exposure. I. Concentration in alveolar air and blood at rest and during exercise. *Work Environ. Health, 9,* 119–130

Auergesellschaft (1955) *Quantitative Detection of Benzene in Air (German Patent DBR 933,711, September 29)*

Baernstein, H.D. (1943) Photometric determination of benzene, toluene and their nitroderivatives. *Ind. Eng. Chem. Anal. Ed., 15,* 251–253

Bailey, A. & Hollingdale-Smith, P.A. (1977) A personal diffusion sampler for evaluating time-weighted exposure to organic gases and vapors. *Ann. Occup. Hyg., 20,* 345–356

Bamberger, R.L., Esposito, G.G., Jacobs, B.W., Podolak, G.E. & Mazur, J.F. (1978) A new personal sampler for organic vapors. *Am. Ind. Hyg. Assoc. J., 39,* 701–708

Baxter, H.G., Blakemore, R., Moore, J.P., Coker, D.T. & McCambley, W.H. (1980) The measurement of airborne benzene vapour. *Ann. Occup. Hyg., 23,* 117–132

Bencsath, F.A., Drysch, K., List, D. & Weichardt, H. (1978) Analysis of volatile air pollutants by charcoal adsorption with subsequent gas chromatographic headspace analysis by desorption with benzyl alcohol. Part I. Method and applications. *Angew. Chromatogr. (Bodenseewerk Perkin-Elmer) No. 32E*

Berlin, M., Gage, J.C., Gullberg, B., Holm, S., Knutsson, P. & Tuner, A. (1980) Breath concentration as an index of the health risk from benzene. *Scand. J. Work Environ. Health. 6,* 104–111

Blake, A.J. & Rose, B.A. (1960) The rapid determination of toluene and styrene vapours in the atmosphere. *Analyst, 85,* 442–445

Bouillot, J. & Berton, A. (1951) Detection of toxic amounts of benzene in factory atmospheres. *Bull. Soc. Chim. Fr.,* p. 317

Brief, R.S., Lynch, J., Bernath, T. & Scala, R.A. (1980) Benzene in the workplace. *Am. Ind. Hyg. Assoc. J., 41,* 616–623

Brown, R.H. & Purnell, C.J. (1979) Collection and analysis of trace organic vapour pollutants in ambient atmospheres. The performance of a Tenax GC adsorbent tube. *J. Chromatogr. 178,* 79–90

Brugnone, F., Perbellini, L., Grigolini, L., Cazzadori, A. & Gaffuri, E. (1976) Alveolar air and blood toluene concentration in rotogravure workers. *Int. Arch. Occup. Environ. Health, 38,* 45–54

Buchet, J.P. & Lauwerys, R. (1973) Measurement of urinary hippuric and m-methylhippuric acids by gas chromatography. *Br. J. Ind. Med., 30,* 125–128

Burghardt, E. & Jeltes, R. (1975) Gas chromatographic determination of aromatic hydrocarbons in air using a semiautomatic preconcentration method. *Atmos. Environ., 9,* 935–940

Caperos, J.R. & Fernandez, J.G. (1977) Simultaneous determination of toluene and xylene metabolites in urine by gas chromatography. *Br. J. Ind. Med., 34,* 229–233

Casarett, L.J. & Doull, J. (1975) *Toxicology. The Basic Science of Poisons,* New York, McMillan, p. 520

Chandler, J.L.R. (1984) Benzene and the one-hit model. *Risk Anal., 4,* 7–8

Checkoway, H., Wilcosky, T., Wolf, P. & Tyroler, H. (1984) An evaluation of the associations of leukemia and rubber industry solvent exposures. *Am. J. Ind. Med.,* **5,** 239–249

Cheremisinoff, P.N. & Morresi, A.C. (1979) *Benzene – Basic and Hazardous Properties,* New York, Marcel Dekker

Cohr, K.H. & Stokholm, J. (1979) Toluene: a toxicologic review. *Scand. J. Work Environ. Health,* **5,** 71–90

Cole, P.A. (1942) Determination of the concentration of benzene and toluene in air. *J. Opt. Soc. Am.,* **32,** 304–306

Cooper, C.V., White, L.D. & Kupel, R.E. (1971) Qualitative detection limits for specific compounds utilizing gas chromatographic fractions, activated charcoal and a mass spectrometer. *Am. Ind. Hyg. Assoc. J.,* **32,** 383–386

Cropper, F.R. & Kaminsky, S. (1963) Determination of toxic organic compounds in admixture in the atmosphere by gas chromatography. *Anal. Chem.,* **35,** 735

Dambrauskas, T. & Cook, W.A. (1963) Methanol as the absorbing reagent in the determination of benzene, toluene, xylene and their mixtures in air. *Am. Ind. Hyg. Assoc. J.,* **24,** 568–575

Dharmarajan, V. & Smith, R.N. (1981) Permeation of toluene through plastic caps on charcoal tubes. *Am. Ind. Hyg. Assoc. J.,* **42,** 691–692

Dietrich, K.R. (1932) Determination of the benzene content of the atmosphere. *Chem. Fabr.,* **11**

Dolin, B.H. (1943) Detection and determination of benzene in the presence of toluene, xylene, and other substances. *Ind. Eng. Chem. Anal. Ed.,* **15,** 242–270

DSIR (1939) *Leaflet No. 4,* London, Department of Scientific and Industrial Research

Elkins, H.B., Pagnoto, L.D. & Comproni, E.M. (1962) The ultraviolet spectrophotometric determination of benzene in air samples adsorbed on silica gel. *Anal. Chem.,* **34,** 1797–1801

Elliott, H.C., Jr (1957) Microdetermination of hippuric acid in urine. *Anal. Chem.,* **29,** 1712–1715

Elliott, H.C. & Walker, A.A. (1964) Fluorometric microanalysis of plasma hippuric acid and comparison of hippurate with p-aminohippurate clearance in dogs. *Proc. Soc. Exp. Biol. Med.,* **116,** 268–270

Ellman, G.L., Burkhalter, A. & Ladou, J. (1961) A fluorometric method for the determination of hippuric acid. *J. Lab. Clin. Med.,* **57,** 813–818

El Masri, A.M., Smith, J.N. & Williams, R.T. (1956) Studies in detoxication, No. 69. The metabolism of alkyl benzenes: n-propylbenzene and n-butylbenzene with further observations on ethylbenzene. *Biochem. J.,* **64,** 50–56

Elster, I., Bencsath, F.A., Drysch, K. & Häfele, H. (1978) Benzolintoxikation beim Betanken von Fahrzeugen. *Sicherheitsingenieur,* February, 17–26

Engstrøm, K., Husman, K. & Rantanen, J. (1976) Measurement of toluene and xylene metabolites by gas chromatography. *Int. Arch. Occup. Environ. Health,* **36,** 153–160

Evans, M., Molyneux, M., Sharp, T., Bailey, A. & Hollingdale-Smith, P.A. (1977) The practical application of the proton diffusion sampler for the measurement of time-weighted average exposure to volatile organic substances in air. *Ann. Occup. Hyg.,* **20,** 357–363

Fabre, R., Truhaut, R. & Peron, M. (1950) Determination of benzene and toluene in complex solvents and in the atmosphere. *Ann. Pharm. Fr., 8,* 613–626

Faust, C.L. & Hermann, E.R. (1966) Charcoal sampling tubes for organic vapor analysis by gas chromatography. *Am. Ind. Hyg. Assoc. J., 27,* 68

Fishbeck, W.A., Langner, R.R. & Kociba, R.J. (1975) Elevated urinary phenol levels not related to benzene exposure. *Am. Ind. Hyg. Assoc. J., 36,* 820–824

Fishbein, L. (1984) An overview of environmental and toxicological aspects of aromatic hydrocarbons, 1. Benzene. *Sci. Total Environ., 40,* 189–218

Fishbein, L. (1985a) An overview of environmental and toxicological aspects of aromatic hydrocarbons, 2. Toluene. *Sci. Total Environ., 42,* 267–288

Fishbein, L. (1985b) An overview of environmental and toxicological aspects of aromatic hydrocarbons, 3. Xylenes. *Sci. Total Environ., 43,* 165–183

Fishbein, L. (1985c) An overview of environmental and toxicological aspects of aromatic hydrocarbons, 4. Ethylbenzene. *Sci. Total Environ., 44,* 269–287

Flek, J. & Sedivec, V. (1975) Metabolism of isomeric xylene in man. *Prac. Lek., 27,* 9–16

Fujii, T., Yokouchi, Y. & Ambe, Y. (1979) Survey and determination of trace components in air by serial mass-fragmentographic runs over the entire mass range. *J. Chromatogr., 176,* 165–170

Gaffney, G.W., Schreier, K., Di-Ferrante, N. & Altman, K.I. (1954) The quantitative determination of hippuric acid. *J. Biol. Chem., 206,* 695–698

Gerarde, H.W. & Guertin, D.L. (1959) A method for the quantitative determination of benzene and certain alkylbenzenes in blood. *Arch. Ind. Health., 20,* 262–267

Ghimenti, G., Gallo, M. & Galli, E. (1978) An extraction method for determination of solvents in biological samples. *Ann. Inst. Super Sanita, 14,* 583–588

Gompertz, D. (1980) Solvents – the relationship between biological monitoring strategies and metabolic handling: a review. *Occup. Hyg., 23,* 405–410

Greenberg, L. (1926) *U.S. Public Health Reports (Reprint 1026)*

Grunder, F.I. & Moffitt, A.E. (1982) Blood as a matrix for biological monitoring. *Am. Ind. Hyg. Assoc. J., 43,* 271–274

Hester, N.E. & Meyer, R.A. (1979) A sensitive technique for measurement of benzene and alkylbenzenes in air. *Environ. Sci. Technol., 13,* 107–109

Hill, R.H. & Fraser, D.A. (1980) Passive dosimetry using detector tubes. *Am. Ind. Hyg. Assoc. J., 41,* 721–729

Holmberg, B. & Lundberg, P. (1985) Benzene: standards, occurrence and exposure. *Am. J. Ind. Health, 7,* 375–383

Holzer, G., Shanfield, H., Slatkis, A., Bertsch, W., Juarez, P. & Mayfield, H. (1977) Collection and analysis of trace organic emissions from natural sources. *J. Chromatogr., 142,* 755–764

Howard, P.J. & Durkin, P.R. (1974) *Sources of Contamination, Ambient Levels and Fate of Benzene in the Environment (EPA 560/5-75-005),* Washington DC, U.S. Environmental Protection Agency

Hubbard, B.R. & Silverman, L. (1950) Rapid method for the determination of aromatic hydrocarbons in air. *Arch. Ind. Hyg. Occup. Med., 2,* 49–55

Hunter, D. (1978) *The Diseases of Occupations,* 6th ed., London, Hodder and Stoughton, p. 492

IARC (1979) *IARC Monographs on the Evaluation of the Carcinogenic Risk of Chemicals to Humans,* Vol. 19, *Some Monomers, Plastics and Synthetic Elastomers and Acrolein,* Lyon, International Agency for Research on Cancer, pp. 231–274

IARC (1982a) *IARC Monographs on the Evaluation of the Carcinogenic Risk of Chemicals to Humans,* Vol. 29, *Some Industrial Chemicals and Dyestuffs,* Lyon, International Agency for Research on Cancer, pp. 93–148

IARC (1982b) *IARC Monographs on the Evaluation of the Carcinogenic Risk of Chemicals to Humans,* Vol. 28, *The Rubber Industry,* Lyon, International Agency for Research on Cancer, pp. 192, 332

Ikeda, M. & Ohtsuji, H. (1969) Significance of urinary hippuric acid determination as an index of toluene exposure. *Br. J. Ind. Med., 26,* 244–246

Infante, P.,F. & White, M.C. (1985) Projections of leukemia risk associated with occupational exposure to benzene. *Am. J. Ind. Med., 7,* 403–414

Infante, P.F., Rinsky, R.A., Wagoner, J.K. & Young, R.J. (1977) Leukemia in benzene workers. *Lancet, ii,* 76–78

Irvine, D. (1984) Benzene. *Risk Anal., 4,* 3–4

Jacobs, M.B. (1941) *The Analytical Chemistry of Industrial Poisons, Hazards and Solvents,* New York, Interscience, p. 416

Jentzsch, D. & Fraser, D.A. (1981) A laboratory evaluation of long-term detector tubes: benzene, toluene, trichloroethylene. *Am. Ind. Hyg. Assoc. J., 42,* 810–822

Jonsson, A. & Berg, S. (1978) *Report to Statens Naturvädsverk,* Sweden, University of Stockholm

Kobayaschi, Y. (1952) Gas analysis with detector tubes. II. Determination of minute quantities of benzene in air. *J. Chem. Soc. Jpn, 55,* 544–546

Kokko, A. (1982) *Statistics on Industrial Hygiene Measurements in 1977–80* [in Finnish], Report 59, Helsinki, Institute of Occupational Health, p. 82

Kol'kovsky, P. (1967) A new color reaction for the vapor of some aromatic hydrocarbons. *Russ. J. Anal. Chem., 22,* 403–404

Kol'kovsky, P. (1969) Indicator-tube method for the determination of benzene in air. *Analyst, 94,* 918–920

Konosu, H, & Mashiko, Y. (1965) Industrial analysis of optical methods. XI. Design of nondispersive vacuum ultraviolet photometer and its application to technical gas analysis. *Nippon Kagaku Zaisshi, 1,* 47–53

Konosu, H., Mashiko, Y. & Sato, M. (1972) Technical analyses by optical methods. XIX. Design of a nondispersive vacuum ultraviolet photometer and its application to technical gas analysis. *Nippon Kagaku Zaisshi, 1,* 47–53

Kreuzer, L.B., Kenyon, N.D. & Patel, C.K.N. (1972) Air pollution. Sensitive detection of 10 pollutant gases by carbon monoxide and carbon dioxide lasers. *Science, 177,* 377–379

Krynska, A. (1971) Use of the test solution reacting with benzene for determination of other aromatic hydrocarbons in air. *Pr. Cent. Inst. Ochr. Pr., 21,* 175–183

Küh, G. (1957) (*German Patent (D.B.R.), 102,480, February 2*)

Kupel, R.E. & White, L.D. (1971) Report on modified charcoal tube. *Am. Ind. Hyg. Assoc. J., 32,* 456

Kusnetz, H.L., Saltzman, B.E. & LaNier, M.E. (1960) Calibration and evaluation of gas detecting tubes. *Am. Ind. Hyg. Assoc. J., 21,* 361–373

Laskin, S. & Goldstein, B.D., eds (1977) *Benzene Toxicity: A Critical Evaluation,* New York, American Petroleum Institute

Laurian, P. (1938) Identification and determination of small quantities of benzene. Determination of benzene vapors in the atmosphere. *J. Pharm. Chim., 27,* 561–577

Lautenberger, W.J., Kring, E.V. & Morello, J.A. (1980) A new personal badge monitor for organic vapors. *Am. Ind. Hyg. Assoc. J., 41,* 737–747

Lauwerys, R. (1976) *Review of the Biological Monitoring Methods for Evaluating Exposure to Benzene,* Paris, 9–11 November, International Workshop on Toxicology of Benzene (unpublished)

Lauwerys, R.R. (1979) *Industrial Health and Safety, Human Biological Monitoring of Industrial Chemicals. 1. Benzene (CEC Report EUR 6570/11979),* Luxembourg, Commission of the European Communities

Lauwerys, R.R. (1983) *Industrial Chemical Exposure Guidelines for Biological Monitoring,* Davis, CA, Biomedical Publications

Leichnitz, K. (1977) Use of detector tubes under extreme conditions (humidity, pressure, temperature). *Am. Ind. Hyg. Assoc. J., 38,* 701–711

Levadie, B. & Harwood, J.F. (1960) An application of gas chromatography to analysis of solvent vapors in industrial air. *Am. Ind. Hyg. Assoc. J., 21,* 21–24

Louw, C.W., Richards, J.F. & Faure, P.K. (1977) The determination of volatile organic compounds in city air by gas chromatography combined with standard addition, selective substraction, and infrared spectrometry and mass spectrometry. *Atmos. Environ., 11,* 703–715

Maffett, P.A., Doherty, R.F. & Monkman, J.L. (1956) A direct method for the collection and determination of micro amounts of benzene or toluene in air. *Am. Ind. Hyg. Assoc. J., 17,* 186–188

Maltoni, C., Conti, B. & Cotti, G. (1983) Benzene: a multipotential carcinogen. Results of long-term bioassays performed at the Bologna Institute of Oncology. *Am. J. Ind. Med., 4,* 589–630

Mansur, R.H., Pero, R.F. & Krause, L.A. (1959) Vapor phase chromatography in quantitative determination of air samples collected in the field. *Am. Ind. Hyg. Assoc. J., 20,* 175

McMichael, A.J., Spirtas, R., Kupper, L.L. & Gamble, J.F. (1975) Solvent exposure andd leukemia among rubber workers: an epidemiologic study. *J. Occup. Med., 17,* 234–239

Merian, E. (1982) The environmental chemistry of volatile hydrocarbons. *Toxicol. Environ. Chem., 5,* 167–175

Merian, E. & Zander, M. (1982) Volatile aromatics. In: Hutzinger, G., ed., *Handbook of Environmental Chemistry,* Vol. 3, Part B, *Anthropogenic Compounds,* Berlin (West), Springer-Verlag, pp. 117–161

Mikulski, P., Wiglusz, R., Bublewsla, A. & Uselis, J. (1972) Investigation of exposure of ship painters to organic solvents. *Br. J. Ind. Med., 29,* 450–453

Mueller, F.X. & Miller, J.A. (1979) Determination of airborne organic vapor mixtures using charcoal tubes. *Am. Ind. Hyg. Assoc. J., 40,* 380–386

NAS (1976) *Health Effects of Benzene. A Review,* Washington DC, National Academy of Sciences

NIOSH (1973) *Criteria for a Recommended Standard: Occupational Exposure to Toluene (DHEW [NIOSH])*, Washington DC, National Institute for Occupational Safety and Health, pp. 75–87

NIOSH (1974) *Criteria for a Recommended Standard: Occupational Exposure to Benzene (DHEW [NIOSH])*, Cincinnati, OH, National Institute for Occupational Safety and Health

NIOSH (1975) *Criteria for a Recommended Standard: Occupational Exposure to Toluene (DHEW [NIOSH])*, Cincinnati, OH, National Institute for Occupational Safety and Health

NIOSH (1977a) *Revised Recommendation for an Occupational Exposure Standard for Benzene (DHEW [NIOSH])*, Cincinnati, OH, National Institute for Occupational Safety and Health

NIOSH (1977b) *Manual of Analytical Methods*, 2nd ed., Part II, *Standards Completion Program Validated Methods*, Vol. III (*DHEW [NIOSH]*), Cincinnati, OH, National Institute for Occupational Safety and Health, pp. S311–1 to S311–8

Novak, J., Vasak, V. & Janak, J. (1965) Chromatographic method for the concentration of trace impurities in the atmosphere. *Anal. Chem., 37,* 660–666

OSHA (1981) Occupational exposure to benzene: permanent standard. *Fed. Regist., 46,* 4889–4893

Ogata, M., Tomokuni, K. & Takatsuka, Y. (1969) Quantitative determination in urine of hippuric acid and m- or p-methyl hippuric acid metabolites of toluene and m- or p-xylene. *Br. J. Ind. Med., 26,* 330–334

Ogata, M., Tomokuni, K. & Takatsuka, Y. (1970) Urinary excretion of hippuric acid and m- or p-methyl hippuric acid in the urine of workers exposed to vapors of toluene and m- or p-xylene as a test of exposure. *Br. J. Ind. Med., 27,* 43

Otson, R., Williams, D.T. & Bothwell, P.D. (1983) Charcoal tube technique for simultaneous determination of selected organics in air. *Am. Ind. Hyg. Assoc. J., 44,* 489–494

Ott, M.G., Townsend, J.C., Fishbeck, W.A. & Langner, R.A. (1978) Mortality among individuals occupationally exposed to benzene. *Arch. Environ. Health, 33,* 3–10

Otterson, E.J. & Guy, C.U. (1964) A method of atmospheric solvent vapor sampling on activated charcoal in connection with gas chromatography. *Trans. 26th Annu. Meet. Am. Conf. Gov. Hyg.,* pp. 37–42

Ovrum, P. (1956) Determination of atmospheric benzene concentration by displacement following absorption on silica gel. *Br. J. Ind. Med., 13,* 210–213

Pagnotto, L.D. & Lieberman, L.M. (1967) Urinary hippuric acid excretion as an index of toluene exposure. *Am. Ind. Hyg. Assoc. J., 29,* 129–134

Patzelova, V. Jansta, J. & Dousek, F.P. (1978) Some sorption properties of a new type of active carbon. *J. Chromatogr., 148,* 53–59

Pellizzari, E.D. (1982) Analysis for organic vapor emission near industrial and chemical waste disposal sites. *Environ. Sci. Technol., 16,* 781–785

Piecewicz, J.F., Harris, J.C. & Levins, P.L. (1979) *EPA Reports (EPA 600/7-79-216, September)*, Cincinnati, OH

Pilar, S. & Graydon, W.F. (1973) Benzene and toluene distribution in Toronto atmosphere. *Environ. Sci. Technol., 7,* 628–631

Piotrowski, J.K. (1977) Xylenes. In: *Exposure Tests for Organic Compounds in Industrial Toxicology (NIOSH Publ. No. 77–144)*, Cincinnati, OH, National Institute of Occupational Safety and Health, pp. 55–57

Poggi, G., Giusiani, M., Palagi, U., Paggiaro, P.L., Loi, A.M., Dazzi, F., Siclari, C. & Baschieri, L. (1982) High-performance liquid chromatography for the determination of the urinary metabolites of toluene, xylene, and styrene. *Int. Arch. Occup. Environ. Health, 50,* 25–31

Posner, E. (1928) Determination of hydrocarbon vapors in air by means of active charcoal. *Z. Anorg. Allg. Chem., 174,* 190–294

Purcell, W.P. (1978) Benzene. In: Kirk, R.E. & Othmer, D.F., eds, *Encyclopedia of Chemical Technology,* 3rd Ed., Vol. 3, New York, John Wiley and Sons, pp. 744–771

Raymond, A. & Guichon, G. (1974) Gas chromatographic analysis of C_8–C_{18}-hydrocarbons in Paris air. *Environ. Sci. Technol., 8,* 143–148

Reid, F.H. & Halpin, W.R. (1968) Determination of halogenated and aromatic hydrocarbons in air by charcoal tube and gas chromatography. *Am. Ind. Hyg. Assoc. J., 29,* 390–396

Rieder, H.P. (1957) Bestimmung von Benzosäure neben Hippursäure mit Hilfe einer differential-spectrophotometrischen Methode. *Clin. Chim. Acta, 2,* 497–501

Rinsky, R.A., Young, R.J. & Smith, A.B. (1981) Leukemia in benzene workers. *Am. J. Ind. Med., 2,* 217–245

Roper, C.P. (1971) An evaluation of perchloroethylene detector tubes. *Am. Ind. Hyg. Assoc. J., 32,* 847–849

Runion, H.E. & Scott, L.M. (1985) Benzene exposure in the United States, 1978–1983: an overview. *Am. J. Ind. Med., 7,* 385–393

Rushing, D.E. (1958) Gas chromatography in industrial hygiene and air pollution problems. *Am. Ind. Hyg. Assoc. J., 19,* 238

Saltzman, B.E. (1962) Basic theory of gas indicator tube calibration. *Am. Ind. Hyg. Assoc. J., 23,* 112–126

Samimi, B.S. (1983) Calibration of Miran gas analyzers: extent of vapor loss within a closed loop calibration system. *Am. Ind. Hyg. Assoc. J., 44,* 40–45

Sato, A. (1971) Gas chromatographic determination of benzene, toluene, and *m*-xylene in blood by an equilibration method. *Jpn. J. Ind. Health, 13,* 173–179

Sato, A. & Fujiwara, Y. (1972) Elimination on inhaled benzene and toluene in man. *Jpn. J. Ind. Health, 14,* 224

Sato, A., Nakajima, T. & Fujiwara, Y. (1975) Determination of benzene and toluene in blood by means of syringe-equilibration method using a small amount of blood. *Br. J. Ind. Med., 32,* 210–214

Schrenk, H.H., Pearce, S.J. & Yant, W.P. (1935) *Report of Investigation 13287,* Washington DC, US Dept. of Interior, Bureau of Mines

Sefton, M.V., Kostas, A.V. & Lombardi, C. (1982) Stain length passive dosimeters. *Am. Ind. Hyg. Assoc. J., 43,* 820–824

Seifert, B. & Abraham, H.J. (1982a) Indoor air concentrations of benzene and some other aromatic hydrocarbons. *Ecotoxicol. Environ. Saf., 6,* 190–192

Seifert, B. & Abraham, H.J. (1982b) Use of passive samplers for the determination of gaseous organic substances in indoor air at low concentration levels. *Int. J. Environ. Anal. Chem, 13,* 237–253

Sherwood, R.J. (1976) *Criteria for Occupational Exposure to Benzene,* Paris, 9–11 November, International Workshop on Toxicology of Benzene (unpublished)

Siegel, D., Müller, F. & Neuschwander, K. (1974) Fully automatic measurement of hydrocarbons and emissions. Selective measurement of C_1–C_5 and total C_6 hydrocarbons and benzenes. *Chromatographia, 7,* 399–406

Slob, A. (1973) A new method for determination of mandelic acid excretion at low level styrene exposure. *Br. J. Ind. Med., 30,* 390–393

Smith, B.S. & Pierce, J.O. (1970) The use of plastic bags for industrial air sampling. *Am. Ind. Hyg. Assoc. J., 31,* 343–348

Smyth, H.F. (1929) Determination of small amounts of benzene vapors in air. *J. Ind. Hyg., 11,* 338–348

Smyth, H.F. (1931) Determination of small amounts of benzene vapors in air. *J. Ind. Hyg., 13,* 227–230

Snyder, C.A. (1977) Benzene toxicity: A critical evaluation: Analytical techniques. *J. Toxicol. Environ. Health (Suppl. 2),* 5–22

Snyder, C.A. & Kocsis, J.J. (1975) Current concepts of chronic benzene toxicity. *CRC Crit. Rev. Toxicol., 3,* 265

Snyder, C.A., Ehrlichman, M.N., Goldstein, B.D. & Laskin, S. (1977) An extractive method for the determination of benzene in tissue by gas chromatography. *Am. Ind. Hyg. Assoc. J., 38,* 272–278

Steger, E. & Kahl, H. (1969) Infrared spectroscopic analysis of gaseous atmospheric impurities. *Chem. Technol., 21*(8), 483–488

Stephens, E.R. (1973) *Hydrocarbons in Polluted Air, Summary Report,* Riverside, CA, Statewide Air Pollut. Res. Cent, Univ. California

Tabershaw, I.R. & Lamm, S.H. (1977) Letter to the Editor. *Lancet, ii,* 867–868

Tompkins, F.C., Jr. & Goldsmith, R.L. (1977) A new personal dosimeter for the monitoring of indoor pollutants. *Am. Ind. Hyg. Assoc. J., 38,* 371–377

Truhaut, R. & Murray, R. (1978) International Workshop on Toxicology of Benzene, Paris, 9–11 November 1976. *Int. Arch. Occup. Environ. Health, 41,* 65–76

Tsani-Bazaca, E., McIntyre, A., Lester, J. & Perry, R. (1982) Ambient concentrations and correlations of hydrocarbons and halocarbons in vicinity of an airport. *Chemosphere, 11,* 11–23

Umberger, C.J. & Fiorese, F.F. (1963) Colorimetric method for hippuric acid. *Clin. Chem., 9,* 91–96

Urone, P. & Smith, J.E. (1961) Analysis of chlorinated hydrocarbons with the gas chromatograph. *Am. Ind. Hyg. Assoc. J., 22,* 36

Utidjian, H.M.D. & Weaver, N.K. (1974) Criteria for a recommended standard. Occupational exposure to toluene. *J. Occup. Med., 16,* 107

Van Raalte, H.G.S. (1982) A critical look at hazards from benzene in workplace and community air. *Regul. Toxicol. Pharmacol., 2,* 67–76

Van Raalte, H.G.S. & Grasso, P. (1982) Hematological, myelotoxic, clastogenic, carcinogenic and leukemogenic effects of benzene. *Regul. Toxicol. Pharmacol., 2,* 153–176

Van Raalte, H.G.S., Grasso, P. & Irving, D. (1984) Tackling a very difficult problem. *Risk Anal., 4,* 1–2

Van Roosmalen, P.B. & Drummond, I. (1978) Simultaneous determination by gas chromatography of the major metabolites in urine of toluene, xylene and styrene. *Br. J. Ind. Med., 35,* 56–60

Van Tassel, S., Amalfitano, N. & Narang, R.S. (1981) Determination of arenes and volatile haloorganic compounds in air at microgram per cubic meter levels by gas chromatography. *Anal. Chem., 53,* 2130–2135

Veulemans, H. & Masschelein, R. (1979) Experimental human exposure to toluene. III. Urinary hippuric acid excretion as a measure of individual solvent uptake. *Int. Arch. Occup. Environ. Health, 43,* 53–62

Vigalok, R.V., Gabitova, R.K., Anoshina, N.P., Palikov, N.A., Maidachenko, G.G. & Vigdergauz, M.S. (1976) Study of liquid-crystal adsorbents for gas chromatography of aromatic isomers. *Zh. Analit. Khim., 3*(4), 644–648

Vigliani, E.C. (1976) Leukemia associated with benzene exposure. *Ann. N.Y. Acad. Sci., 271,* 143–151

Wallace, L.A., Zweidinger, R., Erickson, M., Cooper, S., Whitaker, D. & Pellizzari, E.D. (1982) Monitoring individual exposure: measurements of volatile organic compounds in breathing-zone air, drinking water, and exhaled breath. *Environ. Int., 8,* 269–282

Wallace, L., Pellizzari, E., Hartwell, T., Perritt, K. & Ziegenfus, R. (1987) Exposures to benzene and other volatile compounds from active and passive smoking. *Arch. Environ. Health* (in press)

West, P.W., Sen, B. & Gibson, N.A. (1958) Gas-liquid chromatographic analyses applied to air pollution sampling. *Anal. Chem., 30,* 1390–1397

White, L.D., Taylor, D.G., Mauer, P.A. & Kupel, R.E. (1970) A convenient optimized method for the analysis of selected solvent vapors in the industrial atmosphere. *Am. Ind. Hyg. Assoc. J., 31,* 225–232

White, M.C., Infante, P.F. & Chu, K.C. (1982) A quantitative estimate of leukemia mortality associated with occupational exposure to benzene. *Risk Anal., 2,* 195–203

Whitman, N.E. & Johnston, A.E. (1964) Sampling and analysis of aromatic hydrocarbon vapors in air: a gas liquid chromatographic method. *Am. Ind. Hyg. Assoc. J., 25,* 646

WHO (1973) Report of WHO Expert Committee. Environmental and health monitoring in occupational health. *WHO tech. Rep. Ser., No. 53,* p. 20

WHO (1981) Recommended health based limits in occupational exposure to selected organic solvents. *WHO tech. Rep. Ser., No. 664,* pp. 7–24

WHO (1982) *Environmental Health Criteria No. 20, Selected Petroleum Products,* Geneva, p. 26

Williams, N.H. (1965) Gas chromatographic techniques for the identification of low concentrations of atmospheric pollutants. *Anal. Chem., 37,* 1723–1732

Wilson, H.K. & Ottley, T.W. (1981) The use of a transportable mass spectrometer for the direct measurement of industrial solvents in breath. *Biomed. Mass Spectrom., 8,* 606–610

Withey, R.J. & Martin, L. (1974) A sensitive micro method for the analysis of benzene in blood. *Bull. Environ. Contam. Toxicol., 12*(6), 659–664

Wolf, P.H., Andjelkovich, D., Smith, A. & Tyroler, H. (1981) A case-control study of leukemia in the U.S. rubber industry. *J. Occup. Med., 23,* 103–108

Wood, R.W., Rees, D.C., McCormich, J.P. & Kilpper, R.W. (1981) Determination of toluene in blood and tissues by vapor phase equilibrium chromatography. *Toxicologist, 1,* 77

Yant, W.P., Pearce, S.J. & Schrenk, H.H. (1936) *A Microcolorimetric Method for the Determination of Toluene (Report Investigations No. 3323)*, Washington DC, US Dept. of Interior, Bureau of Mines, pp. 12

Yin, S-N, Li, Q., Liu, Y., Tian, F., Du, C. & Jin, C. (1987) Occupational exposure to benzene in China. *Br. J. Ind. Med., 44,* 192–195

Yuan, W. & Ma, Z. (1981) Rapid ultraviolet spectrophotometry for determination of benzene, toluene and xylene in the air. *Zhonghua Yufangyixue Zazhi, 15,* 251–252 (*Chem. Abstr., 96,* 167713d)

CHAPTER 8

SAMPLING AND ANALYSIS OF INDUSTRIAL AIR

R.H. Brown

Health and Safety Executive, Occupational Medicine and Hygiene Laboratory,
403 Edgware Road, London NW2 6LN, UK

MONITORING STRATEGY

Introduction

The objectives of air sampling are to measure pollutant levels, identify specific pollutant sources, improve process control and ensure compliance with any relevant hygiene standard (Leidel *et al.*, 1977; CEFIC, 1983; Leichnitz, 1983; Health & Safety Executive, 1984a).

Exposure analysis

Prior to the start of a monitoring exercise, a hazard inventory should be compiled, listing all chemicals or products containing benzene/toluene/xylene, irrespective of level. Workplaces should be evaluated for their potential for worker exposure to these chemicals. Any exposure data obtained previously from the workplace, or similar installations, should be examined and the possibility of replacing the product concerned with a less hazardous substitute should be considered.

Depending on the specific objectives of the survey, it may be desirable to undertake personal monitoring in which a sampling device is worn on the body, with the sampling head located near the breathing zone, or area/fixed-location monitoring. The two types of measurement may not correlate well, as discussed elsewhere.

For personal monitoring, the time of sampling should be appropriate for the actual period of exposure; i.e., it would normally be for a full shift. Specific short-term activities which break containment, such as sampling or drum filling, should be evaluated separately. Area monitoring for process control might be done by a series of short-term "instantaneous" measurements or by continuous monitoring. For a relationship between short- and long-term monitoring, see Leichnitz (1980).

Number of samples

If a correct exposure analysis has been performed, it should be possible to identify those individuals most at risk. Alternatively, a purely statistical approach can be made

(Leidel *et al.*, 1977; Eller, 1984), in which it can be assured that a representative selection of workers is monitored (e.g., for a group of 50 workers, 18 must be monitored to ensure, at the 90% confidence level, that at least one individual from the 10% most highly exposed is monitored).

Frequency of sampling

An initial survey should provide sufficient data to establish the personal exposure pattern, and the results might be expressed as, e.g., a log-normal distribution on probability paper (Brief *et al.*, 1980). A minimum of about 10 data points will be required. Further surveys should be conducted if there is any variation in work patterns or operating practices or major environmental change (e.g., wind and temperature). When the addition of new data makes little difference to the established exposure pattern, a lower frequency of monitoring can be established to check on long-term trends.

For compliance testing, the frequency of repeat monitoring may be more precisely defined, and usually depends on how close the measurements are to the limit value. For example, in the German regulation TRG S 402 (Bundesanstalt für Arbeitsschutz und Unfallforschung, 1986), the maximum interval between measurements is 64 weeks if the observed concentration is less than a quarter of the limit value, but 16 weeks if the observed concentration is more than half, but does not exceed, the limit value.

Boundary-fence monitoring

Boundary-fence monitoring is usually carried out to determine the maximum concentration of a pollutant outside the plant limits. Concentration levels at the boundary are determined as a function of space, time, ambient weather and plant operating conditions and a prediction is made of the actual concentration distribution in the community environment. The prediction must allow for emissions which might pass over the factory fence at a height above a feasible monitoring position.

Reporting guidelines

The monitoring report concerning any operation or selection of workers should include enough detail to cover all the variables involved and to define completely the situation, conditions and limitations which apply to the results.

SHORT-TERM MONITORING TECHNIQUES

Introduction

These techniques, sometimes called "snap" or "spot" measurements, give an almost instantaneous measurement of a concentration at one point in the factory environment. Subsequent laboratory analysis is not usually necessary, so that an immediate assessment of the hazard can be made. However, these methods may not be of high accuracy, so that a statistically meaningful number of readings should be taken if compliance with a hygiene standard is to be assessed (Leidel *et al.*, 1977; Brief *et al.*, 1980; CEFIC, 1983; Gentry & Jones, 1984).

Gas indicator tubes

Gas indicator tubes are available for benzene/toluene/xylene, but are not specific to any one aromatic hydrocarbon (Leichnitz, 1983, 1985; Detectawl, undated). Nevertheless, they provide a rapid, inexpensive and simple method for evaluating levels of either benzene, toluene or xylene when they are found singly in the industrial environment. However, they give only an approximate measurement (accuracy about ± 25%) and are not suitable for mixtures of these compounds. Tubes should be stored and used according to the manufacturer's recommendations.

Specificity to benzene may be conferred by the use of a Tenax pre-tube to retain higher aromatics. Both colour comparison tubes and stain-length tubes are available.

The colour comparison tube is based on the reaction of aromatic hydrocarbons with formaldehyde to produce, in the case of benzene, diphenyl methane. The product is then oxidized by sulfuric acid to a reddish-brown quinoid compound. Benzene, toluene and xylene are indicated with approximately equal sensitivity.

The stain-length tubes are based on the reduction of iodine pentoxide by aromatic hydrocarbons in the presence of sulfuric acid to produce free iodine. In this case, the sensitivity is different for each of the three hydrocarbons.

Colorimetric method

The aromatic hydrocarbons may be determined by reaction with an acidified aqueous solution of paraformaldehyde (Health & Safety Executive, 1972). An air sample is draw through the solution contained in a bubbler (impinger) by means of a portable sampling pump. Analysis may be visual or spectrophotometric. Specificity to benzene may be conferred by the use of an acidified selenious acid solution in a preceding bubbler.

The test is rapid (about 10 min), but relatively insensitive; the detection limit for benzene is about 16 mg/m^3 (5 ppm). The method gives only an approximate indication of the concentration level, the precision, expressed as the coefficient of variation (CV), being about 20%.

Gas sampling

Direct sampling of air containing benzene/toluene/xylene has been carried out by means of glass or plastic gas-tight syringes, plastic bags, metal boxes, evacuated cans and many other vessels. A careful choice of container material must be made to minimize adsorption losses. Analysis is usually performed by gas chromatography (GC).

Advantages and disadvantages

Detector tubes are commercially available, inexpensive and very convenient. Because of excellent quality control, calibration (e.g., by reference to a standard vapour atmosphere) is not usually necessary, but the measurements should nevertheless be regarded as approximate. The colorimetric method is less convenient and requires freshly-made reagents.

Direct gas sampling is convenient, but laboratory facilities or a portable gas chromatograph will be required for on-site analysis. A (portable) apparatus for the generation of standard atmospheres is desirable for calibration, although liquid-phase standards can be employed.

INTEGRATED MEASUREMENTS

Introduction

Most exposure limits are based on the measurement of integrated time-weighted-average (TWA) exposure, i.e., the determination of an average concentration over a specified time, usually between 10 min and 8 h. Such measurements require a continuous sampling device operating at a uniform rate, and an analytical procedure for the collected vapour. Older methods (see Chapter 5) have used cryogenic trapping, bubblers or large adsorbent tubes containing a variety of adsorbents such as silica gel, charcoal, alumina or Molecular Sieve. Sampling is effected by means of a pump and analysis is performed by GC, although liquid chromatography and ultraviolet spectrophotometry have occasionally been used. More recently, the National Institute for Occupational Safety and Health (NIOSH) has introduced a small charcoal tube which can be used with a low-flow-rate pump and is much more convenient (see below). The NIOSH method, however, uses a desorption solvent and many analysts prefer a thermal desorption technique.

To cover the wide boiling range, a two-stage adsorption technique may be employed for the separation of benzene/toluene/xylene from petroleum vapour. Capillary GC is then used for the resolution of multiple components. More recently still, diffusive sampling methods have been introduced, but these, whilst offering many potential advantages, are only recently gaining wider acceptance.

Both pumped and diffusive sampling devices require the services of an analytical laboratory for the subsequent (usually GC) analysis. Since samples are normally taken over 8 h, there is often no particular advantage in attempting to analyse on-site. Direct gas sampling and continuous monitoring methods (below) can be used or adapted for TWA measurement.

Charcoal tubes

The method introduced by NIOSH (White *et al.*, 1970) uses a small (100 mg) charcoal tube to adsorb organic vapours, a back-up (50 mg) section to check for breakthrough, and a (personal) low-flow-rate sampling pump. Collected benzene/toluene/xylene is desorbed with carbon disulfide and the resulting solution is analysed by GC.

The method developed by the originators is described in NIOSH method 1501 (Eller, 1984). It has also been adopted as a (non-exclusive) recommended method in countries other than the USA, for example by the UK Health and Safety Executive (1983a,b), and is under discussion as a draft for an international standard by the International Organisation for Standardisation. It is reproduced in a modified form as Method 1 in this volume. The method is appropriate for the determination of benzene, toluene and/or xylene in the approximate concentration range 1–1 000 mg/m^3 (about 0.2 to 200 ppm) in 12-L air samples.

A collaborative test (Larkin et al., 1973), which included benzene and xylene, indicated that the precision (CV), including between-laboratory and day-to-day variance, was about 13% under conditions where pump error was about 9%.

In a field trial (Walkin et al., 1985), the charcoal tube method was compared with an independent diffusive tube method (Health & Safety Executive, 1985) for measuring occupational exposure to benzene; the results obtained by the two methods could not be distinguished statistically.

Several quality assurance schemes have been developed which apply to the charcoal tube method. One of these is the National Institute for Occupational Safety and Health Proficiency Analytical Testing (PAT) Program (NIOSH, 1984) and the associated Laboratory Accreditation Program of the Americal Industrial Hygiene Association (1985). Another is the Health and Safety Executive AQUA scheme. Details of these programs may be obtained from the Chief, Quality Assurance Section, Monitoring and Control Research Branch, Division of Physical Sciences and Engineering, NIOSH, 4676 Columbia Parkway, Cincinnati, Ohio 45226; The Laboratory Accreditation Coordinator, AIHA, 475 Wolf Ledges Parkway, Akron, Ohio 44311-1087; and Dr N. West, HSE, Occupational Medicine & Hygiene Laboratories, London.

A problem may arise from the occurrence of benzene as a common trace contaminant in carbon disulfide, which is used in the charcoal tube method. A procedure for the preparation of clean carbon disulfide is described in Method 1.

Thermal desorption

Because of the high toxicity and inflammability of carbon disulfide and the labour-intensive nature of the solvent desorption procedure, a useful alternative is to desorb the collected benzene/toluene/xylene vapour thermally (Baxter et al., 1980; Brief et al., 1980; Saunders, 1982). This is not practical with charcoal as adsorbent, as the temperature needed for desorption would result in some decomposition of the analytes. Porous polymer adsorbents are therefore used instead, in particular Tenax, Porapak Q and Chromosorb 106. Of these, Tenax has the lowest thermal blank (typically less than 0.1 µg/g of adsorbent, when properly conditioned), but only modest adsorption capacity compared with carbon.

The thermal desorption method conventionally uses larger tubes than the NIOSH method described above; usually 200–500 mg adsorbent are used, depending on type. Desorption can be made fully automatic and analysis is usually carried out by GC. Some desorbers also allow automatic selection of sample tubes from a multiple-sample carousel. For most applications, the whole collected sample is transferred to the GC, resulting in greatly increased sensitivity compared with the solvent desorption method.

The method has been adopted as a (non-exclusive) recommended method in some countries, including the UK (Health & Safety Executive, 1983c, 1984b), and is reproduced in a somewhat modified form in Method 2 of this volume. Method 2 is appropriate for the determination of benzene, toluene and/or xylene in the approximate concentration range 0.5–50 mg/m^3 (about 0.1 to 10 ppm) in 5-L air samples. The analytical precision (CV) of the method (Baxter et al., 1980; Health & Safety Executive, 1983c) is about 5% in laboratory trials, and the pump error is expected to be in the range 5–10%.

In a field trial (Walkin et al., 1985), the pumped tube method was compared with an independent diffusive tube method for measuring occupational exposure to benzene (Health & Safety Executive, 1985); the results of the two methods could not be distinguished statistically. The mean precision of the pumped thermal desorption method was 13% and that of the diffusive method, 11%.

A quality control study of the thermal desorption method has been conducted by Coker and Simms[1]. The precision of the method, including inter-laboratory variance, was found to be about 22% (16% for "specializing" laboratories).

Petroleum applications

Petroleum typically contains about 1% benzene, 15% toluene and 10% xylene, and is a major source of factory and environmental aromatic hydrocarbons (Brief et al., 1980; Kearney & Dunham, 1986). The presence of a large excess of aliphatic hydrocarbons demands a sampling and analytical procedure which is more complex than those mentioned above. The method recommended by CONCAWE (1986) for sampling petroleum vapours uses two adsorption tubes in series: a carbonaceous adsorbent to collect lower-boiling materials (down to propane) and a porous polymer for the higher-boiling components. The method specifies an OV 1701 capillary column because this is one of the few columns known to resolve n-hexane from methyl-tert-butyl ether; the latter is a recently introduced octane enhancer.

The method is under discussion by the International Organisation for Standardisation as a general method for the determination of hydrocarbons in the workplace atmosphere. There are two versions of the method as described by CONCAWE (1986): one with a single adsorption tube containing two packings and one with two separate tubes which are used in series. For simplicity, the two-tube method is reproduced here, with minor changes, as Method 3, but this can readily be adapted to a single-tube method.

Diffusive sampling

Diffusive sampling relies on the physical process of diffusion, as opposed to a pump, to control the rate of sampling of an airborne pollutant. Reliable diffusive samplers

---

[1] Coker, D.T. & Simms, M.C. (1983) personal communication

must therefore satisfy three basic conditions: (1) they must maintain a "zero sink" at the sorbent surface, (2) they must have a defined static zone (usually an air gap) and (3) their geometrical shape should be such that boundary-layer effects are minimized. Not all available samplers satisfy these criteria and, in any case, condition (1) is a function of the capacity of the sampler adsorbent and the properties of the vapour to be collected.

In the case of benzene, the 3M badge (Joki, 1980) and the Perkin-Elmer tube (Brown *et al.*, 1981) have been found to be satisfactory by some authors. Many other designs may be equally good.

It is too early to say whether such samplers will eventually gain universal acceptance; perhaps the recent introduction of recommended validation protocols (Health & Safety Executive, 1983d; Cassinelli *et al.*, 1987) will resolve the issue.

Diffusive methods have been accepted as (non-exclusive) recommended methods in the UK (Health & Safety Executive, 1985). Their range of applicability is broadly similar to that of pumped methods, and their precision is at least as good.

Advantages and disadvantages

The charcoal tube method has been thoroughly validated and enjoys wide international acceptance. However, it is becoming increasingly apparent that thermal desorption methods and diffusive methods are at least as good and may well be more reliable. Charcoal tube methods usually employ carbon disulfide as the desorption solvent, which is potentially hazardous because of its toxicity and inflammability. Moreover, difficulties can arise in the analysis of mixtures if compounds other than aromatic hydrocarbons are present, as different desorption solvents may be required for different analytes and it is not normally possible to desorb the tube twice. The desorption efficiency of the analyte of interest may also be affected by the presence of co-pollutants, particularly water vapour.

The most commonly noted objections to thermal desorption procedures are the necessity to clean the adsorbent thoroughly and the "one-shot" nature of the technique. Many institutions routinely re-analyse a proportion of their samples (e.g., by GC-mass spectrometry) and, for thermal desorption, this necessitates taking two samples. The technique does require additional apparatus (i.e., a reliable thermal desorber), but the extra expense is justified for many by considerations of convenience and sensitivity.

Diffusive methods too, have had their share of criticism. Some early designs suffered from boundary-layer effects and, even now, "badge" samplers (e.g., 3M and DuPont) are suitable only for personal monitoring where a minimal amount of air movement can be assured. There have also been doubts, probably unfounded, concerning the ability of the samplers to give an accurate integrated measurement when confronted with rapidly changing concentrations. In the author's view, the only serious disadvantage is the lack of extensive calibration data; this is a consequence of the relatively large amount of effort needed to establish such data over the operating range of the samplers.

ANALYTICAL TECHNIQUES

Most of the methods used for monitoring benzene/toluene/xylene in the workplace involve GC. This technique enables the benzene, toluene and xylene to be separated from one another and from any other components before they are quantified. Many different types of gas chromatograph are available commercially, but all consist basically of a sample injection mechanism, a separating column and a detector.

Samples taken on charcoal tubes are usually analysed by solvent desorption and an aliquot of the solution introduced into the GC *via* an injection port by means of a microlitre liquid syringe.

Porous polymer adsorption tubes are generally analysed by thermal desorption, which requires specialized equipment for sample injection. Such equipment is available commercially. Thermal desorption avoids the presence of a large solvent peak, which may obscure the analyte of interest, particularly with packed-column chromatography. Complex analyses are best done by capillary chromatography. When using a capillary column, care must be exercised not to overload it and, in general, a sample splitting device will be needed either at the head of the column or, if thermal desorption is used, in the desorption apparatus. It is of considerable advantage to have a fully automatic thermal desorber, with computer control of desorber, gas chromatograph and data handling, if the full potential of thermal desorption is to be gained.

CONTINUOUS MONITORING DEVICES

Introduction

Many devices offer the possibility of time-resolved measurement (Brief *et al.,* 1980; Gentry & Jones, 1984). These are generally fairly expensive instruments, but have direct read-out. Flammable gas detectors are non-specific, very insensitive for this application and not particularly stable. Portable GC detectors, flame-ionization (FID) or photoionization (PID), are more useful and are much more sensitive, but unless combined with a gas chromatograph (when they become intermittent rather than continuous) they are not specific. The FID is selective for molecules containing C-H and has a practical detection limit of about 5 mg/m^3 (~ 1 ppm). The PID is about 25 times more sensitive (for benzene) and has a larger dynamic range than the FID. It also offers some discrimination against aliphatic hydrocarbons if a lamp of appropriate ionization potential (10.3 eV) is used.

Safety concerns are of particular importance with flammable gas detectors, and such devices should be used in accordance with local safety regulations.

The only specific, continuous monitor of note is the portable infra-red analyser.

Exposimeters

Exposimeters are self-contained, portable meters which contain a heated catalytic sensor, usually a platinum filament or metal oxide "pellistor". Any flammable vapour (below its lower explosive limit) will burn on the filament, changing the temperature and hence the resistance of the latter. This change is measured electrically. The response of the instrument to different vapours differs greatly, although its response to flammable vapours varies very approximately with the weight per cent of the vapour in air. Most flammable gas detectors have a detection limit of around 500 mg/m^3 (~ 100 ppm) and precision (CV) of about 20%.

Portable GC detectors

The response of a flame-ionization detector in a gas chromatograph arises from ions generated in the flame during combustion of the column effluent. These ions may be monitored by measuring the current passing between two polarized electrodes adjacent to the flame. The same principle may be used in a portable instrument, in which air is sampled directly from the atmosphere and passed to a flame-ionization detector. The response is linear with concentration over 4 or 5 orders of magnitude, the limit of detection is about 5 mg/m^3 (~ 1 ppm) and the precision is about 10%.

The FID instrument measures total organic vapour. An obvious modification includes a GC column, in which case several vapours may be measured independently, but the instrument then becomes intermittent rather than truly continuous. Another modification employs a photoionization or other GC detector, when some selectivity of measurement may be obtained.

Infra-red analysers

Benzene, toluene and xylene may be measured with a reasonable degree of specificity with a portable infra-red analyser, fitted with a long-path-length cell. Benzene, toluene and xylene interfere with each other to some extent (cross sensitivity), and chlorobenzene interferes as well. The detection limit is about 5 mg/m^3 (~ 1 ppm) and the precision about 10%. It is necessary to remove CO_2 with an ascarite scrubber.

Advantages and disadvantages

The expense and bulk of continuous monitoring instruments make their usage limited. The advantage of on-site, continuous measurement is offset by the relative difficulty of using such devices for personal monitoring and by the inability to monitor at more than one place at a time. Since benzene, toluene and xylene in most industrial applications occur in a complex mixture of other organic compounds, the infra-red method is probably the most useful.

The possibility of installing sampling lines to a central instrument (as has been done for vinyl chloride) may be worth considering in some applications.

TYPICAL APPLICATIONS

Brown *et al.* (1981) describe the use of pumped porous-polymer adsorption tubes and diffusive porous-polymer tubes for the measurement of benzene vapour during tanker operations.

Joki (1980) describes the use of 3M Organic Vapour Monitors and charcoal tubes for the evaluation of exposure to benzene during benzene manufacture at three Shell locations. Berlin and Tunek (1984) review measurements of personal occupational exposure to benzene in Sweden during 1978. Dowd and Doyle (1984) review the literature on ambient concentrations and population exposure to benzene, toluene and xylene during 1980–82, and include data on petroleum refinery boundary and service station locations. The study by Clark *et al.* (1984) is also concerned primarily with ambient measurements, and provides a useful comparative study of a portable gas chromatograph/photoionization detector and the pumped porous-polymer adsorption tube method.

DIRECTORY OF EQUIPMENT AND SUPPLIERS

Equipment

Charcoal adsorption tubes
  MDA, SKC, Vinten, Sipin, Draeger
Thermal desorption tubes
  Perkin-Elmer, Century, EMS, Thorn EMI, AMA
Thermal desorber
  Perkin-Elmer, Chrompack, Quantitech, Spantech, SYPOL, Thorn EMI, Dani, Carlo-Erba, AMA
Carbon disulfide
  Merck, BDH, Rathburn
Diffusive samplers
  Dräger, 3M, DuPont, MSA, MDA, Perkin-Elmer
Gas bags
  SKC, Dräger, Sipin
Evacuated canisters
  SKC, Dräger, Sipin
Detector tubes
  Dräger, MSA, Gastec, Kitigawa
Gas chromatographs
  Varian, Hewlett-Packard, Perkin-Elmer, Carlo-Erba, Dani, Philips Analytical, Siemens, Shimadzu, Tracor, MSE
GC accessories
  Chromatography Services, Field Instruments Phase Separations, Chrompack
Exposimeters
  Dräger, SYPOL, Field Instruments, Vinten
Portable FID
  Quantitech, Vinten
Portable PID
  HNU, Photovac
Portable GC
  HNU, Vinten

Personal sampling pumps
  Dräger, Rotheroe-Mitchell, Sipin, SKC, MDA, DuPont
Infra-red analysers
  Foxboro

Addresses of suppliers

AMA GmbH,
Fichtestrasse 27,
4010 Hilden, FRG
tel (02103) 60494

BDH Chemicals Ltd.,
Broom Road,
Poole, Dorset, B12 4NN
UK
tel (0202) 745520

Carlo Erba Strumentazione SpA,
Strada Rivoltana,
20090 Rodana Mi,
Italy
tel (02) 95059.1

Chromatography Services Ltd.,
Carr Lane Industrial Estate,
Hoylake, Merseyside,
UK
tel (051) 632 5884

Chrompack International B.V.,
PO Box 3,
4330 Middleburg EA,
The Netherlands
tel (01180) 11251

Dani SpA,
Via Rovani 10,
20052 Monza (Milan),
Italy
tel (039) 323993

Draegerwerk AG,
Postfach 1339,
Moislinger Allee 53/55,
D 2400 Lübeck 1, FRG
tel (451) 8821

E.I. DuPont de Nemours & Co. Ltd.,
Clinical and Instrument Systems,
Concord Plaza,
Wilmington, DE,
USA
tel (302) 772 5451

Field Instruments Co. Ltd.,
374–378 Ewell Road,
Surbiton, Surrey, KT6 7BB
UK
tel (01) 299 6262

The Foxboro Co.,
Bristol Park,
Foxboro, MA,
USA
tel (617) 543 8750

Gastec Corp.,
Kitazawa Building,
2-23-10 Higashi,
Shibuya-Ku, Tokyo 150,
Japan
tel (03) 499 4498

Hewlett-Packard Co.,
Analytical Group,
Mailstop 30B3, PO Box 01301,
Palo Alto, CA 94303,
USA
tel (415) 857 5731

HNU Systems, Inc.,
160 Charlemont Street,
Newton, MA 02164,
USA
tel (617) 964 6690

Kitagawa,
Komyo Rikagaku K.K.,
660 Miyauchi,
Nakahara-Ku,
Kawasaki 211,
Japan
tel (044) 751 5511

3M (Minnesota Mining and
Manufacturing Co.),
3M Center,
St Paul, MN 551.44.1000,
USA
tel (612) 733 5454

MDA Scientific, Inc.,
405 Barclay Blvd.,
Lincolnshire, IL 60069,
USA
tel (312) 634 2800

E. Merck,
Frankfurter Str. 250,
Postfach 4119,
D 6100 Darmstadt, FRG
tel (06151) 72 2868

Mine Safety Appliances Co.,
Advanced Systems Div.,
PO Box 429,
Pittsburgh, PA 15230,
USA
tel (412) 538 3510

MSE Scientific Instruments,
(Div. of Fisons PLC),
Manor Royal,
Crawley, West Sussex RH10 2QQ
UK
tel (0293) 31100

Perkin-Elmer Ltd.,
Post Office Lane,
Beaconsfield, Bucks, HP9 1QA
UK
tel (04946) 6161

Phase Separations,
Deesside Industrial Estate,
Queenferry, Clwyd CH5 2LR
UK
tel (0244) 816444

Philips Analytical,
Eindoven,
The Netherlands
tel (040) 785 213

Photovac Inc.,
Unit 2, 134 Doncaster Road,
Thornhell, Ontario,
Canada L3T 1L3
tel (416) 881 8225

Quantitech Ltd.,
75 Garamond Drive,
Wymbush, Milton Keynes,
Bucks, MK8 8DD,
UK
tel (0908) 564141

Rathburn Chemicals Ltd.,
Caberston Road,
Walkerburn, Peeblesshire EH43 6AU
UK
tel (089687) 329

Rotheroe & Mitchell Ltd.,
Victoria Road,
Ruislip, Middlesex HA4 0YL
UK
tel (01) 422 9711

Shimadzu Scientific Instruments, Inc.,
7102 Riverside Road,
Columbia, MD 21046,
USA
tel (301) 997 1227

Siemens AG,
Abt. Analysentechnik, E68A,
Postfach 211080,
D 7500 Karlsruhe 21, FRG
tel (0721) 5951

Sipin International,
5 Portway Gardens,
Aynho, Banbury, Oxon OX13 3AR,
UK

SKC, Inc.,
334 Valley View Road,
Eighty Four, PA 15330,
USA
tel (412) 941 9701

Spantech Products Ltd.,
Spantech House, Lagham Road,
South Godstone, Surrey RH9 8HB
UK
tel (0342) 893239

SYPOL,
Market House, Market Square,
Aylesbury, Bucks, HP20 1TN
UK
tel (0296) 5715

Thorn EMI, Ltd.,
Bury Road,
Ruislip, Middlesex, HA4 7TA
UK
tel (08956) 30771

Tracor Instruments,
6500 Tracor Lane, Bldg. 27–7,
Austin, TX 78725,
USA
tel (512) 929 2023

Varian Associates, Inc.,
611 Hansen Way,
Palo Alto, CA 94303,
USA
tel (415) 493 4000

Vinten Instruments Ltd.,
Jessamy Road,
Weybridge, Surrey KT13 9LE
UK
tel (0932) 55721

REFERENCES

Americal Industrial Hygiene Association (1985) *Laboratory Accreditation,* Akron, OH

Baxter, H.G., Blakemore, R., Moore, J.P., Coker, D.T. & McCambley, W.H. (1980) The measurement of airborne benzene vapour. *Ann. occup. Hyg., 23,* 117–132

Berlin, M. & Tunek, A. (1984) *Benzene.* In: Aitio, A., Riihimäki, V. & Vainio, H., eds, *Biological Monitoring and Surveillance of Workers Exposed to Chemicals,* Washington DC, Hemisphere Publications, pp. 67–81

Brief, R.S., Lynch, J., Bernath, T. & Scala, R.A. (1980) Benzene in the workplace. *Am. Ind. Hyg. Assoc. J., 41,* 616–623

Brown, R.H., Charlton, J. & Saunders, K.J. (1981) The development of an improved diffusive sampler. *Am. Ind. Hyg. Assoc. J., 42,* 865–869

Bundesanstalt für Arbeitsschutz und Unfallforschung (1986) *Assessment and Evaluation of Poisonous or Health Hazardous Working Materials in the Air of Work Areas,* Dortmund

Cassinelli, M.E., Hull, R.D., Crable, J.V. & Teass, A.W. (1987) *Protocol for the evaluation of passive monitors.* Comm. Eur. Communities, Technical Report EUR 10555, pp. 190–202

CEFIC (1983) *CEFIC Criteria Document on Benzene,* Brussels, European Council of Chemical Manufacturers' Federations

Clark, A.I., McIntyre, A.E., Lester, J.N. & Perry, R.A. (1984) Comparison of photoionisation detection gas chromatography with a Tenax GC sampling tube procedure for the measurement of aromatic hydrocarbons in ambient air. *Int. J. Environ. Anal. Chem., 17,* 315–326

CONCAWE (1986) *Method for Monitoring Exposure to Gasoline Vapours in Air,* Den Haag

Detectawl (undated) *Gastec Precision Gas Detector System (Gastec "Blue Book")*

Dowd, R.M., Doyle, B.G. & Loyd, A.C. (1984) A review and evaluation of recent literature on ambient concentrations, emissions, modelling and population exposure to benzene, toluene and xylene. In: *Proc. 77th Ann. Meet. Air Pollut. Control Assoc., San Francisco, CA., June 1984,* Vol. 6

Eller, P.M., ed. (1984) *NIOSH Manual of Analytical Methods,* 3rd Ed., Cincinnati, OH, US Department of Health and Human Services Publ. 84–100

Gentry, S.J. & Jones, T.A. (1984) *Basic Principles of On-the-spot Sampling and Monitoring Techniques for Toxic Gases (Health & Safety Executive Internal Report No. IR/L/CS/84/5),* Sheffield

Health & Safety Executive (1972) *Benzene: Toluene & Xylene: Styrene (Methods for the Detection of Toxic Substances in Air Series No. 4),* London

Health & Safety Executive (1983a) *Benzene-in-air (Methods for the Determination of Hazardous Substances Series No. 17),* London

Health & Safety Executive (1983b) *Toluene-in-air (Methods for the Determination of Hazardous Substances Series No. 36),* London

Health & Safety Executive (1983c) *Benzene-in-air (Methods for the Determination of Hazardous Substances Series No. 22),* London

Health & Safety Executive (1983d) *Protocol for Assessing the Performance of a Diffusive Sampler (Methods for the Determination of Hazardous Substances Series No. 27)*, London

Health & Safety Executive (1984a) *Monitoring Strategies for Toxic Substances (Guidance Note EH 42)*, London

Health & Safety Executive (1984b) *Toluene-in-air (Methods for the Determination of Hazardous Substances Series No. 40)*, London

Health & Safety Executive (1985) *Benzene-in-air (Methods for the Determination of Hazardous Substances Series No. 50)*, London

Joki, H.M. (1980) *Passive Dosimeters I. An Evaluation of the 3M Brand OVM for Benzene Exposure (Shell Technical Progress Report WRC 113–80)*, Houston, TX

Kearney, C.A. & Dunham, D.B. (1986) Gasoline vapour exposures at a high volume service station. *Am. Ind. Hyg. Assoc. J., 47*, 535–539

Larkin, R.L., Crable, J.V., Catlett, L.R. & Seymour, M.J. (1973) Collaborative testing of a gas chromatographic charcoal tube method for seven organic solvents. *Am. Ind. Hyg. Assoc. J., 38*, 543–553

Leichnitz, K. (1980) Vergleich von Kurzzeit- und Langzeitmethoden zur Beurteilung der Schadstoffsituation am Arbeitsplatz. *Staub-Reinhalte-Luft, 40*, 241–243

Leichnitz, K. (1983) *Detector Tube Measuring Techniques*, Landsberg, Ecomed

Leichnitz, K. (1985) *Prüfröhrchen-Taschenbuch (Detector Tube Handbook)*, Lübeck, Draegerwerk AG

Leidel, N.A., Busch, K.A. & Lynch, J.R. (1977) *Occupational Exposure Sampling Strategy Manual*, Cincinnati, OH, US Department of Health and Human Resources Publ. 77–173

NIOSH (1984) *NIOSH Proficiency Analytical Testing (PAT) Program*, Cincinnati, OH, National Institute for Occupational Safety and Health, US Department of Health and Human Resources Publ. 83–121

Saunders, K.J. (1982) Techniques for atmospheric analysis. In: Albaiges, J., ed., *Analytical Techniques in Environmental Chemistry, 2*, Oxford, Pergamon Press, pp. 287–296

Walkin, K.T., Saunders, K.J. & Fields, B. (1985) *Back-up Data Report: Diffusive Tube Method for Benzene (MDHS 50) (Health & Safety Executive Internal Report IR/L/AO/85/12)*, London

White, L.D., Taylor, D.G., Mauer, P.A. & Kupel, R.E. (1970) A convenient optimized method for the analysis of selected solvent vapors in the industrial atmosphere. *Am. Ind. Hyg. Assoc. J., 31*, 225–232

CHAPTER 9

SAMPLING AND ANALYSIS OF AMBIENT AND INDOOR AIR

B. Seifert

Institute for Water, Soil and Air Hygiene,
Federal Health Office,
Berlin-Dahlem, FRG

SAMPLING STRATEGY

Introduction

The objectives of ambient and indoor air analyses are to measure concentration levels of pollutants, identify their sources and control compliance with air quality standards or guidelines. Analytical results depend mainly on three factors; (i) the sampling procedure, (ii) the analytical procedure, (iii) the sampling strategy. The importance of sampling strategy is sometimes largely underestimated. Besides the selection of the sampling site, both the frequency and duration of sampling will have an important influence on the reported result and will therefore be discussed in detail below.

Selection of the sampling site(s)

As for other air pollutants, the concentrations of benzene, toluene and xylenes in air vary both in time and space. The degree of variation depends on a number of factors, one of the most important being the quality of the emission source. For ambient air analyses, the two major types of sources to be considered are stationary sources (e.g., cokeries, refineries, gasoline stations) and line sources (e.g., traffic). In addition to the strength of the source and its variation with time, and to the dispersion of pollutants due to meteorological conditions, the distance of the source from the monitoring site will have a pronounced influence on the result of a measurement. Depending on the aim of the latter, area- or point-related analyses should be carried out.

Fett and Lahmann (1971) have devised an excellent strategy for recording the influence of a stationary source on the pollutant level in ambient air. Figure 1 gives the position of the sampling sites around the emitter. Sampling is carried out at the

Fig. 1. Sampling scheme for ambient air measurements in the vicinity of a source (according to Fett & Lahmann, 1971)
The distance between the sampling sites is determined by the stack height and the quantity of emitted pollutants.

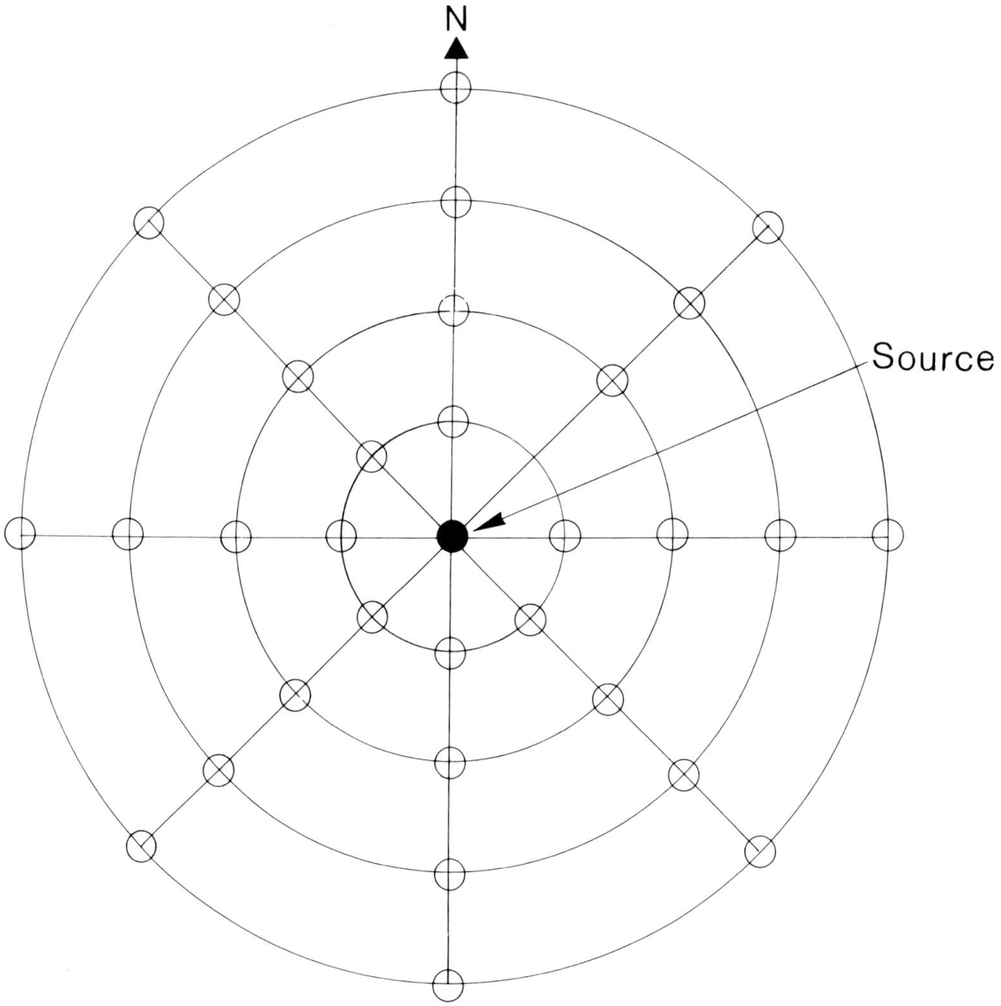

sites in the lee of the source (taking into account the wind direction during the sampling period), as significant pollutant concentrations are to be expected only at these sites. It may prove useful to add a number of measurements up-wind of the source, to determine the general level of aromatic hydrocarbons in the area.

Concentrations of aromatic hydrocarbons in ambient air may also be measured in order to determine the level of exposure of the population due to mobile sources, e.g., in a street with dense traffic. Due to the concentration gradient which has been observed for pollutants from automotive exhaust, e.g., CO and NO_x (Lahmann & Prescher, 1978), the inlet of the sampling line should be placed at about breathing height, in the middle or at the edge of the pedestrian walk.

With regard to the determination of air pollutants in indoor environments, literature concerning the selection of monitoring sites is scarce. The difficulty in selecting suitable sites arises from the variety of sources contributing to the final pollutant concentration. Since indoor measurements generally aim at characterizing occupant exposure levels, the monitoring site should be installed in the room where people spend the largest amount of time (generally the bedroom) or, to be on the safe side, where the highest concentrations are likely to be encountered. To facilitate the decision, a number of preliminary analyses may be necessary before starting the main study. Generally, it would also be useful to establish a source inventory.

The foregoing considerations concern measurements of the general pollutant level. If individual exposure is to be determined, personal sampling will be required. The monitoring site should then be mobile and vary according to the spaces which the individual occupies in the course of a day.

Frequency of sampling

For the sampling scheme described by Fett and Lahmann (1971), measurements have to be carried out under conditions of varying wind directions. To obtain an annual mean concentration, one- or two-day sampling series every two weeks (i.e., about 30 sampling days) have proved sufficient.

In the case of indoor environments, the source characteristics may have a stronger influence on the measured concentration, since the number of measurements has generally to be restricted to a much greater extent than in outdoor air studies. A classification of the different types of sources has been given by Seifert and Ullrich (1986). To overcome the principal difficulties, Seifert (1984a,b) has proposed the collection of one long-term sample (1–2 weeks) under the conditions normally encountered in the room, or one short-term sample (< 1 to 2 h) in the closed room, 2 to 3 h after window ventilation. The result would give the average concentration to be expected in the room. An additional short-term measurement under worst-case conditions (i.e., the room tightly closed for at least 24 h) would permit an estimate of the highest probable concentration. Similarly, a measurement in the well-ventilated room would indicate the lowest concentration to be expected. It is clear that this sampling strategy represents the minimum requirement for adequate characterization of the air quality in a room.

Duration of sampling

Since, in many cases, 30- or 60-min averages are specified for air quality standards related to health effects, these sampling intervals would be chosen preferentially to control compliance with the standards. However, attempts have been made to shorten this interval without introducing a bias.

If spot sampling is carried out (e.g., by using sample bags filled within an extremely short time), it has been recommended (VDI, 1979) to take five 'instantaneous' samples within every 30-min interval to check compliance with the standard. Frohne and Reis (1980), when analysing data sets from the determination of airborne aromatic hydrocarbons near a refinery, came to the conclusion that two such samples could be sufficient, provided that a fairly stable concentration level could be expected, with the coefficient of variation for five subsequent spot measurements not exceeding 40%. At a concentration level far below the level of the standard, even one sample could be satisfactory.

If the pollutant has to be concentrated on a sorbent, the only limiting factor with regard to the duration of sampling is the breakthrough volume. Although it is not possible to give a definite figure for this parameter, periods of time between a few minutes and several hours will normally be used in outdoor studies.

In studies devoted to indoor air, a longer sampling time is often required (see preceding section). The sampling interval may then be extended to one week or two. Such long-term sampling can be achieved with either active or passive sampling devices. If, on the other hand, short-term sampling has to be carried out in indoor air studies, procedures used for the workplace could also serve for the non-industrial indoor environment. Assuming a normal distribution of the pollutant concentration, several short-term samples taken at random will lead to the same average as one long-term sample covering the same period of time, as has been demonstrated by Leichnitz (1980) for toluene measurements over 4 h. However, in the case of larger temporal fluctuations of the concentration, repeated short-term sampling will underestimate the average.

Reporting guidelines

When reporting results, the rationale for the choice of the monitoring site should be given, as well as its precise description (height above ground, distance from potential sources). The date, time and duration of sampling should also be included. In addition, the meteorological conditions prevailing during sampling should be recorded for outdoor air measurements. The sampling report for indoor air measurements should contain information concerning the history of the room before starting to sample (ventilation status, sources) and, if possible, the ventilation rate, temperature and relative humidity.

SHORT-TERM SAMPLING TECHNIQUES

Introduction

Short-term sampling techniques lead to information which concerns only the very few seconds or minutes during which sampling takes place. Furthermore, such 'grab' sampling will generally only be possible in cases where concentrations high enough to permit direct analysis of the air sample can be expected.

Grab sampling

Aromatic hydrocarbons and other volatile organic compounds may be sampled by collecting the air to be investigated in a suitable vessel. Preferred materials for rigid vessels are glass (VDI, 1979; Nelson & Quigley, 1982) and stainless steel (Harsch, 1980; Rudolph et al., 1981). For reasons of practicability in the field, bags made from plastic materials are also used (c.f. Axelrod & Lodge, 1976). In both cases, it is important to choose materials which exclude losses of the analyte due to irreversible adsorption on the inner walls. Kudo et al. (1980) reported that polytetrafluoroethylene bags give the best results.

With rigid vessels, the air to be analysed is sampled by pumping it through the vessel for some time before closing the inlet and the outlet, or by opening the evacuated vessel at the sampling site. Bags are filled by pumping the sample air into them.

If the pollutant concentration is high enough, an aliquot of the air sample can be analysed directly by gas chromatography (GC). At lower concentrations, it is possible to draw the total air sample through an adsorption tube to concentrate the pollutants and to carry out the analysis as described below.

Indicator tubes

Unlike grab sampling, the use of indicator tubes excludes the need for analysis of the air mixture in the laboratory.

Using a small pump, the air sample is drawn through a commercially-prepared tube. The length of the resulting coloured zone indicates the concentration of the pollutant to which the tube is sensitive. Every stroke of the pump represents a fixed volume, generally 100 mL (Leichnitz, 1981). The air flow-rate depends on the pump characteristics and the packing (i.e., the resistance) of the tube. Pumps generally need between 3 and 40 s for one stroke (Drägerwerk AG, 1985).

For the determination of benzene, indicator tubes are available which are based on the formation of a brownish quinoid compound by reaction with formaldehyde in the presence of sulfuric acid. The working range of the most sensitive version of these tubes starts at the relatively high concentration of 0.5 ppm (~ 1.6 mg/m^3), and a relative standard deviation of 20–30% has been indicated for this level (Drägerwerk AG, 1985). Other aromatic hydrocarbons such as toluene and xylenes are also indicated.

The existing indicator tubes for toluene and o-xylene are even less suited for most ambient and indoor air measurements, since their working range starts only at several ppm.

Advantages and disadvantages

From the viewpoint of speed of analysis and expense, indicator tubes are certainly the most appropriate tool for determining benzene, toluene and xylenes in air. However, they are not specific and generally not sensitive enough to be used in routine ambient and indoor air analyses.

Grab sampling is also a rapid and inexpensive means of collecting samples. The subsequent analysis, however, requires a fully equipped chromatographic laboratory and skilled staff. On the other hand, the possibility of pre-concentration of the pollutants before the GC analysis represents an advantage, since it broadens the working range considerably.

INTEGRATED SAMPLING TECHNIQUES

Introduction

Due to restrictions in instrumentation and manpower, collecting integrated rather than time-resolved samples is often the only means of controlling outdoor and indoor air quality. However, from the point of view of health effects, this restriction does not represent a major drawback if the pollutants show long-term rather than acute effects. Since such is the case for benzene, and probably the other aromatic hydrocarbons, integrated sampling would be appropriate to check compliance with air quality standards, which may be defined on the basis of a 24-h up to a one-year average.

Integrated sampling may be carried out with or without the use of a pump. In the first case, the air is forced through a sorbent ("active" sampling), whereas, in the second case, the pollutants are trapped by permeation or diffusion processes ("passive" sampling). Both methods require an additional analytical step in the laboratory.

Adsorption tubes

In the combination sorbent/pump/gas meter, which is generally used for active sampling of volatile hydrocarbons, the sorbent plays the most important part. However, exact measurement of the sample volume should not be neglected.

To concentrate the pollutants, most authors have made use of adsorption tubes filled with charcoal (Mieure & Dietrich, 1973; Bertsch *et al.*, 1974; Burghardt & Jeltes, 1975; PedCo Environmental, 1978), silica gel (Sherwood, 1971; Gage *et al.*, 1977) and a number of sorbents used in GC, such as Tenax GC, Porapak or XAD resins (Gallant *et al.*, 1978; Ullrich & Seifert, 1978; Brown & Purnell, 1979). Brooks *et al.* (1979) have used an adsorption tube containing a mixture of several sorbents.

A number of disadvantages, such as the catalytic activity of charcoal which may give rise to secondary reactions, the adsorption of water vapour by silica gel and the thermal instability of Tenax GC at temperatures above 250 °C, limit the applicability of these sorbents. Melcher *et al.* (1978) have published criteria which permit the evaluation of such sorbents. However, it should be borne in mind that these criteria may not apply to tubes stored before analysis, as migration of adsorbed substances may occur within the tube during storage.

One of the most important considerations in long-term sampling with adsorption tubes is to guarantee quantitative adsorption, even over a longer period of time. The collection efficiency is generally expressed by the breakthrough volume, which is a function of other parameters; e.g., the nature of the sorbent, the properties and the concentration of the pollutant, the geometry of the adsorption tube, the air flow rate, the humidity and the temperature at which the sorbent is held. Breakthrough volumes for numerous compounds on Tenax-GC have been listed by Brown and Purnell (1979). As a general rule, losses are likely to have occurred if more than 25% of the total amount of a collected compound is found adsorbed on the last third of the tube packing (Melcher *et al.*, 1978).

Since the temperature may have a considerable impact on the collection efficiency, especially for compounds with boiling points below 100 °C, attempts have been made to keep the adsorption tube at low temperatures during sampling (Ullrich & Seifert, 1978). However, the use of such procedures is restricted by the need for cumbersome equipment and the fact that water vapour is also trapped. The availability of mixed-sorbent tubes has reduced the necessity to sample at temperatures below the ambient level (Averill & Purcell, 1978; Brooks *et al.*, 1979).

Depending on the sorbent used, the trapped hydrocarbons are desorbed thermally or by liquid (solvent) extraction.

Sampling with subsequent thermal desorption

On heating the sorbent, the pollutants are desorbed into the carrier gas stream. To obtain optimal separation, the compounds are again concentrated on a cooled trap installed in front of the GC capillary column, or at the cooled head of the column if packed columns are used. The fact that the whole sample is transferred to the column results in good sensitivity.

With 1-L samples of air, concentrations of benzene, toluene and xylenes down to 0.1 µg/m^3 can be determined. The upper limit of the working range depends on the analytical instrument. If the sample is not split, generally not more than 100 ng per sample can be tolerated if good performance of the GC column is desired. Assuming a 1-L air sample, the resulting upper concentration limit would be 100 µg/m^3.

For 10 samples of calibration gas mixtures containing 31, 66 and 16.8 µg/m^3 of benzene, toluene and *m*-xylene, respectively, on a mixed sorbent (Tenax-GC, Carbosieve S), subsequent GC analysis on a CP-Sil8 capillary column gave relative standard deviations of 9, 3 and 5%, respectively (VDI, 1985).

A comparative study of various techniques for determining aromatic hydrocarbons at levels below 40 µg/m^3 has shown that thermal desorption appears to be less reproducible and accurate than solvent desorption (Dahmann *et al.*, 1985). However, the thermal desorption technique was represented by a much smaller data set and does not readily permit working with an internal standard. In addition, slight variations of the blank between single runs cannot be excluded for aromatic hydrocarbons, since the porous polymers used as adsorbents (Tenax-GC, XAD resins) are chemically based on an aromatic structure.

Sampling with subsequent solvent desorption

There are various situations which require repetitive analyses of a sample. Such repetition, which is generally unusual when using thermal desorption (although not impossible if the sample is split and the waste is collected on an adsorbent tube), can be readily carried out using a solvent to desorb the pollutants. The adsorption tube/solvent system generally used is charcoal/carbon disulfide. The standardized (NIOSH) charcoal tubes (see Chapter 8) which have been developed for analysing workplace atmospheres are also suitable for non-occupational environments. With these tubes, the adsorbent is removed from the tube after sampling, then extracted with the solvent.

Besides NIOSH tubes, home-made adsorption tubes filled with charcoal can be used (VDI, 1984a,b). These tubes offer the advantage of being re-usable, because the trapped compounds are eluted while the sorbent remains in the tube. For work with home-made tubes, it should be borne in mind that different batches of the same brand of charcoal may vary in their collection and recovery properties. The frequent running of blanks is therefore of the utmost importance. Flushing the tubes with methanol/diethylether from time to time results in better performance (VDI, 1984a). It is also necessary to check the purity of the carbon disulfide, which has frequently been found to contain benzene. The purification can be achieved by distillation (VDI, 1984b) or other means (Riddic & Bunger, 1970).

As charcoal tubes are used exclusively at ambient temperatures, the breakthrough volume has to be carefully determined. At a benzene concentration of 30 $\mu g/m^3$, NIOSH tubes would permit the sampling of about 100 L of air without loss of benzene. This corresponds to a 1-h sample. For the tubes described in the VDI guideline, a 5% loss of benzene has been reported for a 120-L air sample, whereas toluene and the higher aromatic hydrocarbons showed breakthrough losses below 1% (VDI, 1984a).

Passive sampling

In the course of the last decade it has become more and more evident that only a small portion of human exposure outside the workplace area can be predicted using data from fixed outdoor-air monitoring stations. Although personal monitoring devices had been introduced at workplaces as early as about 1960 (Namiesnik *et al.,* 1984), such devices have as yet only been used in a few smaller studies to measure the exposure of the general public (e.g., WHO, 1982a,b). The main reason for this restriction was the need for a pump, which resulted in a relatively high cost per sampling unit and caused the latter to be noisy and relatively heavy.

With the above disadvantages in mind, another type of personal sampler, the passive sampler, was developed. A passive sampler collects the pollutant by permeation or diffusion processes. Although the best-known passive sampler is probably that for nitrogen dioxide (Palmes *et al.,* 1976), a number of passive samplers for organic substances, including benzene, toluene and xylenes, have become available in recent years.

Passive samplers have been described and tested (Bamberger *et al.,* 1978; Abraham & Seifert, 1981; Sefton *et al.,* 1981; Coutant & Scott, 1982; Seifert & Abraham, 1983;

Namiesnik *et al.*, 1984), and have also been compared with each other and with active sampling with charcoal (Hickey & Bishop, 1981; Voelte & Weir, 1981; van der Wal, 1981). Since most of the inter-comparison measurements were carried out at concentrations much higher than 1 mg/m^3, little was learned about the performance of passive samplers at the concentration levels generally found in ambient and indoor air. From the results of two European inter-comparison programmes (de Bortoli *et al.*, 1984, 1986), however, it can be concluded that volatile organic substances, including aromatic hydrocarbons, can be determined with a reproductibility of about 20% at concentrations between 30 and 300 μg/m^3. For non-polar compounds, such as *o*-xylene, a close agreement between the results of OVM-3500 passive samplers (3M Company) and those obtained from active sampling with thermal desorption could be obtained.

At the concentration levels encountered in ambient and indoor air, passive samplers for volatile organic compounds would have to be exposed for a much longer time than the 8 h normally foreseen for occupational studies. An appropriate time interval may be two weeks.

Advantages and disadvantages

When comparing sampling with an adsorption tube to sampling with a passive device, it appears that better reproducibility and more accurate results are obtained with the former. Provided an exact calibration of the pump and a careful determination of the breakthrough volume can be guaranteed, results which are accurate to within ± 10% can be achieved for concentrations found in ambient and indoor air.

When sampling is followed by thermal desorption, the sample is totally consumed during the analysis, so that no replicates are possible. Despite this drawback, the thermal desorption technique is often used in practice if, in addition to benzene, toluene and xylenes, the simultaneous quantitative trapping of organic substances down to at least C$_3$ is desired. In this case, sampling with charcoal and subsequent solvent desorption is not appropriate, since the cited substances cannot be trapped quantitatively due to their low breakthrough volume on charcoal.

Although liquid desorption has a number of advantages, its use is limited by the availability of a sufficiently pure solvent. Carbon disulfide, in particular, which is used in the majority of procedures, has been found to be contaminated by benzene.

Passive samplers are advantageous if a low-cost, low-noise and easy-to-handle sampling procedure is needed. In such a situation, they are in many cases superior to adsorption tubes for determining personal exposure or contamination of the air in non-occupational areas. One of the disadvantages of passive samplers may be the need for relatively long exposure periods, resulting in low time-resolution of the measured concentrations. However, this aspect is of minor importance if carcinogenic substances such as benzene are to be analysed. For the determination of benzene, toluene and xylenes in ambient and indoor air, measurements which are accurate to within ± 20% can be expected with passive samplers.

Table 1.   Repeatability and reproducibility from tests using VDI guidelines to determine aromatic hydrocarbons in test gases (from Dahmann *et al.*, 1985)

Substance	Concentration (μg/m³)	Repeatability (r)[a] (%)		Reproducibility (R)[b] (%)	
		solvent desorption	thermal desorption	solvent desorption	thermal desorption
Benzene	10–30	16–80	20–50	75–200	120–330
Toluene	1–3	20–50	25–135	100–500	140–450
p-Xylene	10–30	17–60	20–60	65–315	130–320

[a] $r = 100 \sqrt{2}\, t\, s_r/\bar{x}$
[b] $R = 100 \sqrt{2}\, t\, s_R/\bar{x}$
where $\bar{x}$ = arithmetic average
t = Student's factor
s_r = within-laboratory standard deviation
s_R = between-laboratory standard deviation

ANALYTICAL TECHNIQUES

Following the sampling procedure, the separation and determination of benzene, toluene and xylenes are generally carried out by GC. Although packed GC columns may be used (VDI, 1984b), the majority of procedures prescribe the use of capillary columns. Information concerning packed and capillary columns which are particularly useful for separating aromatic hydrocarbons has been collected (Umweltbundesamt, 1982).

A flame-ionization detector is generally used with the GC column, and shows a linear dynamic range of up to 10^6. The lowest detectable amount of substance is of the order of 0.1 ng. Standard solutions are used to determine the response of the detector. Benzene has a higher response than the other aromatic hydrocarbons discussed here.

The analytical procedure, including the sampling step, should be calibrated with test gases of known concentrations. For concentrations between $1\ \mu g/m^3$ and $100\ \mu g/m^3$, such test gases can be generated using permeation systems (VDI, 1980).

To check the analytical procedures described in VDI guidelines for the determination of organic compounds (VDI, 1979, 1984a,b, 1985), three inter-laboratory tests were conducted (Frohne *et al.*, 1981, 1983; Dahmann *et al.*, 1985) using calibration gas mixtures containing benzene, toluene and *p*-xylene at concentrations below $100\ \mu g/m^3$. The average concentrations reported by the participating laboratories were generally in good agreement with the true (given) values. As could be expected, the repeatability (within one laboratory) was much better than the reproducibility (between different laboratories). The observed repeatabilities and reproducibilities for the last of these tests (Dahmann *et al.*, 1985), in which 23 laboratories participated and extremely low concentrations were chosen, are summarized in Table 1.

CONTINUOUS MONITORING

At workplaces, real-time monitoring of aromatic hydrocarbons is often carried out with infra-red analysers (see Chapter 8). For ambient or indoor air studies, such analysers are not sensitive enough because they cover only the low parts-per-million to percent concentration range. In addition, these instruments do not permit the separate determination of benzene, toluene and xylenes, but indicate the sum of all the aromatic compounds present.

Similarly, non-methane hydrocarbon analysers (which are mostly equipped with flame-ionization detectors), although somewhat more sensitive, do not permit discrete determinations of single substances unless they are used in combination with a GC column. This would mean, however, that the data are no longer generated in a real-time mode.

To date, the most sensitive detector for aromatic hydrocarbons is the photoionization detector (PID). Automatic instruments using a PID are commercially available and can be used as quasi-continuous monitors for benzene, toluene and xylenes. The instruments inject a known volume of air (grab sample, with about 1 s sampling time) onto a GC column. The total time for one analytical cycle is of the order of several minutes (Nutmagul *et al.*, 1983). With PID/GC combinations, the detection limit for aromatic hydrocarbons varies between 0.6 and 1.3 pg (Hester & Meyer, 1979; Clark *et al.*, 1984). Using a 1-mL injection volume, this would permit the determination of around 1 $\mu g/m^3$. This low limit of detection makes PID/GC systems particularly useful for most outdoor and indoor applications. Satisfactory results were reported from outdoor air studies in California, USA (Hester & Meyer, 1979), London, UK (Clark *et al.*, 1984) and Berlin (West), FRG (Häntzsch, 1986).

DIRECTORY OF EQUIPMENT

See Chapter 8.

REFERENCES

Abraham, H.J. & Seifert, B. (1981) Passivsammler nach dem Diffusionsprinzip als Hilfsmittel zur Bestimmung der individuellen Schadstoffbelastung in Aussen- und Innenluft. In: Leschber, R. & Rühle, H., eds, *Aktuelle Fragen der Umwelthygiene. Schriftenreihe Verein für Wasser-, Boden- und Lufthygiene No. 52,* Stuttgart, Gustav Fischer, pp. 363–380

Averill, W. & Purcell, J.E. (1978) Concentration and GC determination of organic compounds from air and water. *Chromatogr. Newslett.,* **6,** 30–32

Axelrod, H.D. & Lodge, J.P. (1976) Sampling and calibration of gaseous pollutants. In: Stern, A.C., ed., *Air Pollution,* Vol. III, 3rd Ed., New York, Academic Press, pp. 145–182

Bamberger, R.L., Esposito, G.G., Jacobs, B.W., Podlak, G.E. & Mazur, J.F. (1978) A new personal sampler for organic vapors. *Am. Ind. Hyg. Assoc. J.,* **39,** 701–708

Bertsch, W., Chany, R.C. & Zlatkis, A. (1974) The determination of organic volatiles in air pollution studies. Characterisation of profiles. *J. Chromatogr. Sci., 12,* 175–184

Bortoli, M. de, Knöppel, H., Mølhave, L., Seifert, B. & Ullrich, D. (1984) *Interlaboratory Comparison of Passive Samplers for Organic Vapours with Respect to their Applicability to Indoor Air Pollution Monitoring: A Pilot Study,* Commission of the European Communities, Report EUR 9450 EN, Luxembourg

Bortoli, M. de, Mølhave, L., Thorsen, M.A. & Ullrich, D. (1986) *European Interlaboratory Comparison of Passive Samplers for Organic Vapour Monitoring in Indoor Air,* Commission of the European Communities, Report EUR 10487, Brussels

Brooks, J.J., West, D.S., David, D.J. & Mulik, J.D. (1979) *A Combination Sorbent System for Broad Range Organic Sampling in Air,* U.S. Environmental Protection Agency, Report 600/g–79–032

Brown, R.H. & Purnell, C.J. (1979) Collection and analysis of trace vapour pollutants in ambient atmospheres. The performance of a Tenax-GC adsorbent tube. *J. Chromatogr., 179,* 79–90

Burghardt, E. & Jeltes, R. (1975) Gas-chromatographic determination of aromatic hydrocarbons in air using a semi-automatic preconcentration method. *Atmos. Environ., 9,* 935–940

Clark, A.I., McIntyre, A.E., Lester, J.N. & Perry, R. (1984) A comparison of photoionisation detection gas chromatography with a Tenax GC sampling tube procedure for the measurement of aromatic hydrocarbons in ambient air. *Int. J. Environ. Anal. Chem., 17,* 315–326

Coutant, R.W. & Scott, D.R. (1982) Applicability of passive dosimeters for ambient air monitoring of toxic organic compounds. *Environ. Sci. Technol., 16,* 410–413

Dahmann, D., Frohne, J.-C. & Manns, H. (1985) Dritte VDI-Vergleichsmessung Aromaten. *Staub-Reinhalt. Luft, 45,* 359–362

Drägerwerk AG (1985) *Prüfröhrchen Taschenbuch. Luftuntersuchungen und technische Gasanalyse mit Dräger-Röhrchen,* Lübeck

Fett, W. & Lahmann, E. (1971) Zur Bewertung der Immissionen in der Umgebung einer Einzelquelle. *Staub-Reinhalt. Luft, 31,* 200–205

Frohne, J.-C. & Reis, J. (1980) Zur Ermittlung von Immissionskenngrössen mit Momentprobenverfahren. *Staub-Reinhalt. Luft, 40,* 522–529

Frohne, J.-C., Reis, J. & Werner, W. (1981) VDI-Ringversuch «Immissions-messungen Aromaten». *Staub-Reinhalt. Luft, 41,* 8–13

Gage, J.C., Lagesson, V. & Tunek, A. (1977) A method for the determination of low concentrations of organic vapors in air and exhaled breath. *Ann. Occup. Hyg., 20,* 127–134

Gallant, R.F., King, J.W., Levins, P.L. & Piecewicz, J.F. (1978) *Characterization of Sorbent Resins for Use in Environmental Sampling,* U.S. Environmental Protection Agency, Report 600/7–78–054, March 1978

Häntzsch, S. (1986) Kfz-bedingte Immissionen in Berlin – Aktueller Stand. In: Seifert, B., ed., *Luftverunreinigungen durch Kraftfahrzeuge in der Bundesrepublik Deutschland. Stand und Trend. Schriftenreihe Verein für Wasser-, Boden- und Lufthygiene,* Stuttgart, Gustav Fischer, pp. 29–48

Harsch, D.E. (1980) Evaluation of a versatile gas sampling container design. *Atmos. Environ.*, *14*, 1105–1107

Hester, N.E. & Meyer, R.A. (1979) A sensitive technique for measurement of benzene and alkylbenzenes in air. *Environ. Sci. Technol.*, *13*, 107–109

Hickey, J.L.S. & Bishop, C.C. (1981) Field comparison of charcoal tubes and passive vapor monitors with mixed organic vapors. *Am. Ind. Hyg. Assoc. J.*, *42*, 264–267

Kudo, M., Tanaka, N. & Kimura, J. (1980) Retention of organic solvent vapors in plastic bags. II. *Sangyo Igaku*, *22*, 278–279 (*Chem. Abstr.*, *94*, 196697r (1981))

Lahmann, E. & Prescher, K.-E. (1978) Räumliche und zeitliche Verteilung von Stickstoffoxiden in städtischer Luft. *Ges. Ing.*, *99*, 32–36

Leichnitz, K. (1980) Vergleich von Kurzzeit- und Langzeitmethode zur Beurteilung der Schadstoffsituation an Arbeitsplätzen. *Staub-Reinhalt. Luft*, *40*, 241–243

Leichnitz, K. (1981) *Prüfröhrchen-Messtechnik*, Landsberg/Lech, Ecomed-Verlagsgesellschaft

Melcher, R.G., Langner, R.R. & Kagel, R.O. (1978) Criteria for the evaluation of methods for the collection of organic pollutants in air using solid sorbents. *Am. Ind. Hyg. Assoc. J.*, *39*, 349–361

Mieure, J.P. & Dietrich, M.W. (1973) Determination of trace organics in air and water. *J. Chromatogr. Sci.*, *11*, 559–570

Namiesnik, J., Gorecki, T., Kozlowski, E., Torres, L. & Mathieu, J. (1984) Passive dosimeters – an approach to atmospheric pollutants analysis. *Sci. Total Environ.*, *38*, 225–258

Nelson, P.F. & Quigley, S.M. (1982) Non-methane hydrocarbons in the atmosphere of Sydney, Australia. *Environ. Sci. Technol.*, *16*, 650–655

Nutmagul, W., Cronn, D.R. & Hill, H.H. (1983) Photoionization/flame-ionization detection of atmospheric hydrocarbons after capillary gas chromatography. *Anal. Chem.*, *55*, 2160–2164

Palmes, E.D., Gunnison, A.F., DiMattio, J. & Tomczyk, C. (1976) Personal sampler for nitrogen dioxide. *Am. Ind. Hyg. Assoc. J.*, *37*, 570–577

PedCo Environmental (1978) *Tentative Method for the Determination of Benzene in the Atmosphere by 24 hrs. Integrated Sampling*, Contract U.S. Environmental Protection Agency No. 68-02-2722, November 1978

Riddic, J.A. & Bunger, W.B., eds (1970) *Technique of Chemistry*, Vol. II: *Organic Solvents*, 3rd Ed., New York, Wiley-Interscience

Rudolph, J., Ehhalt, D.H., Khedim, A. & Jebsen, C. (1981) Determination of C_2–C_5 hydrocarbons in the atmosphere at low parts per 10^9 to high parts per 10^{12} levels. *J. Chromatogr.*, *217*, 301–310

Sefton, M.V., Mastracci, E.L. & Mann, J.L. (1981) Rubber disk passive monitor for benzene dosimeter. *Anal. Chem.*, *53*, 458–461

Seifert, B. (1984a) Planung und Durchführung von Luftmessungen in Innenräumen. *Haustech. Bauphys. Umwelttech. Ges. Ing.*, *105*, 15–18

Seifert, B. (1984b) A sampling strategy for the representative characterisation of the chemical composition of indoor air. In: Berglund, B., Lindvall, T. & Sundell, J., eds, *Indoor Air*, Vol. 4, *Chemical Characterization and Personal Exposure*, Stockholm, Swedish Council for Building Research, pp. 361–366

Seifert, B. & Abraham, H.-J. (1983) Use of passive samplers for the determination of gaseous organic substances in indoor air at low concentration levels. *Int. J. Environ. Anal. Chem., 13*, 237–253

Seifert, B. & Ullrich, D. (1986) Methodologies for evaluating sources of volatile organic chemicals (VOC) in homes. *Atmos. Environ., 21*, 395–404

Sherwood, R.J. (1971) The monitoring of benzene exposure by air sampling. *Am. Ind. Hyg. Assoc. J., 32*, 840–846

Ullrich, D. & Seifert, B. (1978) Gas-chromatographische Analyse von Kohlenwasserstoffen in der Aussenluft nach Probenahme mit dem Tieftemperatur-Gradientenrohr. *Fresenius' Z. Anal. Chem., 291*, 299–307

Umweltbundesamt (1982) *Luftqualitätskriterien für Benzol,* Berichte 6/82, Berlin (West), Erich Schmidt Verlag

VDI (Verein Deutscher Ingenieure) (1979) VDI-Richtlinie 3482, Blatt 3, *Messen gasförmiger Immissionen. Gaschromatographische Bestimmung von aromatischen Kohlenwasserstoffen – Momentprobenahme,* VDI-Handbuch Reinhalt. Luft, Düsseldorf

VDI (Verein Deutscher Ingenieure) (1980) VDI-Richtlinie 3490, Blatt 9, *Messen von Gasen. Prüfgase. Herstellung durch Permeation der Beimengung in einen Grundgasstrom,* VDI-Handbuch Reinhalt. Luft, Düsseldorf

VDI (Verein Deutscher Ingenieure) (1984a) VDI-Richtlinie 3482, Blatt 4, *Measurement of Gaseous Emissions. Gaschromatographic Determination of Organic Compounds Using Capillary Columns. Sampling by Enrichment on Activated Carbon. Desorption with Solvent (Issue German/English),* VDI-Handbuch Reinhalt. Luft, Düsseldorf

VDI (Verein Deutscher Ingenieure) (1984b) VDI-Richtlinie 3482, Blatt 5, *Measurement of Gaseous Emissions. Gaschromatographic Determination of Aromatic Hydrocarbons. Sampling by Enrichment on Activated Carbon. Desorption with Solvent (Issue German/English),* VDI-Handbuch Reinhalt. Luft, Düsseldorf

VDI (Verein Deutscher Ingenieure) (1985) VDI-Richtlinie 3482, Blatt 6, *Messen gasförmiger Immissionen. Gaschromatographische Bestimmung organischer Verbindungen – Probenahme durch Anreicherung – Thermische Desorption (Draft),* VDI-Handbuch Reinhalt. Luft, Düsseldorf

Voelte, D.R. & Weir, F.W. (1981) A dynamic-flow chamber comparison of three passive organic vapor monitors with charcoal tubes under single and multiple solvent exposure conditions. *Am. Ind. Hyg. Assoc. J., 42*, 845–852

van der Wal, J.F. (1981) *Onderzoek naar het Gedrag von Diffusiegasbadges,* Inst. voor Milieuhygiene en Gezondheidstechniek TNO, Report F 1857, Delft

WHO (World Health Organization) (1982a) *Human exposure to Carbon Monoxide and Suspended Particulate Matter in Zagreb, Yugoslavia (WHO Report EFP/82.33),* Geneva

WHO (World Health Organization) (1982b) *Human Exposure to SO₂, NO₂ and Suspended Particulate Matter in Toronto, Canada (WHO Report EFP/82.38),* Geneva

CHAPTER 10

CHEMICAL WASTE DISPOSAL SITES: SAMPLING AND ANALYSIS

R.A. Zweidinger & L.S. Sheldon

Research Triangle Institute
Research Triangle Park, North Carolina 27709, USA

INTRODUCTION

While benzene, toluene and xylenes are liquids at normal ambient temperatures, they all have significant vapour pressures. For this reason, consideration must be given to volatilization and transport in the atmosphere, as well as leaching in soils and transport through aquifers, when developing a sampling plan. Volatility is also important when applying sampling and analysis methods. Some aspects of sampling and analysis which are independent of analyte properties will also be included in the following discussion.

Identifying objectives is one of the first and most important steps in determining the choice of sampling and analytical procedures. In the case of a waste disposal site, one of the primary questions is whether contamination by the analyte of interest is below a predetermined level. In practice, it is not sufficient to show that the average concentration is below a threshold level above which remedial action is required. Rather, it must be demonstrated that the average concentration, plus a certain confidence interval, is below the threshold level (EPA, 1986). The confidence interval is determined by the precision of the measurement, which thus has a direct influence on decisions concerning remedial action. The estimation of the confidence interval includes variability introduced by the sampling strategy and the sampling and analysis methods. These factors and their effect on the confidence interval are discussed below.

SAMPLING STRATEGY

Sampling variability is estimated by using a probability sampling strategy. In the simplest case, probability sampling may involve a three-dimensional grid superimposed on the site. The locations at which samples are collected are determined by a random number table (or generator) and the numbered locations on the grid.

This approach presumes that the contaminant is randomly dispersed throughout the volume (or area) of the site. Where this is not the case, large variances and a broad confidence interval will result. If prior information or preliminary sampling suggests that there are areas of the site which have distinctly different contamination levels, these areas can be sampled and analysed separately to give a stratified random sample.

The choice between simple random sampling and stratified random sampling should be viewed in terms of allocation of resources and remedial actions which might be required. In the case of simple random sampling, the assumption is made that the waste disposal site represents a single population of contamination levels randomly distributed throughout. The variance obtained from a random selection of samples should give an estimate of the variance of contamination levels within the site. As this variance increases, the confidence interval for the average contamination level will also increase, and the average contamination level must be lower before it can be asserted that a particular threshold has not been exceeded at a given confidence level (usually 80% [Ford *et al.*, 1983]). If the variation in contamination level is not randomly distributed, the site may be stratified into "high", "medium", and "low" areas which are randomly sampled. If the contamination levels are indeed different in the designated areas, the variances for each area will be reduced. The narrower confidence interval that results may, in fact, eliminate some or all of the areas from remedial action.

Stratified random sampling, in general, requires a larger number of samples and analyses than simple random sampling, but may result in reduced remedial action. The costs of these two activities must be considered when choosing the sampling strategy.

The number and size of the samples collected may also affect the outcome of the sampling and analysis effort. If the cost of collecting additional samples beyond the planned minimum is not severe, then it is generally desirable to collect extra samples. These extra samples may be analysed if the variance and confidence interval are slightly larger than desired, since the additional analyses will tend to reduce both the variance and the confidence interval.

The amount of material collected at each sampling location can also influence the outcome of the effort. The larger the amount of material taken and analysed, the less influence local variation will have on the determination, provided the sample has been well homogenized before aliquots are taken. Another approach is to combine several discrete samples within the location identified on the site grid. The effect of combining the samples is similar to that of collecting a larger volume of sample; each reduces the variance by smoothing out local concentration variations. Unfortunately, both of these approaches may introduce errors caused by volatilization of analytes during combining or aliquoting operations.

Some sites, such as lagoons, are amenable to a modification of random sampling termed "systematic" random sampling. In systematic random sampling, the starting point is randomly selected and subsequent samples are taken at regular intervals along a transect starting at that point. This approach is used where location of the sampling points on a grid would be especially difficult. In the case of a lagoon, a point on the edge would be selected at random and samples would be collected at predetermined intervals along a transect perpendicular to the edge.

Any information which would indicate the existence of areas of higher or lower levels of contamination would, of course, be useful in determining whether to use stratified or simple random sampling. The history and topography of the site may help to decide whether a two-dimensional evaluation would be appropriate or whether depth must also be considered. Depth may be stratified, especially at the intended boundary of the site. If the sampling is stratified by depth, then penetration into the soil and, ultimately, to aquifers can be detected.

Contamination beyond the boundaries of the waste site should be considered, especially with compounds such as benzene, toluene, and xylenes, where migration can occur through several processes (leaching, volatilization, etc.). Obviously, off-site and on-site sampling should involve separate strata. Further stratification may include direction or distance as criteria for defining a stratum. For an introduction to probability sampling, the reader is referred to Cochran (1977).

SAMPLING METHODS

The sample collection procedure must take into account the physical state of the waste to be sampled and the fact that volatility losses can occur while transferring the sample from the collection site to the final container. In the case of benzene, toluene and xylenes, the waste may well be a free-flowing liquid or slurry contained in drums, shallow open-top tanks, pits or similar containers. These wastes are best sampled using a Coliwasa (Composite Liquid Waste Sampler), which incorporates a tube long enough to sample the full depth of the liquid waste (Ford *et al.,* 1983; EPA, 1986). The tube is fitted with a closure that can be operated from the top. This closure is usually a stopper at the end of a rod which runs through the tube and extends beyond it. Once the tube is filled with liquid waste, the stopper is pulled into the tube, which is then withdrawn, and the sample transferred to an appropriate container. If possible, the transfer should be performed using a closed system to prevent volatility losses. Where this is not possible, the transfer should be made as rapidly as possible and the container sealed immediately. The Coliwasa should be constructed from glass, metal or fluorocarbon polymer to avoid sample alterations associated with the use of plastics.

Other commonly used samplers for liquid wastes are weighted bottles and dippers (Ford *et al.,* 1983; EPA, 1986). The weighted bottle consists of a glass or fluorocarbon polymer bottle with a stopper, plus a line to remove the stopper and retrieve the bottle. The clean, empty bottle with stopper in place is lowered to the desired depth; the stopper is jerked free with the line and the bottle retrieved after it has filled with sample. The sampling bottle in this device can serve as the sample container, and a sample with no head-space is thereby obtained, thus minimizing volatility losses. For this reason, the weighted bottle is especially suitable for volatile compounds such as the aromatic solvents.

A third liquid sample collection device consists of a dipper on a pole. The dipper itself is a glass or fluorocarbon beaker, clamped to the end of an aluminum telescoping pole. This sampling device is suitable for collecting surface liquid samples only. The presence of organic films on the surface of the waste presents a special problem for sampling, especially with a dipper. The benzene, toluene or xylenes may be much more concentrated in this organic layer than in the bulk of the waste, and the portion of the organic layer sampled relative to the bulk of the waste can vary, causing substantial sampling error. Care must be taken to collect a representative surface sample. Unfortunately, this device does not provide any mechanism for minimizing volatility losses.

Other devices, such as peristaltic pumps, have been used for environmental applications (Ford *et al.*, 1983). However, these pumps are relatively expensive and must be decontaminated between samples. Decontamination at the site can prove difficult and time consuming. On the other hand, sampling devices such as the Coliwasa, weighted bottle and dipper can be sufficiently inexpensive to use as disposable samplers, thereby removing the need to decontaminate the sampling device in the field.

Solids can be sampled with several different devices, depending upon the nature and consistency of the solid. Readily accessible sludges, moist powders or granules and soils may be sampled with a trier (Ford *et al.*, 1983; EPA, 1986). A trier is a tube cut in half, lengthwise, with one end sharpened. A handle may be affixed to the unsharpened end to assist in its manipulation. The trier is inserted into the material to be sampled, rotated to produce a core, and the core lifted out.

Dry powders and granules may be sampled with a thief, which consists of two concentric tubes with matching slots and a pointed tip (Ford *et al.*, 1983; EPA, 1986). The thief is forced into the sample and the slots are aligned by rotating the inner tube, allowing the sample to flow into the thief. The inner tube is rotated again to close the slots, and the thief with the sample is removed.

An auger is used to sample heavy or packed materials or soils. The auger consists of sharpened spiral blades on a rigid metal shaft. The sharpened lower edges of the blades cut or shave the material and lift it to the surface. The auger may be used in one of two ways: either the shavings can be collected by passing the auger through a hole in a collection pan, such as an aluminium pie pan (Ford *et al.*, 1983), or a hole may be bored to the desired depth with the auger and a thin-walled tube corer used to remove the sample (EPA, 1986). When sampling at several depths, or when precisely-known depths are required, the use of the corer with the auger is advisable. This system can be used to depths of 6 m or more. However, unfavourable conditions such as rocks or borehole walls which collapse may limit the depths attainable.

Solid wastes may be sampled with scoops or shovels when the material is granular or powdered and easily accessible. These sampling tools have been recommended for the collection of sludges or sediment samples, provided the depth of water over the sediment is very small (a few centimeters) (EPA, 1986). The water-sediment interface is disturbed by this method of sampling, and the integrity of the sediment sample may be impaired if there is much mixing with the water column.

Sludges and sediments may be sampled with several other devices. The simplest is a hand corer with a check valve (Ford *et al.*, 1983). This device consists of a tube with the wall on one end sharpened and the other end carrying a check valve which prevents washout by the water column as the sample is withdrawn. The corer may be attached to extension handles which allow the collection of samples below a shallow layer of liquid. When appropriate, care must be taken not to damage the liner of the impoundment when using this type of sampler.

For sampling bottom sludges and sediments in deep water, a gravity corer, which is a variation of the corer with a check valve, may be used (Ford *et al.*, 1983). Weights, and in some cases fins, are added to the corer to facilitate the collection of bottom samples, using gravity to force the corer into the sludge or sediment. The gravity corer is retrieved using a line. The weight can be varied to attain the desired penetration into the bottom material. Again, if the impoundment has a liner, care must be exercised to avoid damage from this sampler.

The Ponar grab sampler is another sampling device for bottom material (Ford *et al.*, 1983). This device consists of a clamshell-like scoop which is lowered slowly until it rests on the bottom. The closure of the two jaws is triggered from above and the sample withdrawn. This device takes bottom samples over a depth of a few centimeters, depending upon the nature of the bottom material. The Ponar sampler is less likely to damage impoundment liners than the corer-type samplers, but is likely to disrupt the water-sediment interface. Furthermore, any depth stratification is lost with this sampler, whereas the corers collect samples which may be separated according to depth.

None of the samplers described above for solid materials is designed to eliminate volatility losses. Again, care should be taken to transfer samples and to seal containers as quickly as possible after collection.

ANALYSIS

The analysis of volatile compounds such as benzene, toluene or xylene(s) is prescribed for waste sites by OSW-846 Method 8020 (gas chromatography (GC) with photoionization detection) or Method 8240 (GC/mass spectrometry) (EPA, 1986). In both methods, sample introduction is accomplished using a purge-and-trap device in which a stream of inert gas is bubbled through the liquid sample (or an aqueous slurry of a solid sample) in a glass purge vessel. The effluent gas is passed through a near-ambient-temperature sorbent trap, where the volatile organic compounds are selectively retained. After a prescribed purge volume, the sorbent trap is placed on-line with the GC system and heated rapidly under flowing carrier gas to transfer the analytes to the GC column. As indicated above, two different detectors may be used for the GC step – mass spectrometry or photoionization detection.

With samples from hazardous waste sites, the levels of analytes may vary over many orders of magnitude. To accommodate this range, methanol or polyethylene glycol may be used to extract the analyte and subsequently dilute the sample. Both solvents are totally miscible with water and small volumes of the methanol or polyethylene glycol extract are dissolved in reagent water for purge-and-trap analysis. Using appropriate dilution factors, samples containing high levels of analyte can be accommodated within the linear range of the GC system.

Every step of the collection, transport, storage and analysis of samples must be designed and executed in a manner that maintains sample integrity. For instance, the choice of sample container can have a significant effect on the results. In addition to the usual considerations of materials compatibility, which for the aromatic solvents usually means glass or fluorocarbon containers, there is the question of head-space. Since benzene, toluene and the xylenes all have significant vapour pressures at ambient temperatures, they may volatilize into the head-space of the containers during transport and storage. When the container is opened for analysis, some of the analyte may be lost. This problem is especially severe for benzene (the saturated head-space may contain hundreds of micrograms of benzene per millilitre), since regulatory levels for this substance are some three to four orders of magnitude lower than for the other aromatic compounds. Volatilization into the head-space may be reduced by adsorption of the analytes by the sample matrix, but this is a sample-dependent phenomenon and cannot be relied upon to maintain sample integrity. For this reason, either the head-space in the sample container must be minimized and/or care must be taken when the container is opened for analysis. The SW-846 methods address part of the problem by requiring that the sample be removed quickly and that a sample container, once opened, be discarded. An obvious consequence of this precaution is the necessity of collecting replicates of each sample in separate containers. Other approaches have also been used. For example, Speis (1980) developed a sampling and analysis system using a hypovial which was sealed immediately after sample collection and served as the purge vessel for the analysis, so that the container was never opened to the atmosphere. There are two drawbacks to this approach which offset the improved sample integrity. One is lower purge efficiency and the other is loss of dynamic range. With the closed system there is no opportunity for diluting the sample, and the analytical system can easily be overloaded.

As with any sampling and analysis endeavour, rigorous quality assurance and quality control procedures must be included and described. There are two areas which must be documented – one is the sampling and the other is the analytical accuracy and precision. In general, the analytical uncertainty is much smaller than the sampling uncertainty, but it must be documented and considered in the data analysis. Guidance on the development of quality assurance/quality control programs is given in the *Interim Guidelines and Specifications for Preparing Quality Assurance Project Plans (QAMS)* (EPA, 1980).

The data interpretation is, in general, determined by the sampling strategy. The level of stratification used in the sampling strategy determines the spatial resolution with which the data may be interpreted. If the strategy was appropriate to the site, the data should accurately define areas which do or do not require remedial action.

REFERENCES

Cochran, W.G. (1977) *Sampling Techniques,* 3rd Ed., New York, NY, Wiley

EPA (1980) *Interim Guidelines and Specifications for Preparing Quality Assurance Project Plan – QAMS–005/80,* Washington DC, Office of Monitoring Systems and Quality Assurance, Office of Research and Development, US Environmental Protection Agency

EPA (1986) *Test Methods for Evaluating Solid Waste – Physical/Chemical Methods – SW–846, Vol. 2, Laboratory Manual,* Third Edition, Washington DC, Office of Solid Waste and Emergency Response, US Environmental Protection Agency

Ford, P.E., Turina, P.J. & Seely, D.E. (1983) *Characterization of Hazardous Waste Sites – A Methods Manual: Volume II. Available Sampling Methods,* EPA–600/ 4–83–040, Springfield, VA, National Technical Information Service

Speis, D.N. (1980) *Determination of Purgeable Organics in Sediment Using a Modified Purge and Trap Technique,* Edison, NJ, US Environmental Protection Agency

CHAPTER 11

SAMPLING AND ANALYSIS OF DRINKING-WATER AND FOOD

D.T. Williams

Environmental Health Directorate
Health and Welfare Canada
Ottawa, Ontario, Canada

INTRODUCTION

In any study involving the sampling or analysis of food or drinking-water, the information to be obtained by the study should be unambiguously defined and the complete study protocol should be planned and coordinated before any samples are collected. Studies which are designed to assess human exposure to specific chemical contaminants in food and drinking-water can be required for a number of purposes and applications, such as to ensure that guidelines or regulations are being met, to obtain data on background levels of chemical contaminants, to respond to specific problems (e.g., spillage or leakage of chemicals) or to evaluate the significance of new or emerging problems. The finding of higher than acceptable concentrations of toxic chemicals in food or drinking-water can lead to a number of actions, such as removal or recall of food products, changes in packaging and storage of food, switching to alternative water supplies and changes in chemicals or processes used in water treatment. The potential impact of these actions is such that only results obtained from a well-defined sampling and analytical protocol are acceptable.

Surveys may be small-scale or extensive in nature and will generally indicate the level of a specific pollutant at a particular time. If the results of the survey are positive, it may then become necessary to determine the change in pollutant concentration over time; this is usually defined as surveillance and monitoring. Surveys and surveillance, which may include a research component, are usually designed to find out more about a problem before a policy or course of action is decided on. Monitoring is normally initiated after the policy or course of action is decided, and is designed to find out how well the policy is working and whether standards are being met (Holdgate, 1979). Except for the frequency of sampling, the sampling protocol will be essentially the same, whether one is dealing with a survey, surveillance or monitoring programme.

SAMPLE COLLECTION

Benzene, toluene and xylene have only occasionally been reported in food and no major surveys have been published. In general, exposure to contaminants in food is determined either by a total diet study or by studies specific to particular food products. Samples for total diet or specific studies are randomly chosen from across the country to approximate a total dietary intake. They are stored, prepared and cooked in the usual manner and then analysed for the contaminants of interest. Statistical calculations (United States national residue monitoring programme) indicate that it is necessary to analyse 300 samples per compound per product in order to detect a 1% incidence of contamination with a 95% degree of confidence (Office of Technology Assessment, 1979). Considering the infrequent occurrence of benzene, toluene and xylene in foodstuffs, such extensive monitoring is inappropriate and emphasis should be placed on foods that appear to have the highest probability of contamination, such as fish and seafoods. There is also a possibility that foods might be contaminated by migration from packaging materials. Appropriate studies may be necessary to determine whether the contaminants were present in the original foodstuff or had been introduced during handling and storage.

It may also be necessary to determine levels of contaminants in food at the point of purchase or prior to cooking. In these cases, the sample should be identical with the bulk of the material from which it is taken, although, in practice, a sample is considered satisfactory if the properties under investigation correspond to those of the bulk material within the limits set by the nature of the test. The samples should be large enough for all intended analyses and they should be collected, transported and stored so that no significant changes occur from the moment of sampling until analysis is completed (Pomeranz & Meloan, 1987). For each specific foodstuff, a judgement must be made concerning the optimal conditions of transportation and storage. However, since the main problem is likely to be loss of benzene, toluene or xylene, due to their volatility, it is generally advisable to keep the samples frozen and to store and transport the foodstuff, if not already suitably packaged, in a clean, airtight, glass container. Many sampling schemes for food recommend that subsamples should be taken and thoroughly mixed to give a composite subsample before analysis (Pomeranz & Meloan, 1978). This may not always be appropriate for benzene, toluene and xylene because of their volatility and it will be necessary to select the most appropriate subsampling procedure for each food product to ensure that losses of the volatile compounds are minimized.

Drinking-water surveillance and monitoring can be carried out for a number of purposes, such as the determination of the quality of raw water entering a treatment plant and the quality of treated water leaving the plant, or at the consumer's tap. The frequency and time of sampling must be chosen for each study, taking account of general principles (Holdgate, 1979; Her Majesty's Stationery Office, 1980) and local knowledge of treatment procedures and variations in water quality. Samples are usually collected at a tap which has been well flushed, unless the study is designed to assess the quality of first-draw samples. Although drinking-water samples can be collected as integrated or composite samples, almost all surveys of benzene, toluene, xylene and other volatile compounds in drinking-water have involved collection of discrete grab samples in glass bottles which are completely filled, then capped with an inert material so that there is no head-space in the bottle. Bellar and Lichtenberg (1979) recommend the use of a brown glass bottle, cleaned by heating at 400 °C for at least 4 h and fitted with a screw cap and a Teflon-faced septum. Benzene and toluene are susceptible to rapid biological degradation under certain environmental conditions (US Environmental Protection Agency, 1984) and it is therefore recommended that samples be acidified to pH <2 by addition of acid at the time of collection, stored and transported at 4 °C and analysed within 14 days. Sampling of groundwater requires special strategies and these have been extensively discussed elsewhere (Van Duijvenbooden, 1981; Wilkinson & Edworthy, 1981). To obtain grab samples from groundwater and some raw water sources, it may be necessary to use a bailer, preferably constructed from Teflon or glass. Water enters the bailer through a hole in the bottom as it is lowered into the water, and is prevented from draining out by a glass marble acting as a plug. The samples are poured into amber glass bottles, avoiding turbulence, and are then treated in the same way as tap water samples (Pettyjohn et al., 1981).

A novel approach, which stabilizes and collects a time-weighted average sample, is simple and inexpensive and requires no power, has been developed by Blanchard and Hardy (1985). Mieure et al. (1976) had shown that organic analytes could be separated from water by means of membranes, then analysed directly by mass spectrometry or concentrated into another solvent. Blanchard and Hardy (1985) extended this approach so that the volatile components, after permeation through a silicone polycarbonate membrane, were adsorbed onto charcoal contained within the sampling device, then desorbed with carbon disulfide and analysed by capillary-column gas chromatography (GC). Twenty-three volatile pollutants, including benzene and toluene, were determined and it was shown that a linear relationship existed between the quantity of volatile pollutants collected and the product of the sampling time and the concentration of the pollutant in the sample.

SAMPLE CONCENTRATION AND ANALYSIS

Columns currently used in GC can withstand the injection of relatively large volumes of water, so that benzene, toluene and xylene can be analysed by direct injection of an aqueous sample if the concentration is high enough. Tepley and Dressler (1980) have analysed benzene, toluene and xylene in water samples at concentrations down to 10 µg/L by direct injection onto the GC column, using steam as the carrier gas. However, for less contaminated water and for most foods it is necessary to concentrate the analytes prior to analysis. This can be achieved by three main procedures: (i) liquid-liquid extraction, (ii) adsorption on some type of adsorbent and (iii) head-space techniques.

Liquid-liquid extraction

Liquid-liquid extraction is widely employed for the analysis of organic substances in water. Various extraction procedures employ different solvents and ratios of organic solvent to water, and extraction may be performed continuously or batchwise. Typically, the extract is concentrated prior to analysis to achieve the desired sensitivity. With benzene, toluene and, to some extent, xylene, however, this could lead to losses, so that most workers have used a microextraction technique for the determination of these compounds. These microextraction procedures require only a single solvent extraction and typically use water:solvent ratios of 100:1, which eliminates the need for a solvent concentration step.

Otson and Williams (1981) evaluated a microextraction technique for 41 volatile and semi-volatile organic pollutants in water, using hexane as the extraction solvent. In order to minimize the number of manipulations and loss of analyte, the hexane extractions were carried out in the sample bottle. The samples were collected in calibrated bottles which were completely filled with water and sealed with a Teflon-faced septum. Removal of 5 mL water from the 120-mL sample bottle and addition of 3 mL hexane allowed adequate mixing of the liquid phases, easy removal of the hexane for subsequent GC analysis and a concentration factor of 115:3. Detection limits for toluene and xylene were 5 and 2 µg/L, respectively, using GC with flame-ionization detection (FID) and recoveries were better than 80%. Benzene could not be determined, since it co-eluted with hexane on the 15 m × 0.5 mm stainless-steel, SCOT, OV-17 column used. Glaze *et al.* (1981) and Thrun and Oberholtzer (1981) used a similar approach, but employed pentane as the extraction solvent, as recommended by Grob *et al.* (1975). Glaze *et al.* (1981) used a 120-mL water sample and 0.5 mL pentane, giving a water:solvent ratio of 240:1, and improved the precision by adding internal standards to the pentane before extraction. The reported detection limits were 1, 0.9 and 0.6 µg/L for benzene, toluene and xylene, respectively, using GC-FID. Despite the use of a 60 m × 0.25 mm, WCOT, SE-54 glass capillary column, they found that benzene and *o*-xylene had retention times similar to those of carbon tetrachloride and bromoform, respectively, and suggested that the use of both FID and electron-capture detectors would overcome this problem. Thrun and Oberholtzer (1981) used a 90-mL water sample and either 1 mL or 5 mL pentane for extraction. At concentrations of ∼440 µg/L, the recoveries for the 1-mL solvent extract were 66, 82 and 89%, and for the 5-mL solvent extract were 91, 100 and 100% for benzene, toluene and xylene, respectively. These recoveries are almost identical to the theoretical values calculated from the known distribution coefficients and solvent ratios. Addition of 14 g sodium sulfate to the water sample before solvent extraction improved the recoveries for the 1-mL extract to 74, 83 and 89% for benzene, toluene and xylene, respectively. Jeltes and Veldink (1967) used nitrobenzene to extract petrol from water and were able to detect benzene, toluene, xylene and other hydrocarbons at levels down to 100 µg/L, using packed-column GC-FID. The poor sensitivity was due to the low ratio (50:1) of water to solvent, although this gave reasonably good recoveries (> 75%) for toluene and xylene. Scheiman *et al.* (1974) reported that a 1:1 mixture of carbon disulfide and dichloromethane efficiently extracted benzene, toluene and xylene from water and that the extract could be concentrated to permit compound identification by capillary column GC-mass spectrometry (GC-MS). Thomason and Bertsch (1983), using a microextraction vessel designed for solvents denser than water, showed that toluene was extracted quantitatively from water by carbon disulfide, using water:solvent ratios of 100:1. Villarreal *et al.* (1984) reported a solvent extraction method for the determination, in beer, of solvent residues from can coatings. Cold beer was stirred with fluorotrichloromethane and an internal standard, and the mixture was then centrifuged and the solvent layer concentrated in a Kuderna-Danish evaporator. The sensitivity of the method was of the order of micrograms per litre for toluene and xylene, using packed-column GC-FID. Donkin and Evans (1984) reported a method for the analysis of hydrocarbons in seawater and mussels, in which steam distillation and extraction were combined in one step. Homogenized wet mussel tissue (6 to 30 g) was held at 80 °C for 1 to 2 h with 400 mL of 0.01 mol/L aqueous sodium hydroxide and 4 mL of hexane in a round-bottom flask, connected to a Dean and Stark apparatus. The solution was then distilled for 0.5 to 2 h at a water condensation rate of about 1 mL/min, and the hexane extract was subsequently analysed by GC. Recoveries of toluene and xylene from mussel tissue fortified at 14 to 90 μg/g were > 80%, with a precision (relative standard deviation, RSD) of < 5%.

Extraction with adsorbents

Although a wide range of organic compounds can be extracted from water by passage through an adsorbent, this technique has not been extensively applied to the sampling and analysis of aromatic hydrocarbons such as benzene, toluene and xylene. Pankow and Isabelle (1982) have shown that adsorption on Tenax (poly-2,6-diphenyl-*para*-phenylene oxide) adsorbent, followed by thermal desorption, is a potentially effective procedure for concentrating benzene, toluene and xylene from water samples containing these compounds at the microgram per litre level. Pankow *et al.* (1985) have extended this approach to permit sampling of groundwater so that volatilization losses and sampler-related contamination are minimized. The sampler consists of a small cartridge, packed with Tenax, a flow restrictor and a tube leading to the ground surface. The device is lowered down a piezometer, and the pressure of the water column forces the sample through the cartridge. When 50 mL of water were passed through the cartridge, the limit of detection using thermal desorption and GC-MS analysis was 90 and 75 ng/L for benzene and toluene, respectively.

Ryan and Fritz (1978) have used XAD-4 macroreticular resin to extract toluene from water, followed by thermal desorption and packed-column GC-FID analysis. Recoveries of toluene were 90% at 1 and 10 μg/L fortification levels, but problems were encountered with impurities arising from the resin. Blok *et al.* (1983) recommend that XAD-2 and XAD-4 resins, which are styrene-divinylbenzene copolymers, should not be used for the extraction of low molecular weight aromatic compounds from water because of the presence of alkylbenzene, styrene and naphthalene impurities in the resin (Hunt & Pangaro, 1982). Care *et al.* (1982) have reported that XAD-2 resin, no matter how rigorously cleaned, continues to excrete a large number of aromatic hydrocarbons such as toluene and alkylbenzenes. Schnare (1979) has shown that xylene is efficiently extracted from water by XAD-2 resin, but that it is difficult to obtain good recoveries from the resin by solvent desorption.

No food products appear to have been analysed for benzene, toluene or xylene using these adsorbent techniques.

Head-space techniques

Techniques of head-space analysis can be separated into two main groups: (i) static head-space techniques, in which an aliquot of the gas phase is analysed after equilibrium has been established between the gas phase and the liquid-solid phase, (ii) dynamic head-space techniques, in which a stream of inert gas is passed through or over the liquid-solid phase and the gaseous effluent is analysed for the compounds of interest (Drozd & Novak, 1979; Ioffe & Vitenberg, 1984). Examples of the dynamic techniques are the gas stripping or purge-and-trap procedure of Bellar and Lichtenberg (1979) and the closed-loop stripping procedure of Grob and Zürcher (1976). General reviews of head-space techniques have been given by Hachenberg and Schmidt (1977), Charalambous (1978), Kolb (1980) and Ioffe and Vitenberg (1984).

(i) Static head-space

The initial liquid or solid phase concentration can be determined from the measurement of the equilibrated vapour phase concentration and the equilibrium partition coefficient (K_i) for the target compound. However, since K_i is rarely known, it is customary to avoid its use by one of three methods: (i) use of the multiple gas phase equilibration method, (ii) use of a reference model with a known amount of the compound in the same matrix as the analyte, (iii) use of the standard additions method, where the gas phase concentration is determined before and after addition of a known amount of the compound to the sample (Drozd & Novak, 1979; McAuliffe, 1980).

The multiple gas phase equilibration method is a simple technique which can be used with water or beverages. A 25-mL sample is taken up in a 50-mL gas-tight syringe, then 25 mL of air or an inert gas are drawn into the syringe, which is then shaken until equilibrium is established. An aliquot of the head-space is analysed by GC and the remaining head-space is carefully discharged. A second 25 mL of air or inert gas are then drawn into the syringe and the analytical process repeated. Two or more successive gas phase equilibrations give all the necessary data for calculating the concentrations in the aqueous phase. A plot of the log of the analyte concentration in each gas phase equilibration *versus* the number of equilibrations produces a straight line. The distribution coefficient can be calculated from the slope of the line, and the analyte concentration in the original sample can be calculated from the slope and the intercept of the line (McAuliffe, 1971, 1980). The method fully allows for matrix effects and is very precise if attention is paid to gas-water volumes and the temperature is kept constant. A precision (RSD) of 0.5% was reported for toluene at 4.2 ppm in water (McAuliffe, 1980).

The traditional static head-space technique involves a gas-tight container, sealed with a septum through which aliquots of the head-space are taken with a gas-tight syringe. Enhancement of vapour phase partitioning can be achieved by increasing the temperature and, for aqueous samples, by addition of an electrolyte (Hachenberg & Schmidt, 1977; Friant & Suffet, 1979). Quantification problems can arise due to adsorption on the relatively large surface of the septum, particularly if it is not Teflon-faced, and on inner surfaces of the syringe. The latter can be heated to suppress adsorption, but this may also lead to errors (Drozd & Novak, 1979). The major problem with regard to quantification is that the matrix cannot always be exactly reproduced in the reference model and, particularly for solid matrices, cannot be adequately fortified with standard amounts of the compounds of interest (Hachenberg & Schmidt, 1977).

Drozd et al. (1978) determined from 2 to 300 ppb of benzene, toluene and xylene in water by heating 50 mL water to 40 °C in a 100-mL sealed container and withdrawing a 1-mL aliquot of the head-space, using a gas-tight syringe heated to 60 °C. The aliquot was cold-trapped on a capillary column and subsequently analysed by GC-FID, using temperature programming. The standard addition method was used for quantification, and the precision (RSD) of the method was reported to be 42, 12 and 14% for benzene, toluene and xylene, respectively. The precision for benzene was poor because of inefficient cold trapping. Drozd and Novak (1978), using a similar method and packed-column GC-FID, reported a precision (RSD) of better than 8% for the determination of 1 to 1 000 μg benzene in 50-mL samples of water and milk. Hollifield et al. (1981) determined toluene in maple syrup by heating 10-mL samples at 90 °C for 2 h in a sealed vial and withdrawing 2 mL of head-space vapour with a gas-tight syringe heated to 90 °C. Analysis was carried out by packed-column GC-FID, and quantification by the standard additions method. The toluene was shown to come from the plastic syrup container by warming sealed unused containers to 40 °C then penetrating the container wall with a can-piercing unit. A head-space sample was then obtained through the septum in the piercing unit, using a hot syringe, and was analysed by GC-MS. Hurst (1975) has also developed a can-piercing device to sample the head-space in sealed food containers.

Wilks and Gilbert (1969) determined toluene in cottonseed oil, using the hot jar method, where the oil was heated at 120 °C for 15 min and a 5-mL head-space aliquot was withdrawn and analysed by packed-column GC-FID. Quantification was effected by means of a calibration curve constructed by analysing oil samples to which known amounts of toluene had been added. Cheese samples were qualitatively analysed after being held at 55 °C for 25 min, but quantification was not possible, since no adequate reference model could be obtained.

Wilks and Gilbert (1969) also noted that evacuation of the jar to 50 cm of mercury prior to heating prevented leakage due to excess pressure in the jar and had no adverse effect on the precision of the method. Stotzka (1980) has employed reduced pressure head-space analysis for the determination of benzene and toluene in water samples and has shown that there is no need to heat the sample when using reduced pressure. In addition, the detection limit is lowered and the equilibration time is decreased. In the analysis of residual solvents in food packaging foils, and to overcome the problem of fortifying solid matrices, Luthi (1980) added cyclohexanone to the head-space vial before carrying out the determination of toluene. Quantification was achieved by means of a calibration curve prepared from data obtained by head-space analysis of cyclohexanone solution, fortified with known amounts of toluene.

(ii) Dynamic head-space (purge-and-trap)

The static head-space technique has relatively high detection limits, since the amount of compound in the head-space depends on the partition coefficient, and only an aliquot of the head-space is taken for analysis. In order to lower the detection limits, dynamic head-space techniques were developed in which the gas phase components were swept from the head-space and collected on an adsorbent, or in a low temperature trap. The purge gas can be bubbled through the sample or passed over its surface. For purgeable organic compounds, including benzene and toluene, the US Environmental Protection Agency (1984) has proposed three methods (Methods 602, 624 & 1624), developed from work of Bellar and Lichtenberg (1979), which involve essentially the same sample preparation and differ mainly in the techniques used to identify and quantify the analytes. Pure nitrogen or helium is bubbled at 40 mL/min for 12 min through a 5-mL water sample, contained in a specially designed vessel at ambient temperature. The purge gas is then passed through an adsorbent trap consisting of 1 cm of 3% OV-1 on Chromosorb W and 23 cm of Tenax. After a 12-min purge time, the adsorbent is dried by maintaining a flow of dry purge gas through it at 40 mL/min for 6 min. The adsorbed organic compounds are then introduced onto the GC column by thermal desorption (the adsorbent trap is held at 180 °C, while backflushing with 20 to 60 mL/min carrier gas for 4 min). This technique has been validated for benzene and toluene, and can also be used for xylene. Using packed-column GC and a photoionization detector (Method 602), the detection limit is about 0.2 µg/L; and, with packed column GC-MS (Methods 624 & 1624), the detection limit is about an order of magnitude higher. Method 1624 differs from Method 624 in that the former involves the addition of deuterated benzene and toluene (20 µg/L) to the water sample to facilitate quantification.

The efficiency of purging depends on the contact of the gas with the water, the total volume of gas used and the partitioning between the gas and liquid phases. The proportion of analyte in the gas phase can be increased by heating the sample and by increasing the volume of purge gas; however, the useful volume of gas is limited by breakthrough of the compounds on the adsorbent trap.

A number of workers have used purge-and-trap methods which differ mainly in the design of the purge apparatus, the volume of sample and purge gas and the nature of the adsorbent. Detection limits of 0.1 µg/L for benzene and toluene, using GC-FID, were reported for both a 5-mL sample (Dowty et al., 1978) and a 100-mL sample (Voznakova et al., 1978).Using packed-column GC-MS and a 25-mL water sample, Munch et al. (1981) reported a detection limit of 0.2 µg/L, which was equivalent to or better than their detection limits using GC-FID. Smillie et al. (1978) reported detection limits as low as 15 ng/L for benzene and alkylbenzenes using packed-column GC-MS and a 1-L water sample, held at 90 °C during purging. The most common trap adsorbents appear to be Tenax (Adlard & Davenport, 1983; Pankow & Rosen, 1984) and 2:1 Tenax:Silica Gel (Dowty et al., 1978; Munch et al., 1981).

Vitzthum and Werkhoff (1978) have reported finding benzene, toluene and xylene in the head-space over black tea, using a purge-and-trap method. Purified helium was swept over dry samples or aqueous suspensions of coffee, tea and cocoa, and the volatile compounds were trapped on Tenax. The adsorbed compounds were transferred to a cold (-60 °C) capillary column by thermal desorption, then analysed by GC-MS.

More sophisticated purge-and-trap techniques have been designed to handle complex food matrices. Withycombe *et al.* (1978) determined benzene, toluene and xylene by purging a slurry of aqueous hydrolysed vegetable protein which was stirred and held at 75 °C. The volatile compounds were collected on Tenax, then thermally desorbed into a U-tube cooled with liquid nitrogen. An aliquot of the residue in the U-tube was sampled using a cold syringe and analysed by GC-MS. Warner *et al.* (1980) determined benzene, toluene and xylene in clams, fish fry, fish eggs and fish liver. Twenty mg to 1 g tissue was refluxed and stirred with 20 mL aqueous 1 mol/L sodium hydroxide while purging with helium. The volatile components were trapped on Tenax, thermally desorbed and analysed by GC. Easley *et al.* (1981) homogenized fish tissue in ice-cold water by ultrasonic cell disruption. The samples were then heated to 70 °C and the volatile compounds purged into a trap containing equal volumes of Tenax, silica gel and activated charcoal. To facilitate quantification, deuterated benzene and toluene were added to the sample before analysis. Recoveries of benzene and toluene were > 75% and the packed-column GC-MS detection limit for these compounds was 10 ng/g for a 1-g fish sample.

Otson and Williams (1982) modified the purge-and-trap method by purging directly onto a Tenax GC column from a 40-mL water sample, held at 40 °C. Detection limits of < 1 µg/L by GC-FID, recoveries of > 75% and a precision (RSD) of < 10% were reported for aqueous concentrations of 4 and 16 µg/L. Saunders *et al.* (1975) designed a special vessel which permitted water to flow in one direction while helium was bubbled through in the reverse direction. The volatile organic compounds were trapped in a liquid nitrogen cooled tube, then transferred thermally to a cooled, 15-m, SCOT column for GC-MS analysis. Benzene, toluene and xylene could be detected at 10–25 ng/L in a 20-L water sample.

Reinert *et al.* (1983) reported two dynamic head-space methods for the determination of volatile organic compounds, including benzene, toluene and xylene, in fish and shellfish tissue samples. In the first method, knife-cut tissue samples were held at 50 °C in 5% aqueous sodium sulfate solution and purged with helium. The volatile compounds were trapped on a carbon adsorbent. Carbon disulfide was used to desorb the volatile organic compounds and the sample extracts were analysed by capillary column GC-FID. At a fortification level of 0.1 µg/g, the recoveries were 45, 52 and 45% for benzene, toluene and xylene, respectively, and the precision (RSD) was < 10%. The second method used an apparatus which allowed both grinding and purging of the tissue sample. The tissue was mixed with anhydrous sodium sulfate, heated to 80 °C, ground to fine particles, then purged with helium. The volatile organic compounds were trapped on a carbon adsorbent, desorbed with carbon disulfide and analysed by capillary column GC-FID. At fortification levels of 0.4 µg/g, the recoveries were 33 and 43% for benzene and toluene, respectively, and 22–42% for xylene, depending on the isomer.

Colenut and Thorburn (1980) analysed water samples by a purge-and-trap method using a carbon adsorbent, followed by desorption with carbon disulfide and GC-FID determination. Recoveries of > 90% were reported for toluene at the microgram per litre and milligram per litre levels.

A dynamic head-space, closed-loop, stripping technique was developed as a general method for the determination of a wide range of volatile organic compounds in water

(Grob, 1973). Grob and Zürcher (1976) improved and standardized the technique, and many laboratories now use a version of that procedure. A 0.5- to 2-L water sample was continuously purged with a small volume of air in a closed system, and the air was circulated continuously through an adsorbent trap containing 1 to 5 mg of a specially prepared carbon. The adsorbed organic compounds were then desorbed with a very small volume (12 to 30 µL) of carbon disulfide. The standard purging time was 2 h, but this can be reduced if only xylenes and more volatile substances are to be determined. The stripping vessel was immersed in a water bath, so that the temperature of the sample could be increased if necessary. Typical temperatures used are 20 °C (Karrenbrock & Haberer, 1984), 35 °C (Marchand & Caprais, 1983) and 40 °C (Grob & Zürcher, 1976; Thomason & Bertsch, 1983). For 18 compounds investigated, Thomason and Bertsch (1983) reported increased recoveries at 40 °C, compared to 25 °C, but at 60 °C zero recoveries were obtained due to water condensation on the carbon adsorbent. A number of solvents have been compared, and carbon disulfide was found to be superior to dichloromethane, methanol, ethyl acetate, hexane and pentane for the desorption of alkyl benzenes (Grob & Zürcher, 1976; Marchand & Caprais, 1983; Curvers et al., 1984). However, if a larger solvent volume could be tolerated, Grob and Zürcher (1976) preferred to use methylene chloride, since it is easier to purify. A good summary of early work using the Grob technique has been given by Coleman et al. (1981). Typical recoveries of benzene, toluene and xylene from 1- to 2-L water samples are 62–77%, with a RSD of 10% at a stripping temperature of 20 °C (Karrenbrock & Haberer, 1984) and 91 ± 6% at 35 °C (Marchand & Caprais, 1983). Detection limits using capillary column GC-FID are about 1 ng/L (Marchand & Caprais, 1983), and are < 50 ng/L using capillary column GC-MS with selected ion monitoring (Karrenbrock & Haberer, 1984). Graydon et al. (1984) have used thermal desorption of the carbon filter instead of solvent extraction, and have identified the volatile organic compounds by GC-MS. Drozd and Novak (1982) used the closed-loop stripping technique for the analysis of volatile compounds in water, but used Tenax as the adsorbent instead of carbon, and employed thermal desorption followed by packed-column GC-FID analysis. Benzene and toluene broke through the Tenax adsorbent fairly quickly, since their retention volumes on Tenax at 40 °C are about 400 mL and 1 000 mL, respectively. Recoveries could be improved by carrying out two strippings in series and summing the results from the two analyses.

IDENTIFICATION AND QUANTIFICATION

Infra-red, ultraviolet and nuclear magnetic resonance spectroscopy, while useful techniques for macro-scale analyses, are of limited use for the analysis of low levels of benzene, toluene and xylene in food or water. However, an infra-red method has been recommended for the determination of total hydrocarbons in water (Rotteri, 1982).

Fourier-transform infra-red coupled with GC has been used to identify benzene, toluene and xylene, but the large quantity (∼ 20 ng injected) required to obtain an adequate spectrum limits its usefulness (Herres, 1984). Zsolnay (1978) found no correlation between ultraviolet spectrophotometric and GC indicators when evaluating petroleum pollution in shellfish, but Murray *et al.* (1983) have used an ultraviolet detector coupled with high-performance liquid chromatography for the semi-quantitative determination of total aromatic compounds in contaminated shellfish. Virtually all identification and quantification of parts per million or lower concentrations of benzene, toluene and xylene have been carried out using GC with either packed or capillary columns. The use of capillary columns has become more prevalent as appropriate instrumentation becomes more readily available and as capillary column technology improves. In particular, the introduction of fused silica columns, with their inertness and strength, and of bonded stationary phases, with their greater stability and lower bleed, have been major advances in capillary column technology. Although narrow bore (0.25 mm i.d.) capillary columns have limited sample capacity, the new "megabore" (0.53 mm i.d.) capillary columns can serve as one-to-one replacements for packed columns. A 30-m megabore column can give better resolution in a shorter time than a 6-foot (1.8 m × 2 mm i.d.) packed column when used for the analysis of benzene, toluene and xylene (Anspec Inc., 1985).

There are three main detectors which can be coupled with GC for the analysis of benzene, toluene and xylene. These are the FID, the photoionization detector (PID) and MS. The FID responds to compounds on the basis of carbon content, is good for quantification and serves as a universal detector, particularly for hydrocarbons (Cox & Earp, 1982). However, its lack of selectivity is also a major weakness. In a quality assurance study of a method for purgeable aromatic compounds in drinking-water, Kingsley *et al.* (1981) found that trichloroethylene had the same retention time as benzene on both packed columns used in the study. The primary column used was a 2.5 m × 2.1 mm stainless-steel column, packed with 0.2% CW 1500 on Carbopack C. The column temperature was raised from 30 °C at 4 °C/min for 18 min, then at 8 °C/min to 175 °C. The confirmatory column was a 3.8 m × 2 mm glass column, packed with 5% SP1000 – 5% Bentone 34 on Supelcoport. The column temperature was held at 45 °C for 8 min, then raised at 10 °C/min to 75 °C. When those samples found to be positive for benzene, toluene and xylene by GC-FID on the two columns were reanalysed by GC-MS, only 44% of the samples were confirmed to contain benzene. Confirmation of toluene and xylene was essentially 100%.

Boland *et al.* (1981) reported similar interference from trichloroethylene in the determination of benzene in drinking-water by GC-FID using the 0.2% Carbowax column, and found a low percentage for GC-MS confirmation. Both studies indicated that as little as 3 ppb trichloroethylene in a 25-mL water sample analysed by the purge-and-trap method would be detected by GC-FID and would interfere with the identification and quantification of benzene by GC-FID. It has been suggested that simultaneous analysis using FID and an electron-capture detector (McCarthy *et al.,* 1980) or an electrolytic conductivity detector (Kingsley *et al.,* 1981) would aid in determining which compounds are present and whether any interference is occurring.

The PID responds on the basis of ionization potential and its sensitivity depends primarily upon carbon content, functional groups and bonding type (Langhorst, 1981). For benzene, toluene and xylene, the PID is at least three to five times more sensitive than the FID (Cox & Earp, 1982), and the instrumental detection limits are about 0.8 pg, 1.2 pg and 4.3 pg, respectively, for benzene, toluene and xylene (Clark *et al.*, 1984). The response for toluene and xylene relative to benzene can be increased by lowering the energy of the PID from 10.2 eV to 9.5 eV (Driscoll, 1982). Method 602 of the US Environmental Protection Agency (1984) specifies the use of a PID for the determination of purgeable aromatic compounds in water using the purge-and-trap technique. The primary column for Method 602 is 1.83 m long × 2.1 mm i.d., stainless steel or glass, packed with 5% SP1200 – 1.75% Bentone 34 on Supelcoport. The column temperature is held at 50 °C for 2 min, then raised at 6 °C/min to 90 °C. The confirmatory column, 2.44 m × 2.54 mm i.d., is packed with 5% 1,2,3-tris-(2-cyanoethoxy)propane on Chromosorb W. The column temperature is held at 40 °C for 2 min, then raised at 2 °C/min to 100 °C. Interference can again be a problem with the PID. Driscoll *et al.* (1980) have suggested connecting the PID and the FID in series and using the ratios of the responses from the two detectors for hydrocarbon identification. Cox and Earp (1982) have made a similar suggestion, except for placing the PID and the FID in parallel, so that each detector can be optimized with respect to make-up gas. Kingsley *et al.* (1983) have used a PID and an electrolytic conductivity detector in series to aid in identification, particularly in differentiating between benzene and trichloroethylene.

Because of the possibility of misidentification and of difficulties in quantification of poorly resolved peaks, many workers now use GC-MS instead of GC-FID or GC-PID for the analysis of benzene, toluene and xylene. A typical approach to the identification and quantification of benzene, toluene and xylene by GC-MS is that reported by Munch *et al.* (1981). GC was performed on a 1.83 m × 2 mm glass column, packed with 0.1% SP1000 on Carbopack C, and the column temperature was raised from 40 °C at 6 °C/min to 220 °C and held at that temperature until completion of the analysis. Mass spectra are acquired every three seconds during the GC run and the data stored in the MS data system. At the end of the sample analysis, the reconstructed ion chromatogram is plotted, peaks are identified by a peak-searching routine and a spectrum is retrieved for each peak. The retrieved spectrum is compared to those in the MS library and the six best matches are indicated. Final identification is made by comparison of retention times and spectra with those of authentic standards. For quantification, an extracted ion current profile (EICP) is plotted using the ion of highest intensity for each compound, and the area under each peak is determined and compared with that of an authentic standard analysed under the same conditions on the same day. The ions selected were $m/z = 78$ for benzene and $m/z = 91$ for toluene and xylene. The precision (RSD < 11%) was comparable to that obtained for GC-FID analyses at similar concentrations, and the MS quantification limits were equal to or lower than the FID limits.

Krasner *et al.* (1981) used a similar approach for GC-MS identification of benzene and toluene in well-water, using ions $m/z = 78$ and $m/z = 92$ for quantification of benzene and toluene, respectively. Method 624-Purgeables (US Environmental Protection Agency, 1984) bases qualitative identification on comparison of EICPs for the primary ion and at least two secondary ions. For positive identification, the ion current for each of the characteristic masses (m/z) must pass through a maximum in the same scan, or in adjacent scans the retention times must fall within 30 s of the retention time of the authentic compound, and the relative peak heights of three characteristic masses in the EICPs must fall within 20% of the relative intensities of these masses in a reference mass spectrum. Kirchmer *et al.* (1983) have statistically evaluated Method 624 and have found that random error is the principal cause of inaccuracy. Method 1624 (US Environmental Protection Agency, 1984) improves on Method 624 by adding isotopically labelled benzene-d_6 and toluene-d_8 to the samples, so that quantification is improved and the percentage recovery is known for each sample.

REFERENCES

Adlard, E.R. & Davenport, J.N. (1983) A study of some of the parameters in purge and trap gas chromatography. *Chromatographia, 17,* 421–425

Anspec Inc. (1985) *Analytical Specialist (Bulletin #12),* Ann Arbor, MI

Bellar, T.A. & Lichtenberg, J.J. (1979) *Semiautomated headspace analysis of drinking waters and industrial waters for purgeable volatile organic compounds.* In: Van Hall, C.E., ed., *Measurement of Organic Pollutants in Water and Wastewater,* Philadelphia, American Society for Testing and Materials, pp. 108–129

Blanchard, R.D. & Hardy, J.K. (1985) Use of a permeation sampler in the collection of 23 volatile organic priority pollutants. *Anal. Chem., 57,* 2349–2351

Blok, V.C., Slater, G.P. & Giblin, E.M. (1983) Comparison of sorption and extraction methods for recovery of trace organics from water. *Water Sci. Technol., 15,* 149–159

Boland, P.A., Kingsley, B.A., Stivers, D.F. & Pomerantz, I.H. (1981) Protocol for the analysis of a broad range of specific organic compounds in drinking water. In: Keith, L.H., ed., *Advances in the Identification and Analysis of Organic Pollutants in Water,* Vol. 2, Ann Arbor, MI, Ann Arbor Science Publishers, pp. 831–838

Care, R., Morrison, J.D. & Smith, J.F. (1982) On the limits of detection of traces of volatile organics in water, using Amberlite XAD-2 resin. *Water Res., 16,* 663–665

Charalambous, G., ed. (1978) *Analysis of Foods and Beverages: Headspace Techniques,* New York, Academic Press

Clark, A.I., McIntyre, A.E., Lester, J.N. & Perry, R. (1984) A comparison of photoionisation detection gas chromatography with a Tenax GC sampling tube procedure for the measurement of aromatic hydrocarbons in ambient air. *Int. J. Environ. Anal. Chem., 17,* 315–326

Coleman, W.E., Melton, R.G., Slater, R.W., Kopfler, F.C., Voto, S.J., Allen, W.K. & Aurand, T.A. (1981) Determination of organic contaminants by the Grob closed loop stripping technique. *J. Am. Water Works Assoc., 73,* 119–125

Colenut, B.A. & Thorburn, S. (1980) Optimization of a gas stripping concentration technique for trace organic water pollutants. *Int. J. Environ. Anal. Chem., 7,* 231–244

Cox, R.D. & Earp, R.F. (1982) Determination of trace level organics in ambient air by high resolution gas chromatography with simultaneous photoionization and flame ionisation detection. *Anal. Chem., 54,* 2265–2270

Curvers, J., Noy, T., Cramers, C. & Rijks, J. (1984) Possibilities and limitations of dynamic headspace sampling as a pre-concentration technique for trace analysis of organics by capillary gas chromatography. *J. Chromatogr., 289,* 171–182

Donkin, P. & Evans, S.V. (1984) Application of steam distillation in the determination of petroleum hydrocarbons in water and mussels (*Mytilus edulis*) from dosing experiments with crude oil. *Anal. Chim. Acta, 156,* 207–219

Dowty, B.J., Antoine, S.R. & Laseter, J.L. (1978) Quantitative and qualitative analysis of purgeable organics by high-resolution gas chromatography and flame ionization detection. In: Van Hall, C.E., ed., *Measurement of Organic Pollutants in Water and Wastewater,* Philadelphia, American Society for Testing and Materials, pp. 24–35

Driscoll, J.N. (1982) Identification of hydrocarbons in complex mixtures using a variable energy PID and capillary column gas chromatography. *J. Chromatogr. Sci., 20,* 91–94

Driscoll, J.N., Marshall, J.K., Jaramillo, L.F., Hewitt, G. & Alongi, V. (1980) Applications of a gas chromatograph employing an integrated photoionization detector. *Am. Lab., 12,* 84–93

Drozd, J. & Novak, J. (1978) Headspace determination of benzene in gas-aqueous liquid systems by the standard additions method. *J. Chromatogr., 152,* 55–61

Drozd, J. & Novak, J. (1979) Headspace gas analysis by gas chromatography. *J. Chromatogr., 165,* 141–165

Drozd, J. & Novak, J. (1982) Determination of trace hydrophobic volatiles in aqueous media by a technique of multiple stripping and trapping in a closed circuit. *Int. J. Environ. Anal. Chem., 11,* 241–249

Drozd, J., Novak, J. & Rijks, J.A. (1978) Quantitative and qualitative head-space gas analysis of parts per billion amounts of hydrocarbons in water. *J. Chromatogr., 158,* 471–482

Easley, D.M., Kleopfer, R.D. & Carasea, A.M. (1981) Gas chromatographic-mass spectrometric determination of volatile organic compounds in fish. *J. Assoc. Off. Anal. Chem., 64,* 653–656

Friant, S.L. & Suffet, I.H. (1979) Interactive effects of temperature, salt concentration, and pH on headspace analysis for isolating trace organics in aqueous environmental samples. *Anal. Chem., 51,* 2167–2172

Glaze, W.H., Rawley, R., Burleson, J.L., Mapel, D. & Scott, D.R. (1981) Further optimisation of the pentane liquid-liquid extraction method for the analysis of trace organic compounds in water. In: Keith, L.H., ed., *Advances in the Identification and Analysis of Organic Pollutants in Water,* Vol. 1, Ann Arbor, MI, Ann Arbor Science Publishers, pp. 267–280

Graydon, J.W., Grob, K., Zürcher, F. & Giger, W. (1984) Determination of highly volatile organic contaminants in water by the closed-loop gaseous stripping technique followed by thermal adsorption of the activated carbon filters. *J. Chromatogr., 285,* 307–318

Grob, K. (1973) Organic substances in potable water and its precursors. Part I. Methods for their determination by gas-liquid chromatography. *J. Chromatogr., 84,* 255–273

Grob, K. & Zürcher, F. (1976) Stripping of trace organic substances from water, equipment and procedure. *J. Chromatogr., 117,* 285–294

Grob, K., Grob, K. & Grob, G. (1975) Organic substances in potable water and in its precursor. III. The closed loop stripping procedure compared with rapid liquid extraction. *J. Chromatogr., 106,* 299–315

Hachenberg, H. & Schmidt, A.P. (1977) *Gas Chromatographic Headspace Analysis,* London, Heyden & Son Ltd.

Her Majesty's Stationery Office (1980) *General Principles of Sampling and Accuracy of Results 1980: Methods for the Examination of Waters and Associated Materials,* London

Herres, W. (1984) *Capillary GC-FTIR analysis of volatiles: HRGC-FTIR.* In: Schreier, P., ed., *Analysis of Volatiles,* Berlin (West), Walter der Gruyter & Co., pp. 183–217

Holdgate, M.W. (1979) *A Perspective of Environmental Pollution,* Cambridge, Cambridge University Press

Hollifield, H.C., Snyder, R.D. & Breder, C.V. (1981) A multiresidue approach to the identification of food packaging-derived volatiles in foods and containers. *J. Chromatogr. Sci., 19,* 514–517

Hunt, G. & Pangaro, N. (1982) Potential contamination from the use of synthetic adsorbents in air sampling procedures. *Anal. Chem., 54,* 369–372

Hurst, R.E. (1975) Device for sampling headspace from canned food. *Anal. Chem., 47,* 1221–1223

Ioffe, B.V. & Vitenberg, A.G. (1984) *Headspace Analysis and Related Methods in Gas Chromatography,* Toronto, John Wiley & Sons

Jeltes, R. & Veldink, R. (1967) The gas chromatographic determination of petrol in water. *J. Chromatogr., 27,* 242–245

Karrenbrock, F. & Haberer, K. (1984) Determination of volatile organic substances in water by GC/SIM: results of an investigation on the rivers Rhine and Main. In: Angeletti, G. & Bjorseth, A., eds, *Analysis of Organic Micropollutants in Water,* Dordrecht, D. Reidel, pp. 179–188

Kingsley, B.A., Gin, C., Peifer,W.R., Stivers, D.F., Allen, S.H., Brass, H.J., Glick, E.M. & Weisner, M.J. (1981) Cooperative quality assurance program for monitoring contract laboratory performance. In: Keith, L.H., ed., *Advances in the Identification and Analysis of Organic Pollutants in Water,* Vol. 2, Ann Arbor, MI, Ann Arbor Science Publishers, pp. 839–859

Kingsley, B.A., Gin, C., Coulson, D.M. & Thomas, R.F. (1983) Gas chromatographic analysis of purgeable halocarbon and aromatic compounds in drinking water using two detectors in series. In: Jolley, R.L., Brungs, W.A. & Cummings, R.B., eds, *Water Chlorination, Environmental Impact and Health Effects,* Vol. 4, Ann Arbor, MI, Ann Arbor Science Publishers, pp. 593–608

Kirchmer, C.J., Winter, M.C. & Kelly, B.A. (1983) Factors affecting the accuracy of quantitative analyses of priority pollutants using GC/MS. *Environ. Sci. Technol., 17,* 396–401

Kolb, B., ed. (1980) *Applied Headspace Gas Chromatography,* London, Heyden & Son Ltd.

Krasner, S.W., Hwang, C.J., Cohen, R.S. & McGuire, M.J. (1981) Development of a volatile organic analysis technique for the Orange-Los Angeles County reuse study. In: Cooper, W.J., ed., *Chemistry in Water Reuse,* Vol. 2, Ann Arbor, MI, Ann Arbor Science Publishers, pp. 17–31

Langhorst, M.L. (1981) Photoionization detector sensitivity of organic compounds. *J. Chromatogr. Sci., 19,* 98–103

Luthi, A. (1980) Residual solvents in packaging foils determined by headspace analysis of a solution, with the solvent backflushed. In: Kolb, B., ed., *Applied Headspace Gas Chromatography,* Bristol, Heyden & Son Ltd., pp. 121–125

Marchand, M. & Caprais, J.C. (1983) Gas stripping analysis of volatile hydrocarbons in water: application of the Grob's procedure. *Analusis, 11,* 216–224

McAuliffe, C.D. (1971) GC determination of solutes by multiple-phase equilibration. *Chem. Technol., 1,* 46–51

McAuliffe, C.D. (1980) The multiple gas-phase equilibration method and its application to environmental studies. In: Petrakis, L. & Weiss, F.T., eds, *Petroleum in the Marine Environment,* Washington DC, American Chemical Society, pp. 193–218

McCarthy, L.V., Overton, E.B., Raschke, C.K. & Laseter, J.L. (1980) Analysis of trace levels of volatile organic contaminants in municipal drinking water by glass capillary gas chromatography using simultaneous flame ionisation and electron capture detection. *Anal. Lett., 13(A16),* 1417–1429

Mieure, J.P., Mappes, G.W., Tucker, E.S. & Dietrich, M.W. (1976) Separation of trace organic compounds from water. In: Keith, L.H., ed., *Identification and Analysis of Organic Pollutants in Water,* Ann Arbor, MI, Ann Arbor Science Publishers, pp. 113–133

Munch, D.J., Munch, J.W., Feige, M.A., Glick, E.M. & Brass, H.J. (1981) A scheme for the routine analysis of purgeable compounds by gas chromatography/mass spectrometry. In: Keith, L.H., ed., *Advances in the Identification and Analysis of Organic Pollutants in Water,* Vol. 2, Ann Arbor, MI, Ann Arbor Science Publishers, pp. 713–728

Murray, A.P., Gibbs, C.F. & Kavanagh, P.E. (1983) Estimation of total aromatic hydrocarbons in environmental samples by high pressure liquid chromatography. *Int. J. Environ. Anal. Chem., 16,* 167–195

Office of Technology Assessment (1979) *Environmental Contaminants in Food,* Washington DC

Otson, R. & Williams, D.T. (1981) Evaluation of a liquid-liquid extraction technique for water pollutants. *J. Chromatogr., 212,* 187–197

Otson, R. & Williams, D.T. (1982) Headspace chromatographic determination of water pollutants. *Anal. Chem., 54,* 942–946

Pankow, J.F. & Isabelle, L.M. (1982) Adsorption-thermal desorption as a method for the determination of low levels of aqueous organics. *J. Chromatogr., 237,* 25–39

Pankow, J.F. & Rosen, M.E. (1984) The analysis of volatile compounds by purge and trap with whole column cryotrapping on a fused silica capillary column. *J. High Resolut. Chromatogr. Chromatogr. Commun., 7,* 504–508

Pankow, J.F., Isabelle, L.M., Hewetson, J.P. & Cherry, J.A. (1985) A tube and cartridge method for down-hole sampling for trace organic compounds in ground water. *Ground Water, 23,* 775–782

Pettyjohn, W.A., Dunlap, W.J., Cosby, R. & Keeley, J.W. (1981) Sampling ground water for organic contaminants. *Ground Water, 19,* 180–189

Pomeranz, Y. & Meloan, C.E., eds (1987) *Food Analysis: Theory and Practice,* 2nd Edition, New York, NY, Van Nostrand Reinhold Co. Inc.

Reinert, K.H., Hunter, J.V. & Sabatino, T. (1983) Dynamic heated headspace analysis of volatile organic compounds present in fish tissue samples. *J. Agric. Food Chem.*, **31**, 1057–1060

Rotteri, S. (1982) Determination of total hydrocarbons in water. *Int. J. Environ. Anal. Chem.*, **11**, 263–269

Ryan, J.P. & Fritz, J.S. (1978) Determination of trace organic impurities in water using thermal desorption from XAD resin. *J. Chromatogr. Sci.*, **16**, 488–492

Saunders, R.A., Blachly, C.H., Kovacina, T.A., Lamontagne, R.A., Swinnerton, J.W. & Saalfeld, F.E. (1975) Identification of volatile organic contaminants in Washington DC municipal water. *Water Res.*, **9**, 1143–1145

Scheiman, M.A., Saunders, R.A. & Saalfeld, F.E. (1974) Organic contaminants in the District of Columbia water supply. *Biomed. Mass Spectrom.*, **1**, 209–211

Schnare, D.W. (1979) Extraction of organic matter in water – the Carolina method. *J. Water Pollut. Control Fed.*, **51**, 2467–2474

Smillie, R.D., Sakuma, T. & Duholke, W.K. (1978) Low molecular weight aromatic hydrocarbons in drinking water. *J. Environ. Sci. Health*, **A13**, 187–197

Stotzka, W. (1980) Reduced pressure headspace analysis for the determination of volatile components in the lower and sub-ppm range. In: Kolb, B., ed., *Applied Headspace Gas Chromatography*, London, Heyden & Son Ltd., pp. 56–60

Tepley, J. & Dressler, M. (1980) Direct determination of organic compounds in water using steam-solid chromatography. *J. Chromatogr.*, **191**, 221–229

Thomason, M.M. & Bertsch, W. (1983) Evaluation of sampling methods for the determination of trace organics in water. *J. Chromatogr.*, **279**, 383–393

Thrun, K.E. & Oberholtzer, J.E. (1981) Evaluation of the microextraction technique to analyze organics in water. In: Keith, L.H., ed., *Advances in the Identification and Analysis of Organic Pollutants in Water*, Vol. 1, Ann Arbor, MI, Ann Arbor Science Publishers, pp. 253–266

US Environmental Protection Agency (1984) Guidelines establishing test procedures for the analysis of pollutants under the Clean Water Act. *Fed. Regist.*, **51**, 43233–43442

Van Duijvenbooden, W. (1981) Ground water quality in the Netherlands – collection and interpretation of data. *Sci. Total Environ.*, **21**, 221–231

Villarreal, R., Sierra, J.A. & Gonzalez, E. (1984) Method for the determination in beer of solvent residues from can coating. *J. Am. Soc. Brew. Chem.*, **42**, 8–10

Vitzthum, O.G. & Werkhoff, P. (1978) Aroma analysis of coffee, tea and cocoa by headspace techniques. In: Charalambous, G., ed., *Analysis of Foods and Beverages: Headspace Techniques*, New York, Academic Press, pp. 115–133

Voznakova, Z., Popl, M. & Berka, M. (1978) Recovery of aromatic hydrocarbons from water. *J. Chromatogr. Sci.*, **16**, 123–127

Warner, J.S., Riggin, R.M. & Engel, T.M. (1980) Recent advances in the determination of aromatic hydrocarbons in zooplankton and macrofauna. In: Petrakis, L. & Weiss, F.T., eds, *Petroleum in the Marine Environment*, Washington DC, American Chemical Society, pp. 87–103

Wilkinson, W.B. & Edworthy, K.J. (1981) Groundwater quality monitoring system – money wasted? *Sci. Total Environ.*, **21**, 233–246

Wilks, R.A., Jr & Gilbert, S.G. (1969) Measurement of volatiles transferred from plastic packaging films to foods. *Food Technol., 23,* 47–52

Withycombe, D.A., Mookherjee, B.D. & Hruza, A. (1978) Isolation of trace volatile constituents of hydrolysed vegetable protein via porous polymer entrainment. In: Charalambous, G., ed., *Analysis of Foods and Beverages: Headspace Techniques,* New York, Academic Press, pp. 81–94

Zsolnay, A. (1978) Lack of correlation between gas-liquid chromatograph and UV absorption indicators of petroleum pollution in organisms. *Water Air Soil Pollut., 9,* 45–51

CHAPTER 12

BIOLOGICAL MONITORING OF EXPOSURE TO BENZENE, TOLUENE AND XYLENE

R. Lauwerys & J.P. Buchet

Industrial Toxicology Unit
Medical School
Catholic University of Louvain
30.54 Clos Chapelle-aux-Champs
1200 Brussels, Belgium

BENZENE

Introduction

The following biological parameters have been employed for the assessment of exposure to benzene: (1) the ratio between inorganic or organic sulfates in urine, (2) the total (free and conjugated) phenol in urine and (3) the concentration of benzene in blood and exhaled air. Peripheral blood examination and cytogenetic analysis of lymphocytes have also been used, but these techniques, which aim at detecting biological effects of benzene, will not be considered in this chapter.

In view of the short biological half-life of benzene and its polar metabolites, all the biological monitoring methods currently in use can only assess the amount absorbed during a short time interval (recent internal dose). Therefore, the time of sampling in relation to exposure is important. It is possible that techniques might yet be developed which will measure the amount of active metabolites bound to circulating molecules; these techniques may permit the integration of exposure during a longer time interval (e.g., during a few months) and may also allow a better assessment of the target (bone marrow) dose.

When biological monitoring involves sampling and analysing urine, the collection methods and the means of expressing the results should be standardized. The analyses are frequently carried out on spot specimens collected at a well-defined time after the beginning or end of exposure. It is therefore advisable to correct the results for dilution of the urine. Two methods of correction have been used: (a) expression of the results per gram of creatinine, (b) adjustment to a constant density. Whatever the method of collection, analyses performed on very dilute urine specimens (density and creatinine less than 1.010 and 0.4 g/L, respectively) are not reliable. The results of urine analyses can be interpreted only if renal excretion is not impaired (no evidence of kidney dysfunction).

When comparing results for benzene metabolite excretion reported in the literature, it must be kept in mind that different methods of urine collection may have been used, so that results may not be comparable. Furthermore, the different degrees of specificity and sensitivity of the analytical methods selected for urine analysis must also be taken into consideration. In many studies, attempts to correlate the changes of a biological parameter with the intensity of benzene exposure are misleading, due to inaccurate assessment of the exposure (e.g., semi-quantitative determination with detector tubes, too few spot samples and possible skin absorption).

Ratio between inorganic and organic sulfates in urine

In urine, the percentage of inorganic to total sulfates is normally higher than 85% (Teisinger & Bergerova-Fiserova, 1955). Exposure to benzene decreases this ratio, since some metabolites of benzene are eliminated as sulfoconjugates (Yant *et al.,* 1936a,b). However, the sensitivity of this test is too low, as exposure to concentrations of the order of 10 ppm (30 mg/m³) would not significantly influence the ratio (Teisinger & Bergerova-Fiserova, 1955; NIOSH, 1974). The specificity of the test is also low, since numerous hydroxylated organic chemicals are also excreted in urine as sulfoconjugates. This test can no longer be recommended for evaluating benzene exposure.

Concentration of total phenol in urine

Contrary to substituted benzene derivatives (e.g., toluene and xylene), the side chains of which are mainly metabolized, benzene gives rise to phenol. The measurement of urinary (free and conjugated) phenol excretion has therefore been proposed as an exposure index. Excretion of phenol is usually completed within 24–48 h after a single exposure, which represents a biological half-life of less than 12 h (Sherwood & Carter, 1970).

Assuming that 30% of the retained benzene is oxidized to phenol, about 60 mg phenol should be produced in workers with a ventilation of 25 L/min after exposure to 10 ppm benzene for 8 h. Individual variability in pulmonary ventilation and also in the proportion of benzene transformed to phenol (80% according to Sherwood[1]) makes the preceding estimation valid only on a group basis. Several methods have been developed for the analysis of free and conjugated phenol in biological material. As indicated above, interpretation of the results must take the specificity of the analytical methods into consideration. The specificity increases in the order (1) the colorimetric method of Theis-Benedict (diazotized *p*-nitroaniline reagent), (2) the colorimetric method using 4-aminoantipyrine, (3) the colorimetric method of Gibbs (2,6-dichloroquinone chlorimide reagent) and (4) various gas chromatographic

---

[1] Sherwood, R.J., unpublished results presented at the International Workshop on the Toxicology of Benzene, Paris, Nov. 1976

methods. The 4-aminoantipyrine method determines many phenol derivatives (Gottlieb & Marsh, 1946).

The method of Theis-Benedict, which measures not only phenol, but also *o-*, *m-* and *p*-cresol and other hydroxy compounds (Müting *et al.,* 1970), gives phenol concentrations in urine about 30% higher than those obtained with the method of Gibbs (Rainsford & Lloyd Davies, 1965). With the latter method, *o-* and *m*-cresol can interfere (Docter & Zielhuis, 1967; Sherwood & Carter, 1970), but since only the *p*-isomer is normally present in significant quantity in urine (Sherwood & Carter, 1970), interference by the other two is usually minimal. Buchwald (1966) has proposed a modification of the method of Theis-Benedict using a stabilized diazonium salt of *p*-nitroaniline. The author claims that, although *o-* and *m*-cresol interfere, *p*-cresol does so only slightly.

Gas chromatographic methods (van Haaften & Sie, 1965; Lebbe *et al.,* 1966; Bakke & Scheline, 1969; Sherwood & Carter, 1970; Buchet *et al.,* 1972; Dirmikis & Darbre, 1974) are more specific than colorimetric methods. They are not only sufficiently specific, but also very precise when used with an internal standard (Buchet *et al.,* 1972). Whatever method is used, it is necessary to verify that the hydrolysis of conjugated phenol is complete before extraction.

Phenacetin, caffein, saccharin, aspirin and salicylic acid do not affect the excretion of phenol (Walkley *et al.,* 1961; Docter & Zielhuis, 1967). It has been reported that non-exposed subjects show no difference in excretion between the sexes, nor between smokers and non-smokers, and that the concentrations in the morning and afternoon do not differ significantly (van Haaften & Sie, 1965). However, there are several factors which influence phenol excretion, such as dermal application of phenol-containing preparations, exposure to phenol itself, some gastrointestinal disorders favouring the bacterial degradation of tyrosine and phenylalanine (Duran *et al.,* 1973) and ingestion of drugs containing phenylsalicylate (Fishbeck *et al.,* 1975; Lauwerys, 1975; Kociba *et al.,* 1976). Furthermore, the proportion of benzene eliminated as phenol increases after ethanol consumption (Sherwood[1]). Table 1 summarizes studies which have attempted to correlate benzene exposure with urinary phenol excretion. Only results obtained with the colorimetric method of Gibbs or by gas chromatography are presented, since they are comparable. Although the data are derived from different investigations, they clearly indicate that (on a group basis) there is a highly significant correlation ($r = 93$; $p < 0.001$) between exposure to benzene and phenol concentration in urine samples collected at the end of exposure. Phenol concentrations in the urine of non-occupationally exposed subjects do not usually exceed 20 mg/L.

In summary, the relationship between benzene exposure and phenol excretion is shown in Table 2. This relationship can be used if a specific method is employed for phenol determination in urine. A phenol concentration exceeding 20 mg/L at the end of the working period suggests that workers have been exposed to benzene, at least if the Gibbs or a gas chromatographic method is used for phenol determination and if the other factors which increase phenol excretion have been excluded (see above).

---

[1] See footnote, p. 206.

Table 1. Relationship between benzene exposure and phenol in urine (colorimetric method of Gibbs and gas chromatographic technique)

Number of subjects	Benzene concentration (ppm)[a]	Duration of exposure (h)	Integrated exposure (ppm × h)	Concentration of phenol in urine		Time of urine sampling	(B)−(A) (mg/L)	Method of phenol determination	Remarks	References
				before exp. (A) (mg/L)	after exp. (B) (mg/L)					
43	<10	8	–	28 (12–44)	33 (19–74)	Immediately after exposure	5	Gibbs	Atmospheric benzene concentration determined by spot samples during the shift	Rainsford & Lloyd Davies, 1965
10	7–15	8	≈88	52 (24–144)	87 (14–176)		35	Gibbs		
8	12–15	8	≈108	55 (37–98)	100 (60–195)		45	Gibbs		
8	7.5–50 (24)	8	≈192	37 (25–46)	74 (52–124)		37	Gibbs		
7	40–60	8	≈400	60 (41–91)	126 (61–310)		66	Gibbs		
6	10–70	8	≈320	37 (21–56)	129 (50–254)		92	Gibbs		
5	10–70	6	≈240	79 (59–177)	140 (107–210)		61	Gibbs		
5	20–80	8	≈400	68 (52–111)	140 (87–224)		72	Gibbs		
14	25–150	5–6	≈480	39 (19–69)	177 (113–278)		138	Gibbs		
3	>500	1	>500	–	132 (82–188)		–	Gibbs		
10			0.55	5.1 (1.5–14.4)	5.1 (2.1–14.7)		0	Chromatog.	Personal sampler	Berlin et al., 1975
10			1.31	4.9 (0.3–12.5)	6.5 (1.6–23.4)		1.6	Chromatog.	Personal sampler	
10			10.20	8.5 (2.2–32)	15.4 (5.9–39.2)		6.9	Chromatog.	Personal sampler	
1	25	4 1/2	115	≈6	50	End of exposure	44	Chromatog.	Sedentary subject (lab exposure)	Sherwood & Carter, 1970
5	0.52	5.3	2.8	2.8 (1–5)	9.8 (5–18)	End of exposure	7 (4–15)	Chromatog.	Personal sampler	Parkinson, 1971
2	2.15	3	6.45	1.5 (1–2)	5.5 (5–6)		4	Chromatog.	Personal sampler	
2	2.0	4.7	9.4	≈5	12.0 (9–15)	End of exposure	7	Chromatog.	Personal sampler	Sherwood, 1972b
1	20.0	5.7	114.0	≈8	71.0		63	Chromatog.	Personal sampler	
1	100		100	50	50	End of exposure to 16 h after exposure		Chromatog.	Personal sampler	Sherwood, 1976[1]

[a] 1 ppm = 3.25 mg/m³
[1] See footnote p. 206

Table 2.   Relation between benzene exposure and phenol excretion

Benzene exposure (ppm × h) [a]	Phenol concentration in urine at the end of the working day (mg/L) [b]
0	< 20
40	30–35
80	45–50
100	50–55
200	85–90

[a] 1 ppm = 3.25 mg/m³
[b] Corrected for a density of 1.016

When using 20 mg/L as the upper threshold for normality, slight exposure to benzene (e.g., 1 ppm) may be overlooked, since the pre-exposure level may be much lower. In that case, comparison of phenol concentrations between pre- and post-shift samples may be used, since control subjects appear to show no significant difference in urinary phenol concentration between morning and afternoon samples (van Haaften & Sie, 1965). At such a low level of exposure, however, determination of benzene in breath or in blood is better for biological monitoring.

Concentration of benzene in exhaled air

The usefulness of the determination of benzene in exhaled air was extensively investigated by Sherwood (1972a,b) and later by Berlin (1985) and Berlin *et al.* (1980). Elimination curves for benzene in exhaled air, obtained by Sherwood and Carter (1970) and Sherwood (1972a), demonstrated a two (or more)-phase elimination process consisting of a rapid phase with a half-time in the vicinity of 2.6 h and a slow phase with an apparent half-time of one day or more. Similar results were obtained by Berlin (1985). The slow compartment contained about half the body burden of benzene at the end of a 6-h exposure to 5 ppm benzene. It can thus be concluded that some tissue in the body, probably fatty tissue, serves as an accumulator of benzene and that benzene is slowly released up to a week after exposure, thereby prolonging the internal benzene exposure (Berlin, 1985). Benzene concentration in expired air during the work period mainly reflects the exposure just before sampling. Sixteen hours after cessation of exposure, the slow compartment contributes about 75% of the benzene concentration in the exhaled breath (Fishbein, 1984). In view of the kinetics of benzene decay in breath, the concentration in exhaled air 16 h after cessation of exposure will progressively increase during the work week (Sherwood & Carter, 1970; Berlin, 1985). According to Sherwood and Carter (1970), after five days' sedentary daily exposure to 115 ppm-h, the concentration of benzene in breath on the sixth morning of the sixth day would be twice that of the second morning, that is, about 0.4–0.3 ppm. Berlin *et al.* (1980) reported that 16 h after a daily exposure to 40 ppm-h the concentration of benzene in breath amounts to ∼0.01 ppm on day 1 and ∼0.02 ppm on day 5. Concentrations reported by other authors have usually been higher (Lauwerys, 1979), but this may be due to analytical variability. Berlin

(1985) found that the concentration of benzene in the breath of non-occupationally exposed persons is in the range 0.001 to 0.002 ppm for non-smokers and 0.002–0.006 ppm for smokers. The difference is due to the fact that the smoke from a cigarette may contain 60–80 μg of benzene (Newsome *et al.,* 1965; Egle & Gochberg, 1976; Berlin, 1985). The consumption of ethanol may also accelerate benzene elimination in exhaled air (Sherwood[1]).

In summary, the determination of benzene in exhaled air is a valuable method for confirming exposure to benzene. It is highly sensitive and more specific than the determination of phenol in urine. The techniques employed (sample collection, time interval before analysis) in air analysis, however, are more cumbersome than in urine analysis, and many factors influence correlations between integrated exposure to benzene and the concentration of the latter in exhaled air on the morning following exposure.

Concentration of benzene in blood

The measurement of benzene in blood has rarely been studied as a method of evaluating exposure. It is likely, however, that the concentration of benzene in blood shows a similar pattern to that in breath.

In three volunteers exposed to 25 ppm benzene for 2 h, the benzene concentration in blood at the end of exposure was approximately 200 μg/L and decreased to 10 μg/L 15 h after the end of exposure (Sato *et al.,* 1975). In a group of workers exposed to approximately 7 ppm benzene, Cavigneaux and Lebbe (1969) found benzene levels in blood between 100 and 300 μg/L 14–18 h after the end of exposure. The determination of benzene in blood is a useful monitoring method for detecting low level exposure to benzene. Since bone marrow retains 20 times as much benzene as blood at equilibrium, even low levels of benzene in blood may be of toxicological interest (Braier *et al.,* 1981).

Conclusions

Among the tests proposed for evaluating current exposure to benzene, three appear to have some practical application: determination of the total phenol concentration in urine and measurement of the benzene concentration in exhaled air and in blood. However, the limitations of these tests must be kept in mind.

When phenol is measured with a specific method, values exceeding 20 mg/L in urine collected at the end of the work shift indicate exposure to benzene, provided other causes of increased phenol excretion can be excluded. In workers with normally low urinary phenol excretion, slight exposure to benzene (less than 10 ppm-h) may not be detected by measuring phenol in a post-shift urine sample. Increased sensitivity may be obtained by comparing concentrations of phenol in pre- and post-shift urine samples. When benzene exposure is very low (less than 1 ppm, i.e., 0.15 ppm for 8 h), this technique is not sensitive enough for confirming exposure. For integrated exposure exceeding 10 ppm-h, the correlation between phenol excretion and benzene

---

[1] See footnote, p. 206.

exposure is valid, but only on a group basis. In a group of workers exposed to 10 ppm benzene for 8 h it has been estimated that the mean phenol concentration in urine samples collected at the end of the exposure period would amount to 45–50 mg/L (density = 1.016).

The methods for determining benzene concentration in exhaled breath and in blood are very specific and sensitive for confirming exposure to benzene. However, correlations between these concentrations and integrated exposure is complex. Furthermore, as benzene is present in cigarette smoke, its detection in exhaled breath or in blood does not necessarily imply occupational exposure to benzene.

TOLUENE

Introduction

Several tests have been proposed for evaluating toluene exposure, namely hippuric acid in urine, benzoic acid in urine, *o*-cresol in urine, hippuric acid in blood, toluene in blood and toluene in expired air.

Hippuric acid in urine

Hippuric acid is a normal constituent of urine, originating mainly from food containing benzoic acid and benzoates. In non-occupationally exposed workers, the concentration of hippuric acid in spot urine samples rarely exceeds 1.5 g/g creatinine (Buchet & Lauwerys, 1973). In 1942, von Oettingen *et al.* reported that exposure to 50 to 800 ppm of toluene is followed by an increased excretion of hippuric acid, roughly parallel to the intensity of the exposure. Pagnotto and Lieberman (1967) have compared the post-exposure hippuric acid: creatinine ratio with toluene exposure in small groups of individuals with similar exposure. At 100 ppm (375 mg/m^3) toluene they found a group-average value of about 2.8 g hippuric acid/g creatinine for urine samples taken at the end of the work shift. However, a non-specific spectro-photometric technique which also measures methylhippuric acid was used, giving higher values than more specific chromatographic techniques if the subject is also exposed to xylenes. According to Ikeda and Ohtsuji (1969), the group-average hippuric acid concentration in urine at the end of the work shift after exposure to 100 ppm toluene is 2.0 g/L (density = 1.016), or 2.35 g/g creatinine. Individual values (5th and 95th percentiles) range from 1.4 to 3.9 g/g creatinine (Imamura & Ikeda, 1973). It should be noted that the toluene concentrations in air (in the photogravure printing industry) were obtained with detection tubes, and thus represent semi-quantitative spot estimates. The authors recognized that fluctuations of environmental toluene concentrations in the workshop surveyed were possible causes of wide variation in hippuric acid excretion. In seven workers exposed for 7 h to 40.2 ppm toluene (range, 28.6–53.7), Tokunaga *et al.* (1974) found 482 mg (range, 364–719) excess hippuric acid excreted within 24 h of the start of exposure, after subtracting the amount of hippuric acid present when the workers were not exposed. Unfortunately, the background levels of hippuric acid were not given. In 36 workers exposed to a mean toluene concentration of 27 ppm, Angerer (1976) reported an average urinary hippuric acid concentration of 2.04 g/L with a standard deviation (SD) of 1.37 g/L. From data by de Rosa *et al.* (1985), it can be estimated that exposure to 25, 40 and 50 ppm toluene gives mean post-shift urinary hippuric acid excretions of 1, 1.5 and 1.9 g/g creatine, respectively.

Ogata *et al.* (1970) exposed 23 male volunteers for 3 h in the morning and 4 h in the afternoon, or just for 3 h in the morning, to toluene vapour and collected urine for about one day after exposure. On a group basis, an excellent correlation was found between the total amount of hippuric acid excreted (exposure period plus 18 h after exposure) and the total exposure. In a group of five persons exposed to 100 ppm toluene for 7 h, the average hippuric acid concentration in urine collected during the second part of the exposure was about 2.81 g/L, corrected for a density of 1.024, or 1.87 g/L when corrected for a density of 1.016. Ninety percent of the values were included in the range 1–2.75 g/L (corrected for a density of 1.016).

For screening, Ogata *et al.* (1970) have suggested that the presence of amounts of urinary hippuric acid > Q-2SD, where Q is the average quantity excreted by persons exposed to the permissible toluene level, should be taken as evidence that the subject concerned may have been exposed to a concentration greater than the permissible value. This will be the case for about 5% of subjects. Hence, for exposure to a mean level of 100 ppm, the screening (5th percentile) concentration of hippuric acid in urine collected during the second period of the shift should be 1.00 g/L (corrected for a density of 1.016). We have indicated earlier that the upper normal limit for toluene may exceed 1 g/L. Thus, on an individual basis, separation of the exposed from the non-exposed can hardly be done with a single urine analysis for hippuric acid. Imamura and Ikeda (1973) and Engström *et al.* (1976) came to the same conclusion. However, on a group basis, this test appears to be sufficiently sensitive. Furthermore, the sensitivity of the test may be increased by comparing the urinary level of hippuric acid before and after the shift (de Rosa *et al.*, 1985).

The excretion rate of hippuric acid at the end of the exposure period is related more closely to the time-weighted toluene concentration (Wilczok & Bieniek, 1978; Veulemans & Masschelein, 1979; Veulemans *et al.*, 1979). On a group basis, a time-weighted average exposure of 100 ppm corresponds to a hippuric acid excretion rate of 4 mg/min, according to Veulemans *et al.* (1979), and to 2.6 mg/min according to Wilczok and Bieniek (1978). Unfortunately, collection of a timed urine sample is often impractical.

In summary, exposure to 100 ppm toluene for 8 h at rest should theoretically result in an additional total excretion of about 1 g of hippuric acid. At light work, a total of 2 to 3 g of hippuric acid is excreted (Cohr & Stokholm, 1979). In practice, a urine specimen is usually collected at the end of the work day, when the excretion of hippuric acid is at its maximum. In a group of workers exposed to 100 ppm toluene for 8 h, the mean hippuric acid concentration in urine samples collected at the end of exposure is approximately 2.5 g/g creatinine. This test can be used to estimate exposure only for groups of workers. Administration of ethanol inhibits the biotransformation of toluene, with increased excretion of the unchanged solvent in expired air (Dossing *et al.*, 1984). However, if alcohol is taken repeatedly, the metabolism of toluene is increased by induction of the microsomal oxidizing enzyme system in the liver (Waldrom *et al.*, 1983).

Benzoic acid in urine

Bardodej (1968) indicated that it is theoretically preferable to measure total benzoic acid concentration in urine (free + conjugated) because benzoic acid produced after toluene exposure is conjugated not only to glycine, but also to glucuronic acid. However, Engström *et al.* (1976) reported no difference in the estimation of urinary toluene by determining either hippuric acid directly or benzoic acid after hydrolysis.

o-*Cresol in urine*

Only a minor fraction of inhaled toluene vapour is oxidized at the aromatic ring to give cresols, which are eliminated in urine (Angerer, 1979; Woiwode *et al.*, 1979; Woiwode & Drysch, 1981; Apostoli *et al.*, 1982; Hansen, 1982; Andersson *et al.*, 1983; Hasegawa *et al.*, 1983). Since the concentration of o-cresol in normal urine is low (< 0.3 mg/L), it has been proposed as a biological monitoring parameter (Angerer, 1979). Woiwode and Drysch (1981) exposed 10 volunteers to approximately 200 ppm toluene for 4 h and found an average o-cresol concentration of 1.6 mg/L of urine (density = 1.017) immediately after exposure. According to Pfäffli *et al.* (1979), exposure to a time-weighted average toluene concentration of 100 ppm corresponds to a urinary o-cresol concentration of 1 mg/L (urine collected at the end of the work shift). Higher estimates (2.2 mg/L and 3.1 mg/L, respectively) are proposed by Dossing *et al.* (1983) and Angerer (1985). For workers exposed to an average concentration of 40 ppm (150 mg/m^3; range, 26 to 61 ppm), de Rosa *et al.* (1985) found a mean urinary o-cresol concentration of 0.45 mg/g creatinine (range, 0.19–0.71 mg/g creatinine) at the end of the work shift. A correlation (r = 0.66 to 0.70) was found between hippuric acid and o-cresol concentrations in urine (Angerer, 1985; de Rosa *et al.*, 1985). o-Cresol may have somewhat higher discriminatory power than hippuric acid since, after toluene exposure, the relative increase of the former is higher than that of the latter. However, the use of o-cresol is fraught with difficulties: (1) the analytical procedure is time-consuming and requires good instrumentation, (2) the background level is close to that measured after very light exposure, (3) the background level is higher in smokers than in non-smokers (Dossing *et al.*, 1983), (4) there is large inter-individual variability of oxidation on the aromatic ring (Hasegawa *et al.*, 1983), (5) de Rosa *et al.* (1985) showed that, for exposure to toluene levels between 37 and 225 mg/m^3 (10 to 60 ppm), the urinary hippuric acid concentration at the end of the work shift is better correlated with the mean daily exposure to toluene than is the concentration of o-cresol.

Hippuric acid in serum

Angerer *et al.* (1975) described a gas chromatographic method for hippuric acid determination in serum. Ninety-eight rotogravure printers exposed to an average of 101 mg/m^3 (27 ppm) of toluene showed mean (± SD) levels of 4.3 ± 30 mg of hippuric acid per litre of serum and 2.2 ± 1.5 g of hippuric acid per litre of urine. There was a low (r = 0.37) correlation between the hippuric acid concentrations in serum and in urine. A control group showed a mean hippuric acid concentration of 1.9 ± 1 mg/L of serum.

Toluene in blood

Engström *et al.* (1976) found a low, but statistically significant, correlation (r = 0.64; n = 20) between toluene in blood and urinary hippuric acid (blood and urine samples taken at the end of an 8-h working day). On the contrary, Szadkowski *et al.* (1973) found no correlation between toluene concentration in blood and hippuric acid in urine. von Oettingen *et al.* (1942) exposed two volunteers to toluene for 8 h and determined toluene in venous blood at the end of exposure; when exposed to 200 ppm the subjects had concentrations in blood of 4.1 and 7.3 mg/L.

For a control group, Szadkowski *et al.* (1973) reported an upper normal limit for toluene in blood of 150 μg toluene/L ($\bar{X}$ = 53 μg/L; n = 30). An occupationally exposed group showed a very low correlation (r = 0.29) between the toluene concentrations in air and in blood. Apostoli *et al.* (1982), however, found a good correlation (r = 0.88) between environmental toluene exposure measured with personal samplers and toluene levels in blood during exposure. They were unable to detect toluene in blood of non-exposed persons. Their data suggest that, for workers exposed to less than 50 ppm toluene (< 188 mg/m^3), the concentration in blood during exposure is about three times higher than in air. A similar ratio was found by Angerer and Behling (1981) (see below), but the ratio for volunteers at rest seems closer to 1. In six subjects at rest exposed to 375 mg/m^3 (100 ppm) toluene, Åstrand *et al.* (1972) found a mean value of 0.45 mg/L (SD = 0.15) for venous blood during exposure. The concentration increased during exercise (1.35 $\pm$ 0.13 mg/L after an exercise of 50 watts during 20 min). At rest, with exposure to 200 ppm, the concentration was 0.61 mg/L (SD = 0.10). Veulemans and Masschelein (1978) found a constant relation between the rate of uptake of toluene and the toluene concentration in venous blood under steady-state exposure. During exposure to 50, 100 and 150 ppm toluene, at rest, the average venous blood concentration reaches (usually within 50 min) plateau values of about 0.2, 0.4 and 0.6 mg/L, respectively. However, under non-steady-state conditions, no simple relation exists between uptake rate and venous blood concentration. Brugnone *et al.* (1986) found a good correlation (r = 0.84) between blood toluene concentrations in some workers' blood samples, collected at the end of a 7-h work shift, and the mean atmospheric toluene level during those 7 h. For a mean atmospheric level of 188 mg/m^3 (50 ppm), the concentration of toluene in blood averaged 0.50 mg/L. According to Angerer and Behling (1981), an atmospheric toluene concentration of 200 ppm toluene corresponds to a blood level higher than 2.6 mg/L. Apostoli *et al.* (1982) reported that blood toluene concentrations 14 and 62 h after exposure were 19 and 9%, respectively, of those found at the end of the exposure periods. The toluene concentration in blood the day after exposure is influenced by fat depots, which release toluene into the blood many days after exposure. Similar findings have been reported for many other solvents.

Toluene in expired air

Åstrand *et al.* (1972) have shown that the concentration of solvent in alveolar air of volunteers during exposure to toluene is related to the atmospheric concentration of the latter. On exposure to 100 ppm of toluene at rest, the mean concentration in alveolar air was 68 mg/m^3 or 18.1 ppm (standard error [SE] = 5.3 mg/m^3 or 1.41 ppm;

n = 15). This rose to 141 mg/m³ (37.5 ppm) on exposure to 750 mg/m³ (200 ppm) at rest. Values twice as high were reported in persons occupationally exposed to toluene. For example, Brugnone *et al.* (1986) found an alveolar air concentration of about 70 mg/m³ during exposure to 50 ppm. From the regression line slope, the ratio between alveolar and environmental toluene concentration was 0.30. Seventeen hours after exposure, the average alveolar toluene concentration was 4.7% of the afternoon alveolar toluene concentration and was better correlated with the instantaneous environmental toluene concentration measured the previous afternoon at the end of the work shift than with environmental toluene concentration measured continuously during the entire work shift. This finding is consistent with the conclusion of Åstrand *et al.* (1972) that "neither alveolar air samples nor venous blood samples taken at given intervals after the conclusion of a period of exposure can provide sufficiently accurate information on the average amount of solvent in inspired air at a working place or on the magnitude of an individual's uptake".

Conclusion

Analysis of expired air and/or blood during exposure roughly reflects current uptake. Exposure to 100 ppm toluene, at rest, gives rise to average toluene concentrations in venous blood and air of approximately 400 µg/L and 70 mg/m³, respectively. During light physical exercise, the blood concentration may be 1.30 mg/L. Determination of the average hippuric acid concentration in urine samples collected at the end of the work shift is still the most practicable method for evaluating overall hygiene conditions. A group average below 2 g/L (density = 1.016) or 2 g/g creatinine suggests exposure to < 100 ppm toluene. Individual values < 2 g/L, however, *may* result from exposure to toluene levels > 100 ppm; values > 2 g/L, on the other hand, clearly indicate exposure to levels > 100 ppm. Determination of urinary *o*-cresol rather than hippuric acid does not seem to be advantageous.

XYLENE

Introduction

The pulmonary retention of xylene vapours in man at rest is about 60–65% of the quantity inhaled (Sedivec & Flek, 1976a). The proportional retention does not change with the level and the duration of exposure, but with pulmonary ventilation. Experiments on volunteers have demonstrated that liquid xylene is absorbed through the skin (Engström *et al.*, 1977; Lauwerys *et al.*, 1978). In man, approximately 95% of the xylene absorbed is metabolized and only 3–6% is exhaled unchanged with the expired air (Sedivec & Flek, 1976a; Åstrand *et al.*, 1978; Riihimäki *et al.*, 1979a).

Biotransformation of the xylene isomers has been summarized by Ogata *et al.* (1970) and by Flek and Sedivec (1975). Oxidation gives toluic acids (methylbenzoic acids). In man, toluic acids are mainly conjugated with glycine to form *o*-, *m*- and *p*-methylhippuric acids (toluric acids), which are excreted in urine. Probably, no toluylglucuronic acid is formed in man (Sedivec & Flek, 1976a). Aromatic ring hydroxylation gives xylenols, but less than 3% of the xylene dose is excreted as xylenols in man (Flek & Sedivec, 1975; Sedivec & Flek, 1976a; Riihimäki *et al.*, 1979a; Engström *et al.*, 1984). As for any industrial solvent, the metabolites of xylene are relatively rapidly excreted. Usually, the urinary methylhippuric acid concentration reaches a maximum at the end of the exposure period (Sedivec & Flek, 1976a). For volunteers exposed to a mixture of xylene isomers, the excretion curve of total toluic acids is the same as that for exposure to individual isomers. The following biological tests have been used for evaluating exposure to xylene: methylhippuric acid in urine, xylene in blood and xylene in expired air.

Methylhippuric acid in urine

Methylhippuric acid is normally not present in urine. Several authors have correlated the exposure level with the urinary excretion of xylene metabolites. Ogata *et al.* (1970) exposed four or five volunteers to 100 ppm (440 mg/m³) *m*- or *p*-xylene or to 200 ppm *m*-xylene for 7 h and found that total *p*- or *m*-methylhippuric acid excretion during and for 18 h after exposure was linearly related to exposure levels. The integrated exposure (7 h at 100 ppm) to *m*- or *p*-xylene corresponded to a total urinary excretion of about 1.5 g of *m*- or *p*-methylhippuric acid. For the same integrated exposure, the average *m*-methylhippuric acid concentration in urine collected during the second part of the exposure was about 2.63 g/L, corrected for a density of 1.024, or 1.75 g/L when corrected for a density of 1.016. Ninety percent of the values were in the range 0.75–2.75 g/L (corrected for a density of 1.016). Data for *p*-methylhippuric acid were similar. The authors confirmed that the ranges of concentration were considerably decreased by correcting results to a constant urine density. As expected, the standard deviations of excretion rates were still smaller. Ogata *et al.* (1970) have suggested that, in man, the presence of amounts of urinary methylhippuric acid > Q-2SD, where Q is the average quantity excreted by subjects exposed to the permissible xylene level, is indicative of exposure to levels greater than the permissible value. This will be true for about 5% of the subjects tested (Ogata *et al.*, 1970). The screening (5th percentile) levels for *m*- and *p*-methylhippuric acids in urine collected during the second period of the shift should be 0.73 and 0.89 g/L, respectively (corrected for a density of 1.016), after a time-weighted average exposure of 100 ppm.

Sedivec and Flek (1976b) also exposed volunteers to xylene for 8 h and found that the excretion of methylhippuric acid (measured as toluic acid) reached a maximum at the end of exposure, then decreased exponentially. There was a linear relationship between the mean xylene concentration in the air and the amount of metabolite excreted. In persons exposed for 8 h to a constant xylene concentration of about 46 ppm (ventilation, 9 L/min), the concentration of methylhippuric acid in urine for the last 2 h of exposure ranged from 0.88 to 1.65 g/g creatinine. When these concentrations are calculated for the urine excreted during the whole exposure period (8 h), the values range from 0.67 to 1.45 g/g creatinine. The authors studied the correlation between exposure level and the amount of methylhippuric acid excreted during the 8-h shift, using different methods of expressing the quantity of metabolite excreted. The variability of the results decreased in the following order: mg/L > mg/L corrected for specific gravity > mg/g creatinine = mg/unit time > mg/kg body weight = mg/kg ideal body weight > mg/L of air ventilated. Exposure to an average level of 400 mg/m³ (92 ppm) for 8 h gave an average urinary concentration of methyl-hippuric acid in the total-shift urine sample of 2.0 g/g creatinine or 1.5 g/L (density = 1.016), with a range of 1.3 to 2.7 g/g creatinine or 0.7 to 2.3 g/L (density = 1.016). The same authors state that if the atmospheric concentration of vapour is constant, the short-term (last 2 h of exposure), all-shift, or all-day samples of urine can be used with equal success to estimate the exposure level.

Mikulski *et al.* (1972) studied the relationship between urinary metabolite excretion and atmospheric xylene concentration in 51 painters inhaling a mixture of toluene (10–20%) and xylene (80–90%). Unfortunately, they used a method which did not distinguish between hippuric and methylhippuric acids. It is therefore difficult to draw precise conclusions from their data.

In painters exposed to xylene, Engström *et al.* (1978) found a good correlation between the time-weighted average exposure and urinary methylhippuric acid concentration at the end of the work day. Methylhippuric acid levels of 0.665 and 1.28 g/g creatinine corresponded to xylene exposure levels of 50 and 100 ppm respectively. However, the authors remark that these values may be too low because their urine analyses neglected the absorbed *o*-isomer, which represented 10 to 15% of the technical xylene used. In volunteers exposed to about 90 ppm *m*-xylene for 6 h, Riihimäki *et al.* (1979b) found at the end of the exposure a mean urinary methylhippuric acid concentration of 0.85 g/g creatinine at rest and 1.27 g/g creatinine at light work.

The available data suggest that, in a group of workers exposed to 100 ppm xylene, the mean methylhippuric acid concentration in urine from the second part of a 7-h exposure period would amount to about 1.5 to 2 g/g creatinine, with a range of 1.0–3.0 g/g creatinine. Experiments on volunteers given a moderate ethanol dose (0.8 g/kg) prior to 4 h of inhalation of xylene (145 and 280 ppm) have shown that urinary methylhippuric acid declined by about 50%, while blood xylene levels rose about 1.5- to 2.0-fold (Riihimäki *et al.*, 1982). This suggests that ethanol decreases the metabolic clearance of xylene by about one-half during xylene inhalation. Other experiments also demonstrated that combined exposure to *m*-xylene and ethylbenzene results in a mutual inhibition of solvent metabolism (Engström *et al.*, 1984).

Xylene in blood

During exposure, the xylene concentration in blood is proportional to recent uptake (Riihimäki *et al.*, 1979b). In workers doing light physical work, exposure to 100 ppm xylene gave blood concentrations from 3.6 to 4.4 mg/L (*m*- and *p*-xylene) and 2.2 to 3.2 mg/L (*o*-xylene) (Angerer & Lehnert, 1979). Volunteers exposed to 200 ppm xylene and doing light physical work (50 W), or exposed to 100 ppm xylene and doing heavy physical work (150 W), showed concentrations of xylene in venous blood of 6 and 5.2 mg/L, respectively (Åstrand *et al.*, 1978).

In volunteers exposed to 90 ppm xylene, Riihimäki *et al.* (1979b) found the mean concentration of xylene in blood at the end of exposure to be 1.3 mg/L at rest and 2.1 mg/L after light work. The corresponding values 18 h after the end of exposure were 0.06 and 0.16 mg/L, respectivly. They also found that ethanol ingested prior to xylene exposure increases the blood xylene concentration (Riihimäki *et al.*, 1982).

Xylene in expired air

Analysis of exhaled air samples taken during the work day may be used for the estimation of current exposure. Engström *et al.* (1978) found that the xylene concentration in the exhaled air of painters amounted to approximately 8% of the mean level in the ambient air sample collected during the preceding 0.5-h period. The same authors were unable to estimate the average amount of xylene in ambient air from exhaled air samples or venous blood taken at several intervals after the termination of exposure. The ratio between solvent concentration in expired air and environmental air reported by Engström *et al.* (1978) for painters is lower than that (24–36%) found by Åstrand *et al.* (1978) for volunteers.

REFERENCES

Andersson, R., Carlsson, A., Byfalt Nordqvist, M. & Sollenberg, J. (1983) Urinary excretion of hippuric acid and *o*-cresol after laboratory exposure of humans to toluene. *Int. Arch. Occup. Environ. Health, 53,* 101–108

Angerer, J. (1976) Chronische Lösungsmittelbelastung am Arbeitsplatz. IV. Eine dünnschichtchromatographisch-densitometrische Methode zur Bestimmung von Hippursäure im Harn. *Int. Arch. Occup. Environ. Health, 36,* 287–297

Angerer, J. (1979) Occupational chronic exposure to organic solvents. VII. Metabolism of toluene in man. *Int. Arch. Occup. Environ. Health, 43,* 63–67

Angerer, J. (1985) Occupational chronic exposure to organic solvents. II. *o*-Cresol excretion after toluene exposure. *Int. Arch. Occup. Environ. Health, 56,* 323–328

Angerer, J. & Behling, K. (1981) Chronische Lösungsmittelbelastung am Arbeitsplatz. IX. *Int. Arch. Occup. Environ. Health, 48,* 137–146

Angerer, J. & Lehnert, G. (1979) Occupational chronic exposure to organic solvents. VIII. Phenolic compounds – metabolites of alkylbenzenes in man. Simultaneous exposure to ethylbenzene and xylenes. *Int. Arch. Occup. Environ. Health, 43,* 145–150

Angerer, J., Kassebart, V., Szadkowski, D. & Lehnert, G. (1975) Chronische Lösungsmittelbelastung am Arbeitsplatz. III. Eine gaschromatographische Methode zur Bestimmung von Hippursäure im Serum. *Int. Arch. Arbeitsmed., 34,* 199–207

Apostoli, P., Brugnone, F., Perbellini, L., Cocheo, V., Bellomo, M.L. & Silvestri, R. (1982) Biomonitoring of occupational toluene exposure. *Int. Arch. Occup. Environ. Health, 50,* 153–168

Åstrand, I., Ehrner-Samuel, H., Kilbom, A. & Ovrum P. (1972) Toluene exposure. I. Concentration in alveolar air and blood at rest and during exercise. *Work-Environ. Health, 9,* 119–130

Åstrand, I., Engström, J. & Ovrum, P. (1978) Exposure to xylene and ethylbenzene. I. Uptake, distribution and elimination in man. *Scand. J. Work Environ. Health, 4,* 185–194

Bakke, O.M. & Scheline, R.R. (1969) Analysis of simple phenols of interest in metabolism. II. Conjugate hydrolysis and extraction methods. *Anal. Biochem., 27,* 451–462

Bardodej, Z. (1968) Beurteilung der Gefährdung durch Toluol in der Industrie mittels der Hippursäurebestimmung im Harn. *Arbeitsmed. Sozialmed. Arbeitshyg., 3,* 254

Berlin, M. (1985) Low level benzene exposure in Sweden: effect on blood elements and body burden of benzene. *Am. J. Ind. Med., 7,* 365–373

Berlin, M., Fredga, K., Gage, J.C., Lagesson, V., Reitalu, J. & Tunek, A. (1975) *Exposure to Benzene during the Handling of Motor Fuels. Trans. Report 75-06-16,* University of Lund, Sweden, Department of Environmental Health

Berlin, M., Gage, J.C., Gullberg, B., Holm, S., Knudsen, P., Eng, C. & Tunek, A. (1980) Breath concentration as an index of the health risk from benzene: studies on the accumulation and clearance of inhaled benzene. *Scand. J. Work Environ. Health, 6,* 104–111

Braier, L., Levy, A., Dror, K. & Pardo, A. (1981) Benzene in blood and phenol in urine in monitoring benzene exposure in industry. *Am. J. Ind. Med., 2,* 119–123

Brugnone, F., de Rosa, E., Perbellini, L. & Bartolucci, G.R. (1986) Toluene concentrations in the blood and alveolar air of workers during the workshift and the morning after. *Br. J. Ind. Med., 43,* 56–61

Buchet, J.P. & Lauwerys, R. (1973) Measurement of urinary hippuric and *m*-methyl-hippuric acids by gas chromatography. *Br. J. Ind. Med., 30,* 125–128

Buchet, J.P., Lauwerys, R. & Cambier, M. (1972) An improved gas chromatographic method for the determination of phenol in urine. *J. Eur. Toxicol., 1,* 27–30

Buchwald, H. (1966) The colorimetric determination of phenol in air and urine with a stabilized diazonium salt. *Ann. Occup. Hyg., 9,* 7–14

Cavigneaux, A. & Lebbe, J. (1969) *Interprétation des Résultats des Epreuves Biologiques Spécifiques de l'Exposition au Benzène (Cahiers des Notes Documentaires n° 35),* Paris, Institut National de Recherche Scientifique

Cohr, K.H. & Stokholm, J. (1979) Toluene, a toxicologic review. *Scand. J. Work Environ. Health, 5,* 71–90

Dirmikis, S.M. & Darbre, A. (1974) Gas-liquid chromatography of simple phenols for urinalysis. *J. Chromatogr., 94,* 169–187

Docter, J.J. & Zielhuis, R.L. (1967) Phenol excretion as a measure of benzene exposure. *Ann. Occup. Hyg., 10,* 317–326

Dossing, M., Aelum, J.B., Hansen, S.H. & Lundqvist, G.R. & Andersen, N.T. (1983) Urinary hippuric acid and orthocresol excretion in man during experimental exposure to toluene. *Br. J. Ind. Med., 40,* 470–473

Dossing, M., Baelum, J., Hansen, S.H. & Lundqvist, G.R. (1984) Effect of ethanol, cimetidine and propranolol on toluene metabolism in man. *Int. Arch. Occup. Environ. Health, 54,* 309–315

Duran, M., Ketting, D., De Bree, P.K., Van der Heiden, C. & Wadman, S.K. (1973) Gas chromatographic analysis of urinary volatile phenols in patients with gastro-intestinal disorders and normals. *Clin. Chim. Acta, 45,* 314–347

Egle, J.L. Jr & Gochberg, B.J. (1976) Respiratory retention of inhaled toluene and benzene in the dog. *J. Toxicol. Environ. Health, 1,* 531–538

Engström, K., Husman, K. & Rantanen, J. (1976) Measurement of toluene and xylene metabolites by gas chromatography. *Int. Arch. Occup. Environ. Health, 36,* 153–160

Engström, K., Husman, K. & Riihimäki, V. (1977) Percutaneous absorption of *m*-xylene in man. *Int. Arch. Occup. Environ. Health, 39,* 181–189

Engström, K., Husman, K., Pfäffli, P. & Riihimäki, V. (1978) Evaluation of occupational exposure to xylene by blood, exhaled air and urine analysis. *Scand. J. Work Environ. Health, 4,* 114–121

Engström, K., Riihimäki, V. & Laine, A. (1984) Urinary disposition of ethylbenzene and *m*-xylene in man following separate and combined exposure. *Int. Arch. Occup. Environ. Health, 54,* 355–363

Fishbeck, W.A., Langner, R.R. & Kociba, R.J. (1975) Elevated urinary phenol levels not related to benzene exposure. *Am. Ind. Hyg. Assoc. J., 36,* 820–824

Fishbein, L. (1984) An overview of environmental and toxicological aspects of aromatic hydrocarbons. I. Benzene. *Sci. Total Environ., 40,* 189–218

Flek, J. & Sedivec, V. (1975) Metabolism of xylene isomers in man. *Prac. Lek., 27,* 9–16 (in Czech)

Gottlieb, S. & Marsh, P.B. (1946) Quantitative determination of phenolic fungicides. *Ind. Eng. Chem., 18,* 16–19

van Haaften, A.B. & Sie, S.T. (1965) The measurement of phenol in urine by gas chromatography as a check on benzene exposure. *Am. Ind. Hyg. Assoc. J., 26,* 52–58

Hansen, S.H. (1982) Determination of urinary hippuric acid and *o*-cresol, as indices of toluene exposure by liquid chromatography on dynamically modified silica. *J. Chromatogr., 229,* 141–144

Hasegawa, K., Shiojima, S., Koizumi, A. & Ikeda, M. (1983) Hippuric acid and *o*-cresol in the urine of workers exposed to toluene. *Int. Arch. Occup. Environ. Health, 52,* 197–208

Ikeda, M. & Ohtsuji, H. (1969) Significance of urinary hippuric acid determination as an index of toluene exposure. *Br. J. Ind. Med., 26,* 244–246

Imamura, T. & Ikeda, M. (1973) Lower fiducial limit of urinary metabolite level as an index of excessive exposure to industrial chemicals. *Br. J. Ind. Med., 30,* 289–292

Kociba, R.J., Kalnins, R.V., Wade, C.E., Garfield, E.L. & Fishbeck, W.A. (1976) Elevated urinary phenols levels in beagle dogs treated with salol. *Am. Ind. Hyg. Assoc. J., 37,* 183–191

Lauwerys, R. (1975) Biological criteria for selected industrial toxic chemicals: a review. *Scand. J. Work Environ. Health, 1,* 139–172

Lauwerys, R. (1979) *Human Biological Monitoring of Industrial Chemicals. 1. Benzene (Document EUR 6570 EN),* Health and Safety Directorate, Commission of the European Communities, Luxembourg

Lauwerys R., Dath, T., Lachapelle, J.P., Buchet, J.P. & Roels, H. (1978) The influence of two barrier creams on the percutaneous absorption of *m*-xylene in man. *J. Occup. Med., 20,* 17–20

Lebbe, J., Lafarge, J.P. & Ménard, R.A. (1966) Recherche et dosage des monophénols urinaires par chromatographie en phase gazeuse. *Arch. Mal. Prof., 27,* 565–570

Mikulski, P., Wiglusz, R., Bublewska, A. & Uselis, J. (1972) Investigation of exposure of ships' painters to organic solvents. *Br. J. Ind. Med., 29,* 450–453

Müting, D., Keller, H.E. & Kraus,W. (1970) Quantitative colorimetric determination of free phenols in serum and urine of healthy adults using modified diazo-reactions. *Clin. Chim. Acta, 27,* 177–180

Newsome, J.R., Norman, V. & Keith, C.H. (1965) Vapor phase analysis of tobacco smoke. *Tob. Sci., 9,* 102–110

NIOSH (1974) *Occupational Exposure to Benzene. Criteria for a Recommended Standard,* National Institute for Occupational Safety and Health, US Department of Health, Education and Welfare, Washington DC

von Oettingen, W.F., Neal, P.A. & Donahue, D.D. (1942) The toxicity and potential dangers of toluene. *J. Am. Med. Assoc., 118,* 579–584

Ogata, M., Tomokuni, K. & Takatsuka, Y. (1970) Urinary excretion of hippuric acid and *m*- or *p*-methylhippuric acid in the urine of persons exposed to vapours of toluene and *m*- or *p*-xylene as a test of exposure. *Br. J. Ind. Med., 27,* 43–50

Pagnotto, L.D. & Lieberman, L.M. (1967) Urinary hippuric acid excretion as an index of toluene exposure. *Am. Ind. Hyg. Assoc. J., 28,* 129–134

Parkinson, G.S. (1971) Benzene in motor gasoline. An investigation into possible health hazards in and around filling stations and in normal transport operations. *Ann. Occup. Hyg., 14,* 145–153

Pfäffli, O., Savolainen, H., Kalliomaki, P.L. & Kalliokoski, P. (1979) Urinary *o*-cresol in toluene exposure. *Scand. J. Work Environ. Health, 5,* 286–289

Rainsford, S.G. & Lloyd Davies, R.A. (1965) Urinary excretion of phenol by men exposed to vapour of benzene: a screening test. *Br. J. Ind. Med., 22,* 21–26

Riihimäki, V., Pfäffli, P., Savolainen, K. & Pekari, K. (1979a) Kinetics of *m*-xylene in man. General features of absorption, distribution, biotransformation and excretion in repetitive inhalation exposure. *Scand. J. Work Environ. Health, 5,* 217–231

Riihimäki, V., Pfäffli, P. & Savolainen, K. (1979b) Kinetics of *m*-xylene in man. Influence of intermittent physical exercise and changing environmental concentrations on kinetics. *Scand. J. Work Environ. Health, 5,* 232–248

Riihimäki, V., Savolainen, K., Pfäffli, P., Pekari, K., Sippel, H.W. & Laine, A. (1982) Metabolic interaction between *m*-xylene and ethanol. *Arch. Toxicol., 49,* 253–263

de Rosa, E., Brugnone, F., Bartolucci, G.B., Perbellini, L., Bellomo, M.L., Gori, G.P., Signo, M. & Ehiesura Corona, P. (1985) The validity of urinary metabolites as indicators of low exposures to toluene. *Int. Arch. Occup. Environ. Health, 56,* 135–145

Sato, A., Nakajima, T. & Fujiwara, Y. (1975) Determination of benzene and toluene in blood by means of a syringe equilibration method using a small amout of blood. *Br. J. Ind. Med., 32,* 210–214

Sedivec, V. & Flek, J. (1976a) The absorption, metabolism and excretion of xylenes in man. *Int. Arch. Occup. Environ. Health, 37,* 205–217

Sedivec, V. & Flek, J. (1976b) Exposure test for xylenes. *Int. Arch. Occup. Environ. Health, 37,* 219–233

Sherwood, R.J. (1972a) Benzene: the interpretation of monitoring results. *Ann. Occup. Hyg., 15,* 409–421

Sherwood, R.J. (1972b) Evaluation of exposure to benzene vapour during the loading of petrol. *Br. J. Ind. Med., 29,* 65–69

Sherwood, R.J. & Carter, F.W.G. (1970) The measurement of occupational exposure to benzene vapour. *Ann. Occup. Hyg., 13,* 125–146

Szadkowski, D., Pett, R., Angerer, J., Manz, A. & Lehnert, G. (1973) Chronische Lösungsmittelbelastung am Arbeitsplatz. II. Schadstoffspiegel im Blut und Metabolitenelimination im Harn in ihrer Bedeutung als Überwachungskriterien bei toluolexponierten Tiefdruckern. *Int. Arch. Arbeitsmed., 31,* 265–276

Teisinger, J. & Bergerova-Fiserova, V. (1955) Valeur comparée de la détermination des sulfates et du phénol contenus dans l'urine pour l'évaluation de la concentration de benzène dans l'air. *Arch. Mal. Prof., 16,* 221–232

Tokunaga, R., Takahata, S., Onoda, M., Ishi-i, T., Sato K., Hayashi, M. & Ikeda, M. (1974) Evaluation of the exposure to organic solvent mixture. *Int. Arch. Arbeitsmed., 33,* 257–268

Veulemans, H. & Masschelein, R. (1978) Experimental human exposure to toluene. II. Toluene in venous blood during and after exposure. *Int. Arch. Occup. Environ. Health, 42,* 105–117

Veulemans, H. & Masschelein, R. (1979) Experimental human exposure to toluene. III. Urinary hippuric acid excretion as a measure of individual solvent uptake. *Int. Arch. Occup. Environ. Health, 43,* 53–62

Veulemans, H., Van Vlem, E., Janssens, H. & Masschelein, R. (1979) Exposure to toluene and urinary hippuric acid excretion in a group of heliorotagravure printing workers. *Int. Arch. Occup. Environ. Health, 44,* 99–107

Waldrom, H.A., Cherry, N. & Johnston, J.D. (1983) The effects of ethanol on blood toluene concentrations. *Int. Arch. Occup. Environ. Health, 51,* 365–369

Walkley, J.E., Pagnotto, L.D. & Elkins, H.B. (1961) The measurement of phenol in urine as an index of benzene exposure. *Am. Ind. Hyg. Assoc. J., 22,* 362–367

Wilczok, T. & Bieniek, G. (1978) Urinary hippuric acid concentration after occupational exposure to toluene. *Br. J. Ind. Med., 35,* 330–334

Woiwode, W. & Drysch, K. (1981) Experimental exposure to toluene: further consideration of cresol formation in man. *Br. J. Ind. Med., 38,* 194–197

Woiwode, W., Wordarz, R., Drysch, K. & Weichardt, H. (1979) Metabolism of toluene in man: gas chromatographic determination of *o-, m-* and *p*-cresol in urine. *Arch. Toxicol., 43,* 93–98

Yant, W.P., Schrenk, H.H., Sayers, R.R., Horvath, A.A. & Reinhart, W.H. (1936a) Urine sulfate determination as a measure of benzene exposure. *J. Ind. Hyg. Toxicol., 18,* 69–88

Yant, W.P., Schrenk, H.H. & Patty, F.A. (1936b) A plant study of urine sulfate determination as a measure of benzene exposure. *J. Ind. Hyg., 18,* 349–356

METHODS FOR INDUSTRIAL AND AMBIENT AIR

METHOD 1 — DETERMINATION OF BENZENE, TOLUENE AND XYLENE IN INDUSTRIAL AIR BY CHARCOAL TUBE, SOLVENT DESORPTION AND GAS CHROMATOGRAPHY

R.H. Brown

1. SCOPE AND FIELD OF APPLICATION

This method is suitable for the measurement of airborne vapours of benzene, toluene and xylene, or mixtures thereof, over a concentration range of approximately 1 to 1000 mg/m³ (about 0.2 to 200 ppm, v/v) in samples of 12 L of air.

The upper limit of the useful range is set by the adsorptive capacity of the charcoal used (measured as the breakthrough volume; see section 3).

2. REFERENCES

International Organisation for Standardisation (1985) *Draft Method: Workplace Atmospheres – Determination of the Mass Concentration of Vaporous Aromatic Hydrocarbons – Pumped Charcoal Tube/Solvent Desorption/Gas Chromatographic Method (ISO/TC146/SC2/WG4/N47)* and subsequent revisions

Health and Safety Executive (1983a) *Benzene-in-air (Methods for the Determination of Hazardous Substances Series No. 17)*, London

Health and Safety Executive (1983b) *Toluene-in-air (Methods for the Determination of Hazardous Substances Series No. 36)*, London

Eller, P.M., ed. (1984) *NIOSH Manual of Analytical Methods,* 3rd Ed., Cincinnati, OH, US Department of Health and Human Services, Publ. 84–100, Method 1501

3. DEFINITIONS

The breakthrough volume is the volume of a standard mixture of aromatic hydrocarbons in air that can be passed through the charcoal tube before the concentration of eluting aromatic hydrocarbon vapour reaches 5% of the applied test concentration.

In this method, aromatic hydrocarbons refers to benzene, toluene and xylenes, although the method is also applicable to many of their homologues.

4. PRINCIPLE

An air sample of known volume is drawn through a glass or metal tube packed with activated charcoal. The organic vapours are adsorbed on the charcoal and are subsequently desorbed by carbon disulfide. The solution is analysed with a gas chromatograph (GC), equipped with a flame-ionization detector.

5. HAZARDS

Benzene is a recognized human carcinogen. Avoid inhalation or skin contact.

Carbon disulfide vapour is toxic by inhalation or skin contact and is highly flammable. Handle only in a well-ventilated hood.

6. REAGENTS[1]

Use only reagents of analytical reagent grade.

Benzene

Toluene

Xylene

Carbon disulfide[2]   Chromatographic quality. Benzene is commonly found in trace quantities in commercial carbon disulfide. If necessary, remove interfering compounds by percolation through silica gel (dried at 180 °C for 8 h under nitrogen) in a small (600 mm × 20 mm i.d.) glass column. This column will clean about 50 mL of carbon disulfide.

Standard solutions   Prepare standard solutions of aromatic hydrocarbons gravimetrically in carbon disulfide. If necessary, prepare a few standards covering a wide range of concentrations (e.g., 1 mg/L to 1 g/L) in order to determine the approximate range in the carbon disulfide extracts of the samples.

---

[1] Reference to a company and/or product is for the purpose of information and identification only and does not imply approval or recommendation of the company and/or product by the International Agency for Research on Cancer, to the exclusion of others which may also be suitable.

[2] Other desorption solvents may be used provided their desorption efficiencies are adequate.

Working standard solutions	Using a standard solution more concentrated than any of the sample extracts; prepare a series of working standard solutions covering the range of interest by serial dilution with carbon disulfide. Prepare fresh standard solutions with each batch of samples.
Charcoal	Activated coconut shell charcoal, particle size 0.4–0.8 mm (20–40 mesh). Before packing into tubes, heat the charcoal in an inert atmosphere at 600 °C for 1 h. To prevent recontamination, cool in an inert atmosphere or in a dessicator and store under similar conditions until packed into tubes. Suitable tubes prepacked with activated charcoal are also available commercially.

7. APPARATUS[1]

Charcoal sampling tubes	Glass tubes with both ends flame-sealed; 70 mm × 6 mm o.d., 4 mm i.d., containing two sections of activated charcoal. The adsorbing section contains 100 mg of charcoal, the back-up section 50 mg. The sections of charcoal are held in place by small plugs of inert material, e.g., glass wool. The pressure drop across the tube should be not greater than 3 kPa (25 mm of mercury) at the maximum flow rate recommended for sampling (i.e., 200 mL/min). Glass tubes should be held in suitable protective holders to prevent breakage.

NOTE: Instead of commercial two-section tubes, two single-section tubes may be used in series. This arrangement has the advantage that it is not necessary to store tubes at sub-ambient temperatures after sampling.

Polyethylene end-caps	For capping used charcoal tubes. Caps must fit snugly to prevent leakage.
Vials	With polytetrafluoroethylene-lined septum caps, or polyethylene-stoppered, nominal 2-mL capacity or larger.
Precision syringe	10-μL, readable to 0.1 μL

[1] Reference to a company and/or product is for the purpose of information and identification only and does not imply approval or recommendation of the company and/or product by the International Agency for Research on Cancer, to the exclusion of others which may also be suitable.

Table 1.   Sample size and sampling rate

Analyte	Breakthrough volume data			Recommended sample	
	Concentration (mg/m³)	Humidity (RH)	Volume (L)	Volume (L)	8-h rate (mL/min)
Benzene	149	low	>46	12	25
Toluene	2 245	low	12	12	25
Xylene	810	low	34	12	25

Personal sampling pump	Capable of running continuously for 8 h at 20–200 mL/min with flow rate stable to within ± 5%.
Plastic or rubber tubing	About 90 cm long, with diameter ensuring a leak-proof fit to both pump and sample tube or tube holder.
Clips	To hold the sample tube and connecting tubing to the wearer's lapel area.

NOTE: To avoid sampling errors, do not use plastic or rubber tubing upstream of the charcoal.

Gas chromatograph	Fitted with a flame-ionization detector, capable of detecting an injection of 5 ng toluene with a signal-to-noise ratio of at least 5 to 1.
GC column	Verify column suitability by testing two or more columns with different packings to ensure the absence of interference (see section 9.6).

8. SAMPLING

8.1 Calibrate the sampling pump with a representative charcoal tube in line, using an external meter.

8.2 Attach the pump to the charcoal tube with plastic or rubber tubing, placing the back-up section nearest to the pump.

8.3 To minimize chanelling, mount the tube vertically in the worker's breathing zone, for example on his lapel.

8.4 Turn the pump on and adjust the flow rate. Table 1 gives the recommended air sample volumes for the aromatic hydrocarbons covered by this method and the equivalent 8-h sampling rates. For sampling over shorter periods, the flow rate may be increased, but should not exceed 200 mL/min. In all cases, a 10-min sample may be taken at 200 mL/min on a 100 ± 50 mg tube. Tubes containing larger quantities of charcoal may be used to sample larger volumes (see section 12.1).

8.5 Record the time, temperature, flow rate (or register reading) and barometric pressure when the pump was turned on. At the end of the sampling period, record the flow rate or register reading, turn the pump off and record the time, temperature and barometric pressure.

8.6 Disconnect the sample tube and seal both ends with polyethylene end-caps. Place identifying labels on each tube.

8.7 If samples are not to be analysed within 8 h, place them in a sealed metal or glass container and store in dry ice or in a freezer maintained at −20 °C in order to minimize migration of the analyte from the primary to the back-up sections of the charcoal tubes. (If two single-section charcoal tubes are used in series, they should be sealed separately, and it is not necessary to freeze them.)

9.   PROCEDURE

9.1 *Blank test*

Prepare at least three sample blanks using tubes identical to those used for sampling. Subject them to the same procedures as the sample tubes, except that no air is pumped through them. Label these as blanks and analyse them with the samples as described in sections 9.5–9.8.

9.2 *Check test*

Not applicable.

9.3 *Test portion*

Not applicable.

9.4 *Desorption efficiency (D)*

For each batch of charcoal and for each analyte, it is necessary to determine the desorption efficiency over the sample concentration range. This is done by sampling from a standard vapour atmosphere at appropriate concentration, temperature, humidity, etc., under conditions where breakthrough does not occur (see section 12.2), and analysing the samples as described in 9.5–9.8. The desorption efficiency equals the mass recovered from the tube divided by the mass applied. Plot the desorption efficiency (D) values against the tube load levels (mass applied).

If the foregoing method is not practicable, spike the charcoal directly with a known volume of liquid analyte (preferably in solution for accurate measurement) and analyse in the same way. This method does not take account of ambient conditions prevailing during sampling.

NOTE: If the desorption efficiency at the sample load level is less than 0.75, the result is strictly invalid. If a fresh sample cannot be taken and analysed under better conditions, note in the report that the analytical result, corrected for desorption efficiency, is only approximate.

9.5 Sample extraction (desorption)

NOTE: Desorption should be carried out in a clean atmosphere in a fume hood.

9.5.1   Pipette 1.0 mL of carbon disulfide into a 2-mL septum vial and cap immediately.

9.5.2   Score the charcoal tube in front of the first section of charcoal and break open the tube. Remove and discard the glass wool.

9.5.3   Add the first section of charcoal to the desorption solvent in the vial and re-cap. Agitate the vial occasionally over a period of 30 min to ensure maximal desorption.

9.5.4   Extract the back-up section, the sample blank (combine the two sections) and the samples used to determine desorption efficiency (9.4) in the same way (9.5.1–9.5.3).

9.6 GC operating conditions

A variety of chromatographic columns may be used for the analysis of aromatic hydrocarbons in carbon disulfide. The choice will depend largely on the presence of interfering compounds, if any. A suitable choice might be a 2 m × 2 mm i.d. glass column, packed with 15% silicone or polyethylene glycol on silanized, acid-washed Chromosorb W (or an equivalent support). The column should be operated at a temperature similar to the boiling point of the analyte (i.e., about 100 °C) or be temperature-programmed. Use of a capillary column might be advantageous.

Correspondence of retention time on a single column should not be regarded as proof of identity.

9.7 Calibration curve

Inject a known fixed volume (1 to 5 µL) of each working standard solution into the GC. Use a standardized injection technique such that reproducible peak heights or areas are obtained. Prepare a calibration graph of peak height (area) against analyte concentration (µg/mL).

9.8 *Analyte determination*

9.8.1   Inject into the GC the same fixed volume (9.7) of the sample extract (9.5.3) from the first charcoal tube section.

9.8.2   Determine the peak height (area) and read the concentration of the analyte from the calibration graph.

9.8.3   Analyse the back-up section, the sample blank and the desorption effi-ciency samples (9.4) in the same way.

10. METHOD OF CALCULATION

From the results obtained in 9.8, the mass concentration, ρ_a(mg/m³), of the analyte in the air sample is given by

$$\rho_a = (\rho_1 + \rho_2 - \rho_b)v/DV$$

where

ρ_1 = mass concentration of analyte in extract (9.5.3) from first section of charcoal tube (µg/mL)

ρ_2 = mass concentration of analyte in extract from back-up section of charcoal tube (µg/mL)

ρ_b = mass concentration of analyte in extract from sample blank (µg/mL)

v   = volume of carbon disulfide employed in 9.5.1 (mL)

D   = desorption efficiency corresponding to ρ_1

V   = volume of air sampled (L).

11. REPEATABILITY AND REPRODUCIBILITY

A collaborative test of the NIOSH procedure, which is very similar to that described in this method and included benzene and *m*-xylene, indicated that the coefficient of variation, including between-laboratory and day-to-day variance com-ponents, was about 13% under conditions where sampling (pump) error was about 9%. Precision was less good for solvent mixtures and at low concentrations.

12. NOTES ON PROCEDURE

12.1 Sampling efficiency will be 100%, provided the capacity of the charcoal is not exceeded. If this capacity is exceeded, breakthrough of vapour from the first section of charcoal to the back-up section will occur. The breakthrough volume may be determined as described in section 12.2. The breakthrough volume varies with ambient air temperature, humidity, the concentration of sampled vapour and of other contaminants and with sampling flow rate. An increase in any of these parameters causes a reduction in breakthrough volume. Some typical breakthrough volumes, which also vary with analyte type, are given in Table 1. Where high humidity or high concentrations of interfering compounds are suspected, use a larger charcoal tube (400 or 800 mg with 200-mg back-up section).

12.2 *Determination of breakthrough volume*

12.2.1   Assemble a gas train consisting of a dynamic standard atmosphere generator delivering a concentration equivalent to the current exposure limit for the analyte of interest (e.g., 375 mg/m^3 for toluene), a single-section tube containing 100 mg charcoal, a 20–200 mL/min range flow-meter and a flame-ionization detector. (If commercially-available two-section tubes are used, remove the charcoal from the back-up section.)

12.2.2   Pass the gas through the sample train at a known constant rate appropriate for the sampling rate intended. Note the time that the flow was initiated.

12.2.3   When the aromatic hydrocarbon vapour begins to emerge, the detector will show a response. Continue the measurement until a plateau corresponding to the input concentration is reached, or until the response is determined to be caused principally by the applied aromatic hydrocarbon. Determine the time at which 5% of the plateau value had been reached.

12.2.4   Calculate the breakthrough volume by multiplying the flow rate (L/min) by the time elapsed (min) between the point of flow initiation and the point where 5% of the plateau value was reached. Typical values for the breakthrough volumes for the individual aromatic hydrocarbons covered by this method are given in Table 1. Lower values will be obtained for mixtures.

12.2.5   If the dead volume of the system is significant in comparison with the volume calculated in 12.2.4, determine this by repeating steps 12.2.2 to 12.2.4 with an empty tube in the gas train and make a suitable correction.

12.2.6   Determine the effect of moisture on the breakthrough volume by humidifying the gas stream to approximately 80% R.H. Do this by diluting a primary gas stream (e.g., 1500 mg/m^3 toluene) with air at 100% R.H., obtained by passing air through a series of water bubblers. Do not pass the aromatic hydrocarbon atmosphere through water. The humidity specified (80%) is a practical value; it does not imply that the method is invalid at higher humidities, provided due attention is given to the restriction on sampling volumes at high humidity.

12.3 In a field trial, the charcoal tube procedure of the Health and Safety Executive (1983a), which is very similar to that described in this method, was compared with an independent diffusive tube test method for measuring occupational exposure to benzene. The results of the two methods could not be distinguished statistically.

13. SCHEMATIC REPRESENTATION OF PROCEDURE

Sample air with charcoal tube
↓
Extract each section with 1.0 mL
analyte-free carbon disulfide
↓
Determine analyte concentration in each extract
using GC and calibration curve
obtained with standard solutions
↓
Calculate mass concentration of analyte
in air sample, correcting for sample blank
and desorption efficiency

14. ORIGIN OF THE METHOD

National Institute for Occupational Safety and Health
4676 Colombia Parkway
Cincinnati, OH 45226
USA

Contact points: Dr A.W. Teass
National Institute for Occupational Safety and Health

Dr R.H. Brown
Health & Safety Executive
Occupational Medicine & Hygiene Laboratory
403 Edgware Road
London NW2 6LN
UK

METHOD 2 — DETERMINATION OF BENZENE, TOLUENE AND XYLENE IN INDUSTRIAL AIR BY POROUS POLYMER ADSORPTION TUBE, THERMAL DESORPTION AND GAS CHROMATOGRAPHY

R.H. Brown

1.   SCOPE AND FIELD OF APPLICATION

The method is suitable for the measurement of airborne vapours of benzene, toluene and xylenes, or mixtures thereof, over a concentration range of approximately 0.5 to 50 mg/m³(about 0.1 to 10 ppm, v/v) in samples of 5 L of air.

The upper limit of the useful range is set by the adsorptive capacity (breakthrough volume) of the porous polymer used and by the linear range of the gas chromatograph (GC) detector.

2.   REFERENCES

Health and Safety Executive (1983) *Benzene-in-air (Methods for the Determination of Hazardous Substances, Series No. 22), London*

Health and Safety Executive (1984) *Toluene-in-air (Methods for the Determination of Hazardous Substances, Series No. 40), London*

3.   DEFINITIONS

The breakthrough volume is the volume of a standard mixture of aromatic hydrocarbons in air that can be passed through the porous polymer tube before the concentration of eluting aromatic hydrocarbon vapour reaches 5% of the applied test concentration.

In this method, aromatic hydrocarbons refers to benzene, toluene and xylenes, although the method is also applicable to many of their homologues.

4.   PRINCIPLE

A measured volume of air is drawn through a glass or metal tube packed with a porous polymer adsorbent. The aromatic hydrocarbon vapour is adsorbed on the polymer and is subsequently desorbed by heat and transferred with inert carrier gas into a GC, equipped with a flame-ionization detector.

5. HAZARDS

Benzene is a recognized human carcinogen. Avoid inhalation or skin contact.

6. REAGENTS[1]

Use only reagents of recognized analytical reagent grade.

Benzene

Toluene

Xylene

Methanol   Chromatographic quality, free from compounds co-eluting with aromatic hydrocarbons.

Porous polymer adsorbent   Tenax GC (or equivalent), particle size 0.18–0.25 mm (60–80 mesh). Precondition the Tenax by heating in an inert atmosphere at 250 °C for 16 h before packing the adsorbent tubes.

Aromatic hydrocarbon   Gravimetrically, prepare stock standard methanol standard solutions of each of the analytes of interest (see section 12.1). Prepare working standard solutions to cover the range of interest by serial dilution of the stock solutions with methanol. The analyte mass range in 5-μL aliquots of the working standards should exceed the mass range in the air samples to be analysed.

Spiked adsorbent tube   Fit clean adsorbent tube into GC injection unit, standards through which inert gas is passed at 100 mL/min. Heat injection unit to 250 °C and inject 5 μL of working standard solution through the septum. Disconnect the loaded tube and seal with end-caps. Prepare at least three tube standards at each load level. Prepare fresh standards with each batch of samples. The range of analyte loads should exceed the range obtained with the air samples.

---

[1] Reference to a company and/or product is for the purpose of information and identification only and does not imply approval or recommendation of the company and/or product by the International Agency for Research on Cancer, to the exclusion of others which may also be suitable.

7. APPARATUS[1]

Adsorbent tubes

Typically constructed of stainless-steel tubing, 90 mm × 5 mm i.d., 6 mm o.d. Mark one end of the tube by, e.g., a scored ring about 10 mm from the end. Pack the tubes with preconditioned porous polymer to within about 10 mm of each end (about 200 mg Tenax). Retain the polymer by stainless-steel gauzes and/or silanized glass-wool plugs. Prior to use, condition the tubes by heating slowly under flowing inert gas to 250 °C and maintaining that temperature for 10 min. If the thermal desorption blank (9.1) is unacceptable, tubes should be reconditioned. Once a sample has been analysed, the tube may be re-used immediately. However, it is advisable to determine the thermal desorption blank if the tubes are left for an extended period, or if sampling for a different analyte is envisaged. Tubes should be sealed and stored in an airtight container.

Thermal desorption apparatus

See section 9.5.

Adsorbent tube end-caps

Metal fittings with polytetrafluoroethylene or Viton seals.

Precision syringe

10 μL, readable to 0.1 μL.

Personal sampling pump

Capable of running continuously for 8 h at 10–200 mL/min, with flow rate stable to within ± 5%.

Plastic or rubber tubing

About 90 cm long, with diameter ensuring leak-proof fit to both pump and sample tube.

Clips

To hold the sample tube and connecting tubing to the wearer's lapel area.

NOTE: To avoid sampling errors, do not use plastic or rubber tubing up-stream of the adsorbent.

Soap-bubble meter

Or other suitable device for calibrating pump.

---

[1] Reference to a company and/or product is for the purpose of information and identification only and does not imply approval or recommendation of the company and/or product by the International Agency for Research on Cancer, to the exclusion of others which may also be suitable.

Gas chromatograph (GC)	Fitted with a flame-ionization detector, capable of detecting an injection of 5 ng toluene with a signal-to-noise ratio of at least 5 to 1.
GC column	Verify column suitability by testing two or more columns with different packings to ensure the absence of interference (see section 9.6).
Injection facility	For preparing standards. Use a conventional GC injection port for preparing spiked adsorbent tubes. The port can be used *in situ,* which has the advantage that the oven fan can be used to cool the tube, or it can be mounted separately. Retain the carrier gas and heating lines to the injector. If necessary, adapt the back of the injection port to take 6-mm o.d. tubing. This can be done conveniently by means of a compression coupling with a Viton O-ring seal.

8.   SAMPLING

8.1 Calibrate the sampling pump with a representative adsorbent tube in line, using an external meter.

8.2 Attach the pump to the adsorbent tube with plastic or rubber tubing. Connect the marked end of the tube furthest from the pump.

8.3 To minimize chanelling, mount the tube vertically in the worker's breathing zone, for example on his lapel.

8.4 Turn the pump on and adjust the flow rate. The recommended air sample volume for the aromatic hydrocarbons covered by this method is 5 L (8-h sampling rate, 10 mL/min). For sampling over shorter periods, the flow rate may be increased, but should not exceed 200 mL/min. In all cases, a 10-min sample may be taken at 200 mL/min. If the total sample is likely to exceed 1 mg, the sample volume should be reduced accordingly, or electrometer overload may occur. Tubes containing larger quantities of adsorbent may be used to sample larger volumes. See section 12.2.

8.5 Record the time, temperature, flow rate (or register reading) and barometric pressure when the pump was turned on. At the end of the sampling period, record the flow rate or register reading, turn the pump off and record the time, temperature and barometric pressure.

8.6 Disconnect the sample tube and seal both ends with compression seals. Tighten the seals securely. Place identifying labels on each tube. If samples are not to be analysed within 8 h, place them in a sealed metal or glass container.

9.   PROCEDURE

9.1 *Blank test*

Prepare sample blanks using tubes identical to those used for sampling. Subject them to the same procedures as the sample tubes except that no air is pumped through them. Label these blanks and analyse them along with the samples as described in sections 9.5–9.8. The adsorbent tube blank level is acceptable if it is no greater than the equivalent of 100 ng benzene. Typical levels are much less than this.

9.2 *Check test*

Not applicable.

9.3 *Test portion*

Not applicable.

9.4 *Desorption efficiency*

9.4.1   Inject 5-µL aliquots of the working standard solutions directly into the GC and prepare a calibration curve of peak height (area) against micrograms of analyte injected.

9.4.2   Analyse the 'spiked' tube standards as described in sections 9.5–9.8 and prepare a second calibration curve. These two curves should be the same, or nearly so. If the detector response for a tube standard is less than 95% of that for the corresponding liquid standard injected directly, then the desorption parameters should be changed accordingly. See section 12.3.

9.5 *Thermal desorption conditions*

Choose desorption conditions such that desorption from the sample tube is complete and no sample loss occurs in the secondary trap, if used. The following conditions are typical:

Desorption temperature	250 °C
Desorption time	10 min
Transfer line	150 °C
Cold trap low	− 30 °C
Cold trap high	300 °C
Cold trap adsorbent	Tenax.

The desorbed vapour occupies a volume of several millilitres, so that it may need to be concentrated if good chromatographic peak shape and adequate separation are to be obtained. This may be achieved by using a secondary adsorbent and/or a cold trap external to the GC. Many makes of thermal desorption apparatus have this facility incorporated into the desorber. Alternatively, the desorbed sample can be passed directly to the GC where it is concentrated by holding the column initially at low temperature, typically about 40 °C.

9.6 *GC operating conditions*

A variety of chromatographic columns may be used for the analysis of aromatic hydrocarbons. The choice will depend largely on the presence of interfering compounds, if any. A suitable choice might be a 2 m × 2 mm i.d. glass column, packed with 15% silicone or polyethylene glycol on silanized, acid-washed Chromosorb W (or an equivalent support). The column should be operated at a temperature similar to the boiling point of the analyte (i.e., about 100 °C) or be temperature-programmed. Use of a capillary column might be advantageous. Correspondence of retention time on a single column should not be regarded as proof of identity.

9.7 *Calibration curves*

9.7.1   Place a 'spiked' adsorbent tube (section 6) in the thermal desorption apparatus and purge air from the tube to avoid chromatographic artefacts arising from thermal oxidation of the porous polymer or GC packing.

9.7.2   Heat the tube to displace the organic vapours, which are passed to the GC by means of the carrier-gas stream. The gas flow direction at this stage should be the reverse of that used during sampling, i.e., the marked end of the tube should be nearest the GC column inlet (reversing the flow is not important for the aromatic hydrocarbons, but ensures the transfer of higher-boiling organic materials to the chromatograph).

9.7.3   Prepare a calibration curve of peak height (area) against mass of analyte loaded on the tube.

9.8 *Analyte determination*

9.8.1   Analyse the samples and sample blanks as described for the calibration standards in 9.7.1–9.7.2.

9.8.2   Determine the peak heights (areas) and read the mass of each analyte from the appropriate calibration curve.

10. METHOD OF CALCULATION

The mass concentration, ρ_a(mg/m³), of the analyte in the air sample is given by

$\rho_a = (m_s - m_b)/V,$

where

m_s = mass of analyte found in sample tube (μg)

m_b = mass of analyte found in blank tube (μg)

V = volume of air sample (L).

11. REPEATABILITY AND REPRODUCIBILITY

Laboratory tests of the thermal desorption procedure for benzene of the Health and Safety Executive (1983) and that for toluene (Health & Safety Executive, 1984), which are very similar to the procedure described in this method, indicated that repeatability (expressed as a coefficient of variation) was about 6%, assuming that pump error is about 5%.

12. NOTES ON PROCEDURE

12.1 It may be necessary to prepare a few standards covering a wide range of loading levels (say 10 μg to 1 mg) in order to determine the approximate weight range of the samples and hence the weight range of interest.

12.2 Sampling efficiency will be 100%, provided the capacity of the adsorbent is not exceeded. If this capacity is exceeded, breakthrough of vapour from the tube will occur. The breakthrough volume may be measured by sampling from a standard vapour atmosphere while monitoring the effluent air with a flame-ionization detector (a suitable procedure is described in Method 1, section 12.2). The breakthrough volume varies with ambient air temperature, falling by a factor of about 2 for each 10 °C rise. It also varies with sampling flow rate, being reduced substantially at flow rates below 5 mL/min or above 500 mL/min. It is only slightly affected by air humidity. To allow a suitable margin of safety, it is recommended that sample volumes of not more than 70% of the breakthrough volume be taken. For benzene, toluene and xylene, typical breakthrough volumes are about 10, 50 and 250 L, respectively, for 200 mg Tenax.

12.3 Ideally, desorption efficiencies should be determined on tube standards loaded from a standard atmosphere, as the method described may not take account of ambient conditions (e.g., humidity) prevailing during sampling, However, in practice, the method described is much more convenient and, in most cases, is quite adequate.

12.4 In a field trial, the procedure of the Health and Safety Executive (1983) was compared with an independent diffusive tube test method for measuring occupational exposure to benzene. The results of the two methods could not be distinguished statistically. The mean repeatability (expressed as a coefficient of variation) for the pumped thermal desorption results was 13%.

13. SCHEMATIC REPRESENTATION OF PROCEDURE

Sample known volume of air with Tenax GC adsorbent tube
↓
Obtain GC calibration curves using adsorbent tubes
spiked with the analytes of interest
↓
Analyse sample tubes and blank tubes
↓
Identify and quantify analytes
using GC data and calibration curves

14. ORIGIN OF THE METHOD

Health and Safety Executive
Occupational Medicine and Hygiene Laboratory
403 Edgware Road
London NW2 6LN
UK

Contact point: Dr R.H. Brown

METHOD 3 — DETERMINATION OF GASOLINE HYDROCARBONS IN INDUSTRIAL AIR BY TWO-STAGE (CHROMOSORB/CHARCOAL) ADSORPTION, THERMAL DESORPTION AND CAPILLARY GAS CHROMATOGRAPHY

R.H. Brown

1. SCOPE AND FIELD OF APPLICATION

The method is suitable for the measurement of airborne vapours of full-range gasoline over a concentration range of approximately 0.2 to 100 mg/m^3 total hydrocarbons (about 0.04 to 20 ppm, v/v) in samples of 2.5 L of air. The method is also suitable for the measurement of the airborne concentrations of individual components of gasoline mixtures.

The upper limit of the useful range is set by the adsorptive capacity (breakthrough volume) of the adsorbents used and by the linear range of the gas chromatograph (GC) detector.

The method may be used in atmospheres of up to 95% relative humidity.

2. REFERENCES

CONCAWE (1986) *Method for Monitoring Exposure to Gasoline Vapour in Air*, Den Haag

International Organisation for Standardisation (1985) *Draft Method: Workplace Atmospheres — Determination of Hydrocarbon Vapour in Air by Thermal Desorption/Capillary Column/Gas Chromatography (ISO/TC146/SC2/WG4/N52)* and subsequent revisions

Price, J.A. & Saunders, K.J. (1984) Determination of airborne methyl *tert*-butyl ether in gasoline atmospheres. *Analyst, 109,* 829–834

3. DEFINITIONS

The breakthrough volume is the volume of a standard mixture of gasoline hydrocarbons in air that can be passed through the adsorbent tubes before the concentration of eluting gasoline hydrocarbon vapour reaches 5% of the applied test concentration.

Gasoline hydrocarbons in this method refers to aliphatic gasoline components from C_3 (propane) to C_{10} (decane) and aromatic components from benzene to trimethylbenzene. The method may also be applicable to many of their homologues and to some gasoline oxygenates, e.g., methanol and methyl t-butyl ether.

4.   PRINCIPLE

A measured volume of sample air is drawn through two adsorbent tubes in series, the first containing Chromosorb 106 and the second containing charcoal. Most gasoline components are adsorbed on the Chromosorb. Some light hydrocarbons are not fully retained by the Chromosorb, but are retained by the back-up charcoal tube. The collected vapour from each tube is desorbed by heat and is transferred with inert carrier gas into a GC equipped with a capillary column and a flame-ionization detector.

5.   HAZARDS

Benzene is a recognized human carcinogen. Benzene and isopropylbenzene (cumene) are toxic by inhalation, ingestion and skin contact. n-Hexane presents a serious health hazard if incorrectly handled. Avoid inhalation.

6.   REAGENTS[1]

Use only reagents of recognized analytical reagent grade.

The following key petroleum components are used as reference compounds for quantification (e.g., n-hexane is used to calibrate for all aliphatic hexane isomers):

n-Pentane

n-Hexane

n-Heptane

n-Octane

n-Nonane

n-Decane

Benzene

Toluene

---

[1] Reference to a company and/or product is for the purpose of information and identification only and does not imply approval or recommendation of the company and/or product by the International Agency for Research on Cancer, to the exclusion of others which may also be suitable.

o-Xylene

Isopropylbenzene

Cyclohexane	Chromatographic quality, free from compounds co-eluting with gasoline hydrocarbons.
Porous polymer adsorbent	Chromosorb 106 (or equivalent), particle size 0.18–0.25 mm (60–80 mesh). Precondition Chromosorb 106 by heating in an inert atmosphere at 250 °C for 16 h before packing the adsorbent tubes.
Activated charcoal	Acid-washed, Sutcliffe Speakman 607C (or equivalent), particle size 0.18–0.25 mm (60–80 mesh). Precondition the charcoal by heating in an inert atmosphere at 250 °C for 16 h before packing the adsorbent tubes.
Standard solutions	Gravimetrically prepare a stock standard solution containing each of the analytes in cyclohexane (see section 12.1). Prepare working standard solutions to cover the range of interest by serial dilution of the stock solutions with cyclohexane. The analyte mass range in 5-µL aliquots of the working standards should exceed the mass range in the samples to be analysed.
Spiked adsorbent tube standards	Fit a clean Chromosorb 106 tube into the GC injection unit, through which inert carrier gas is passed at 100 mL/min. Inject 5-µL aliquot of working standard solution through the septum. Disconnect the loaded tube and seal with end-caps. Prepare at least three tube standards at each load level. Prepare fresh standards with each batch of samples.

7.   APPARATUS[1]

Adsorbent tubes	Typically constructed of stainless-steel tubing, 90 mm × 5 mm i.d., 6 mm o.d. Mark one end of the tube by, e.g., a scored ring about 10 mm from the end. Pack the tubes with charcoal or Chromosorb 106, as appropriate, to within about 10 mm of each end. Tubes contain typically about 200 mg Chromosorb 106 or 300 mg charcoal. Retain the adsorbents by stainless-steel gauzes and/or silanized glass-wool plugs. Prior to use, condition the tubes by heating slowly under flowing inert gas to 250 °C and maintaining that temperature for 10 min. If the thermal desorption blank (9.1) is unacceptable, tubes should be reconditioned. Once a sample has been analysed, the tube may be re-used immediately. However, it is advisable to check the thermal desorption blank if the tubes are left for an extended period, or if sampling for a different analyte is envisaged. Tubes should be sealed and stored in an airtight container.
Thermal desorption apparatus	See section 9.4 for characteristics of the two-stage thermal desorption apparatus.
Adsorbent tube end-caps	Metal fittings with polytetrafluoroethylene or Viton seals.
Adsorbent tube unions	Metal fittings with polytetrafluoroethylene or Viton seals to connect two adsorbent tubes during sampling.
Precision syringe	10-µL, readable to 0.1 µL.
Personal sampling pump	Capable of running continuously for 8 h at 5–200 mL/min, with flow rate stable to within ± 5%.
Plastic or rubber tubing	About 90 cm long, with diameter ensuring leak-proof fit to both pump and sample tube.
Clips	To hold sample tube and connecting tubing to the wearer's lapel area.

---

[1] Reference to a company and/or product is for the purpose of information and identification only and does not imply approval or recommendation of the company and/or product by the International Agency for Research on Cancer, to the exclusion of others which may also be suitable.

NOTE: To avoid sampling errors, do not use plastic or rubber tubing up-stream of the adsorbent.

Soap-bubble meter	Or other suitable device for calibrating pump.
Gas chromatograph (GC)	Fitted with a flame-ionization detector, capable of detecting an injection of 5 ng toluene with a signal-to-noise ratio of at least 5 to 1.
GC column	A variety of columns may be used. The following has been found to be suitable: 50 m × 0.22 mm fused-silica column, with 0.25 µm unbonded OV 1701 stationary phase.
Injection facility	For preparing spiked adsorbent tube standards. A conventional GC injection port may be used *in situ*, or it can be mounted separately. Retain the carrier gas line to the injector. If necessary, adapt the back of the injection port to take 6 mm o.d. tubing. This can be done conveniently by means of a compression coupling with a Viton O-ring seal.

8.   SAMPLING

8.1 Calibrate the sampling pump with a representative adsorbent tube assembly in line, using an external meter.

8.2 Attach the pump to the adsorbent tube assembly with plastic or rubber tubing. Place the charcoal tube next to the pump (section 4). Connect the marked end of each tube furthest from the pump.

8.3 To minimize chanelling, mount the tube assembly vertically in the worker's breathing zone, for example on his lapel.

8.4 Turn the pump on and adjust the flow rate. The recommended air sample volume for the gasoline hydrocarbons covered by this method is 2.5 L (8-h sampling rate, 5 mL/min). For sampling over shorter periods, the flow rate may be increased, but should not exceed 200 mL/min. In all cases, a 10-min sample may be taken at 200 mL/min. If the total sample is likely to exceed 2 mg (i.e., 1 mg on each tube), the sample volume should be reduced accordingly, or electrometer overload may occur. At temperatures higher than 20 °C, reduce the sample volume by a factor of 2 for each 10 °C rise. See section 12.2.

8.5 Record the time, temperature, flow rate (or register reading) and the barometric pressure when the pump was turned on. At the end of the sampling period, record the flow rate or register reading, turn the pump off and record the time, temperature and barometric pressure.

8.6 Disconnect the sample tube assembly and seal both ends of each tube with compression seals. Tighten the seals securely. Place identifying labels on each tube. If samples are not to be analysed within 8 h, place them in a sealed metal or glass container.

9.   PROCEDURE

9.1 *Blank test*

Prepare sample blanks using tubes identical to those used for sampling. Subject them to the same procedure as the sample tubes except that no air is pumped through them. Label these as blanks and analyse them along with the samples, as described in sections 9.4–9.7. The adsorbent tube blank level is acceptable if it is no greater than the equivalent of 100 ng of benzene for any of the calibration compounds. Typical levels are much less than this.

9.2 *Check test*

Not applicable.

9.3 *Test portion*

Not applicable.

9.4 *Thermal desorption conditions*

Choose desorption conditions such that desorption from the sample tube is complete and no sample loss occurs in the secondary trap, if used. The following conditions are typical:

Desorption temperature	250 °C
Desorption time	5 min
Transfer line	150 °C
Cold trap low	− 30 °C
Cold trap high	300 °C
Cold trap adsorbent	Chromosorb 106, 40 mg
Carrier gas	Helium

The desorbed vapour occupies a volume of several millilitres, so that it will need to be concentrated if good chromatographic peak shape and adequate separation are to be obtained. This is achieved by using a secondary adsorbent and/or cold trap external to the GC.

9.5 *GC operating conditions*

The column should be operated on a temperature programme from 10 °C to 200 °C at 6 °C/min. Thread the capillary column back through the transfer line from the thermal desorption apparatus to the GC so that the capillary is 1–2 mm from the adsorbent in the cold trap. The split valve is conveniently placed at the chromatograph end of the transfer line. A typical split ratio is 100:1. Correspondence of retention time on a single column should not be regarded as proof of identity.

9.6 *Calibration curves*

9.6.1   Prepare a set of calibration curves for the key petroleum compounds as follows: place in the thermal desorption apparatus a Chromosorb 106 tube 'spiked' with each key compound and purge air from the tube to avoid chromatographic artefacts arising from thermal oxidation of the porous polymer or GC packing.

9.6.2   Heat the tube to displace the organic vapours, which are passed to the GC by means of the carrier gas stream. The gas flow at this stage should be the reverse of that used during sampling, i.e., the marked end of the tube should be nearest the GC column inlet.

9.6.3   Using data from at least three standards at each load level, plot the peak height (or area) against the mass of the analyte. The slope of the graph obtained gives the average response factor (height or area/μg analyte) for the given key petroleum compound.

9.6.4   For each key petroleum compound, determine the relative response factor, i.e., the ratio of the average response factor (9.6.3) to that for *n*-heptane. If any of the relative response factors lies outside of the range 1.00 $\pm$ 0.15, check for leaks, splitter functioning, detector gas-flow settings and incomplete recovery.

9.7 *Analyte determination*

9.7.1   Analyse the samples and sample blanks as described for the calibration standards in 9.6.1–9.6.2.

9.7.2   Determine the peak heights (areas) and read the mass of each analyte in the desorbed sample from the appropriate calibration curve (9.6.3). However, little additional error is introduced by using the calibration curve for *n*-heptane for all petroleum hydrocarbons when the relative response factors are within the range 1.00 $\pm$ 0.15. For petroleum hydrocarbons other than the ten key components, use the calibration graph of the nearest analogue, i.e., use the *n*-hexane calibration graph for all aliphatic hexane isomers.

10. METHOD OF CALCULATION

The mass concentration, ρ_a(mg/m^3), of a given analyte in the air sample is given by

$$\rho_a = (m_s - m_b)/V,$$

where

m$_s$ = the sum of the masses of the given analyte found in the Chromosorb and charcoal sample tubes (µg)

m$_b$ = the sum of the masses of the given analyte found in the blank Chromosorb and charcoal tubes (µg)

V = the volume of the air sample (L).

11. REPEATABILITY AND REPRODUCIBILITY

Laboratory tests of the procedure (CONCAWE, 1986), using tubes spiked with the key petroleum compounds as specified in section 6 at levels in the range 0.5 to 500 µg of each compound, indicated a mean repeatability (expressed as a coefficient of variation) of 5%. The reproducibility expressed in the same way was 12%. Assuming a pump error of 5%, the combined sampling and analytical errors are 7% and 13%, respectively.

In a second trial, using tubes spiked with a larger range of analytes, including propane and butane isomers, from a standard atmosphere, mean repeatability and reproducibility, including pump errors, were 12% and 26%, respectively.

12. NOTES ON PROCEDURE

12.1 It may be necessary to prepare a few standards covering a wide range of loading levels (say 10 µg to 1 mg) in order to determine the approximate weight range of the samples and hence the weight range of interest.

12.2 Sampling efficiency will be 100%, provided the capacity of the adsorbent is not exceeded. If this capacity is exceeded, breakthrough of vapour from the tube assembly will occur. The breakthrough volume may be measured by sampling from a standard vapour atmosphere, while monitoring the effluent air with a flame-ionization detector (a suitable procedure is described in Method 1, section 12.2). The breakthrough volume varies with ambient air temperature, falling by a factor of about 2 for each 10 °C rise. It also varies with sampling flow rate, being reduced substantially at flow rates below 5 mL/min or above 500 mL/min. To allow a suitable margin of safety, it is recommended that sample volumes of not more than 70% of the breakthrough volume be taken. For *n*-propane, a typical breakthrough volume is 3.5 L for the tube combination sampling 100 ppm at 20 °C and 50% relative humidity.

13. SCHEMATIC REPRESENTATION OF PROCEDURE

Sample known volume of air with Chromosorb 106
and charcoal adsorbent tubes in series
↓
Obtain GC calibration curves using adsorbent tubes
spiked with analytes of interest
↓
Analyse sample tubes and blank tubes
↓
Identify and quantify analytes
using GC data and calibration curves

14. ORIGIN OF THE METHOD

CONCAWE
Babylon i Kantoren A
Koningin Julianaplein 30–9
2595 AA Den Haag
The Netherlands

Contact points: Mr A. Eyres
CONCAWE

Dr R.H. Brown
Health and Safety Executive
Occupational Medicine and Hygiene Laboratory
403 Edgware Road
London NW2 6LN
UK

METHODS FOR BIOLOGICAL MONITORING

METHOD 4 — BREATH SAMPLING

E.D. Pellizzari, R.A. Zweidinger & L.S. Sheldon

1. SCOPE AND FIELD OF APPLICATION

This technique has been designed to collect breath samples from people exposed to volatile pollutants. The breath samples are collected at (or near) the subjects' residence or workplace. The technique was therefore developed for sampling in a mobile unit (van).

2. REFERENCES

Not applicable

3. DEFINITIONS

Not applicable

4. PRINCIPLE

A Tedlar bag is filled with purified, humidified air which the subject inhales using a special mouthpiece. The subject then exhales into the mouthpiece, filling a second Tedlar bag with breath. The breath from the filled (exhale) bag is then drawn through a Tenax cartridge by a Nutech pump (two cartridges and two pumps in parallel are used for duplicate collections). The Tenax cartridge is then dried over calcium sulfate and stored for analysis.

5. HAZARDS

Methanol, used to rinse part of the equipment is flammable and toxic. It should never be used or stored in the van.

6.   REAGENTS[1]

All reagents used should be analytical reagent grade

Compressed air[2]	0.1 THC grade
Compressed helium	99.9% grade
Distilled water[2]	
Charcoal filters[2]	
Calcium sulfate[2]	Drierite, indicating Drierite, non-indicating, cleaned by heating in a muffle-furnace at 400 °C for 2 h
n-Pentane	
Methanol	Distilled in glass
Tenax GC	2,6-Diphenyl-*p*-phenyleneoxide polymer (Applied Science, State College, PA)
Glass wool	Virgin Tenax (or Tenax to be recycled) must be extracted in a Soxhlet apparatus for at least 24 h with methanol, followed by 24 h with *n*-pentane. Dry the extracted Tenax in a vacuum oven at 100 °C for 24 h at 28 inches of water (7.0 kPa), then purge in a nitrogen box for 24 h. Sieve the Tenax under nitrogen to obtain 40/60 particle size range (all sieving and cartridge preparation must be conducted in a "clean" room).

7.   APPARATUS[1]

Spirometer

The spirometer is a device for the collection of breath samples and is shown in Figure 1. An all-Teflon mouthpiece with Tedlar flap valves and a stainless-steel ball valve is used. A bubbler filled with distilled-deionized water is placed in-line with the air tank to humidify the air for subject comfort. Each Tenax cartridge is connected

---

[1] Reference to a company and/or product is for the purpose of information and identification only and does not imply approval or recommendation of the company and/or product by the International Agency for Research on Cancer, to the exclusion of others which may also be suitable.

[2] These reagents are necessary for sample collection and should be carried in the van at all times.

Fig. 1. Spirometer apparatus

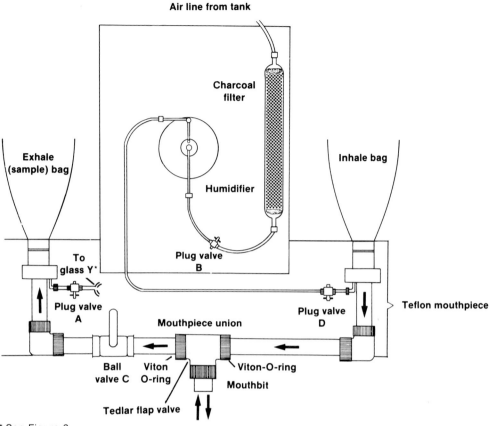

* See Figure 2.

to a separate Nutech 221 sampler equipped with a dry gas meter, so that the amount of air drawn through each cartridge may be accurately measured. The mouthpiece is mounted on an adjustable bar located on the front of the spirometer body. The glass Y, to which the Tenax cartridges are attached, is secured to the frame of the spirometer and the floor.

Tedlar bags	40-L (Nutech Inc.)
Teflon tubing	1/4 inch (6.35 mm) o.d.
Air regulator[1]	(plus one spare air regulator)
Cajon Ultra Torr Union 316[1]	Stainless-steel, with Viton O-rings

---

[1] These materials should be carried in the van at all times. They include materials for sample collection, as well as spare parts for the spirometer and Nutech samplers.

Straight unions	Stainless-steel, 1/4 inch (6.35 mm)
Teflon ferrules	1/4 inch (6.35 mm)
Charcoal filters	See Figure 1

Teflon mouthpiece

Teflon plug valves	1/4 inch (6.35 mm; Cole Palmer-6392–20)
Teflon tubing	1/4 inch (6.35 mm) o.d.
Ball valve with Teflon seats	Stainless-steel, 1 inch (25.4 mm)
Nacom Teflon unions	1 inch (25.4 mm)
Viton O-rings[1]	See 8.5.3
Mouthpiece union, with Tedlar flap valves	
Tedlar flap valves[1]	
Teflon mouthbits[1]	
Solid Teflon mouthbit plug[1]	

Sampling lines

Latex tubing	1/4 inch (6.35 mm) i.d.
Male Quick-Connect	Single-end shut-off (connects sampling line to pump)
Plastic in-line filters (Drierite)	
Cajon Ultra Torr Unions 316[1]	
Stainless-steel needles[1]	1.25 inch (31.75 mm), 21 gauge
Thermogreen septum	Supelco 2-0668
Glass Y's[1]	

---

[1] These materials should be carried in the van at all times. They include materials for sample collection, as well as spare parts for the spirometer and Nutech samplers.

Nutech Model 221 Gas Samplers High-volume gas pump

Auto batteries   12 volts

Humidifier[1]

Flat-bottom boiling flask   500 mL, 24/40 joint

Midget impinger stopper   12/5 ball joint, 24/40 stopper (Lab Glass-6891)

Ground socket joint   12/5 joint (Lab Glass-1041)

Pinch clamps   size 12 (Lab Glass-1045)

Miscellaneous equipment

Large forceps[1]

Small forceps

Empty culture tubes,   with Teflon liner and Teflon-lined screw-caps
Kimax®   2.5 × 15 cm

Glass tubes   10 × 1.5 cm i.d.

Plywood bag press[1]

Small stool

Copper wire

Three-prong clamps   Various sizes

Clamp holders

Small plastic bags

Glass beaker[1]   10 mL

Dummy cartridges[1]   See NOTE, section 8.7.3

Stopwatch/calculator[1]

Noseclip[1]

---

[1] These materials are necessary for sample collection and should be carried in the van at all times.

Mercury thermometer[1]

Kimwipes®[1]   8 × 5 inches

Aluminium foil

Binder clips   2-inch (50.8 mm; to seal Tedlar bags, see 8.2.3)

NOTE: Wash all glassware in 'Isoclean'/water, rinse with deionized-distilled
      water, acetone and air-dry. Heat glassware to 450–500 °C for 2 h to
      ensure that all organic material has been removed prior to use.

      Sonicate Teflon liners in methanol, then pentane, for approximately
      15 min each, then dry in a vacuum oven.

      Rinse the Teflon mouthbits in methanol and air-dry for at least 12 h
      before use.

      Methanol is inflammable and toxic and should at no time be used or
      stored in the van. The mouthbits must be cleaned only in a designated
      area of the workroom. Never allow the mouthbits to soak in methanol
      longer than 5 min. Air-dry and store in an upright position on a Kim-
      wipe® or clean towel.

8. SAMPLING

8.1 *Preparation of sampling cartridges*

   8.1.1   Prepare the sampling cartridges by packing a glass tube (10 cm × 1.5 cm
           i.d.) with 6 cm of 40/60 mesh Tenax GC, using a glass wool plug.

   8.1.2   Condition prepared cartridges at 270 °C with a purified helium flow of
           30 mL/min for > 120 min. (Prior to entering the Tenax GC cartridge, the
           helium is purified by passing through a liquid N_2-cooled trap.)

   8.1.3   Transfer the conditioned cartridges to Kimax® (2.5 cm × 15 cm) culture
           tubes.

   8.1.4   Seal immediately, using Teflon-lined screw-caps, and allow to cool. Store
           the cartridges in a sealed field collection can.

8.2 *Preparation of Tedlar bags*

   NOTE: The 40-L Tedlar bags used are designed to fit the Teflon mouthpiece of
         the spirometer. Tedlar is a brittle material and should never be folded or

---

[1] These materials are necessary for sample collection and should be carried in the van at all times.

creased, since this may cause it to crack or split. 'Inhale' and 'exhale' bags, although identical, should always remain segregated in order to minimize cross contamination.

8.2.1 Label each bag either 'inhale' or 'exhale' (one inhale bag is usually required for three exhale bags).

8.2.2 Attach the in-line charcoal filter to the helium tank and fill the bags with helium from the charcoal filter (do not over-inflate the bags).

8.2.3 Seal the mouth with a two-inch binder-clip (do not fold the mouth of the bag when sealing with the binder clip), then set aside the helium-filled bags for at least 2 h.

8.2.4 Remove the binder clip, place the bag in the wooden bag press and allow the helium to flow out under the weight of the press.

8.2.5 Repeat the bag purging (8.2.2–8.2.4) at least two more times (six times in the case of new Tedlar bags).

8.2.6 At least 30 min before leaving for sample collection, refill each bag with helium and seal the mouth with a two-inch binder clip. Carry the inflated bags to the van and hang on the hooks provided.

NOTE: The Tedlar bags are easily damaged by grit, sand or sharp objects. They must be inspected for small holes or cracks. If the bag has been used frequently and the mouth is very wrinkled or cracked, it may be trimmed back, provided it will still fit the mouthpiece.

8.3 *Purging of humidifier water*

NOTE: This operation may be performed at any time prior to filling the first inhale bag with humidified air. (Freshly-purged water may be used for up to one week before being replaced, if it is kept sealed in the humidifier and purged each day before use.) Purge the humidifier water for at least 15 min each time it is changed, or when additional water is added. Proceed as follows:

8.3.1 Install the in-line glass charcoal filter (Fig. 1).

8.3.2 Attach the air regulator to the gas cylinder and assemble the humidifier apparatus as shown in Figure 1.

8.3.3 Half-fill the humidifier flask with distilled water.

8.3.4 Refer to Figure 1 and open plug valves B and D (the Tedlar bags are not attached).

8.3.5   Close the shut-off valve on the regulator, then slowly open the com-
         pressed air cylinder.

8.3.6   Gradually open the shut-off valve until a steady bubbling through the
         water is observed. Adjust the pressure (regulator diaphragm) to 21 kPa
         (3 psi).

8.3.7   After 15 min, turn off the air supply at the regulator and close plug valves
         B and D. (Plug valve B must be closed whenever water is stored in the
         humidifier. If left open, water from the humidifier will saturate the
         charcoal filter and render it inactive.)

8.3.8   Close the air cylinder valve, remove the regulator and cap the tank.

8.4 *Equipment assemblage*

When the van reaches its destination, the equipment should be made ready for the
collection of the breath sample. Proceed as follows:

8.4.1   Assemble the mouthpiece as shown in Figure 1 and place the Teflon
         mouthbit in the mouthpiece.

8.4.2   Check the two Tedlar flap valves (in the mouthpiece union) by breathing
         in and out through the mouthpiece. Replace if damaged (i.e., if air flow
         is obstructed). The flap valves operate in only one direction. They must
         be installed so that air will flow from the inhale to the exhale bag only.

8.4.3   Attach all of the Teflon lines (using stainless-steel unions and Teflon
         ferrules), including the line from the exhale side of the mouthpiece to the
         glass Y.

8.4.4   Secure the glass Y to a support rod, approximately two feet above the gas
         cylinder, using a small three-prong clamp and copper wire.

8.4.5   Attach two Cajon Ultra Torr unions to the glass Y as depicted in
         Figure 2.

8.4.6   Place the spirometer upright, secure it with the compressed air cylinder
         and attach the gas inlet line to the air regulator.

         NOTE: The van should not be driven with the regulator attached to the
               gas cylinder. Sudden movements may fracture the regulator
               stem or cylinder valve which could lead to serious injury. The
               cylinder valve should be protected by the cap at all times when
               not in use.

8.5 *Inhale bag filling procedure*

8.5.1   Using the bag press, expel all of the helium from the inhale bag.

8.5.2   Immediately install the inhale bag on the right side of the spirometer
         mouthpiece (hang the bag by the grommet from the hook on the
         spirometer body).

Fig. 2. Tenax cartridge and glass Y assembly

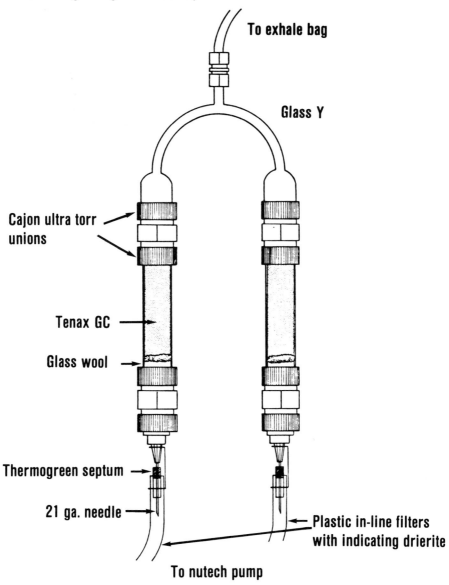

To exhale bag

Glass Y

Cajon ultra torr
unions

Tenax GC

Glass wool

Thermogreen septum

21 ga. needle

**Plastic in-line filters
with indicating drierite**

To nutech pump

8.5.3   Carefully roll the two large O-rings over the mouth of the bag, thus
         sealing the bag against the Teflon mouthpiece.

8.5.4   Place the solid Teflon mouthbit plug in the mouthpiece, open valves B
         and D and close valves A and C.

8.5.5   Attach the air regulator to the air cylinder and carefully bleed air through
         the humidifier into the inhale bag. (Never open the air cylinder before

closing the shut-off valve on the regulator. A sudden surge of air may destroy the humidifier. Keep the back pressure relatively low, controlling the air flow with the shut-off valve.)

8.5.6   Once the inhale bag is full, turn off the air supply and close valve D, then close the air cylinder valve and the air regulator shut-off valve.

8.5.7   Close plug valve B only after turning off the air supply (otherwise, the in-line back pressure may force the stopper from the humidifier, contaminating the air within and possibly destroying the humidifier).

8.6 *Preparation of the Nutech 221 samplers*

NOTE: Two samplers are operated simultaneously, splitting the collected breath sample into two equal portions and drawing it through two parallel Tenax cartridges. Each sampler is powered by a standard 12-volt automotive battery.

8.6.1   While the inhale bag is being filled, connect the Nutech samplers to the batteries and determine if they are both operational (make sure the sampler number and correction factor are displayed on the front panel).

8.6.2   Attach a sampling line to each Nutech sampler, using the male Quick-Connect fitting, and fill the in-line filter of the sampling line with indicating Drierite.

8.6.3   Inspect the sampling line 21-gauge needles daily for blockage.

8.7 *Tenax cartridge installation*

8.7.1   When the participant has arrived, remove the top pad of glass wool (using forceps) from a culture tube containing a Tenax cartridge and lay it on a clean Kimwipe®.

8.7.2   Using a clean Kimwipe®, remove the Tenax cartridge and connect the void end to the Cajon fitting of the sampling line leading to the Nutech 221 sampler.

8.7.3   Carefully connect the other end of the Tenax cartridge to the fitting on the glass Y. Label the cartridge.

NOTE: A standard breath sample consists of only one Tenax cartridge; therefore, an unused or 'dummy' cartridge is placed in line with the second Nutech sampler. If duplicate samples are to be collected from a participant, a clean Tenax cartridge is used in place of the dummy Tenax cartridge. If a dummy Tenax cartridge is used, place a distinctive marking on it so that it cannot be mistaken for the breath sample.

8.8 *Breath collection*

NOTE: The subjects must be cautioned to breathe at a normal rate, otherwise they may hyperventilate.

8.8.1   Place an exhale bag on the left side of the spirometer by repeating steps 8.4.1 to 8.4.3, inclusive.

8.8.2   Instruct the participants to breathe only through the mouth, to keep their lips sealed around the mouthbit, and not to stop before the exhale bag is full.

8.8.3   Have the participants put on the noseclip so that no air can pass through the nose.

8.8.4   Remove the solid Teflon plug from the mouthpiece and install a clean mouthbit.

8.8.5   Begin the breath collection by having the participants exhale, then place their lips on the mouthbit.

8.8.6   Open ball valve C and instruct the participants to begin breathing. (Start timer to determine duration of breath collection.)

NOTE: Observe the participants for a moment and remind them to breathe at a normal rate and to maintain a good seal on the mouthbit with their lips.

8.8.7   Using large forceps, remove the bottom pad of glass wool from the culture tube (8.7.1) and place it on a clean Kimwipe®.

8.8.8   Fill a 10-mL beaker to the 5-mL mark with non-indicating Drierite, pour the Drierite into the culture tube and replace the bottom pad of glass wool. Cap the tube and retain for step 8.9.6.

8.8.9   When the exhale bag is full, close valve C and tell the participants to stop breathing into the mouthbit. (Stop timer and record duration of exhalation.)

8.8.10   Remove the mouthbit and place the solid Teflon plug in the mouthpiece.

8.9 *Cartridge loading procedure*

8.9.1   Open plug valve A

8.9.2   Record temperature and the serial number, correction factor and meter reading for the Nutech sampler which will be used to collect the sample (assuming duplicate samples are not required), then begin pumping the breath sample through each Tenax cartridge.

8.9.3   Using the needle valve on the Nutech sampler, adjust the flow rates so that a back pressure of 150 to 175 torr is observed on each sampler (it is imperative that the pressure drop not exceed 175 torr (0.23 atm), or loss of target compounds may result). A normal sample collection (30 L divided evenly between two cartridges) should take approximately 15 min.

8.9.4   Using the needle valves on the samplers, adjust the flow rates (1 L/min) to be as equal as possible while maintaining approximately equal vacuum readings.

8.9.5   When a total of 30 L have been pumped, turn off both samplers and record the pumping time. Record the final dry gas meter reading from the Nutech sampler and close plug valve A.

8.9.6   Using a clean Kimwipe®, carefully remove the Tenax cartridge from the Cajon fittings and place it in the culture tube containing 2–3 g calcium sulfate and store for 24 h to day sample. Then transfer to a culture tube for long-term storage and add the top pad of glass wool (using forceps) on the Tenax cartridge and cap the culture tube (do not allow excess glass wool to lie over the top edge of the culture tube, preventing the cap from forming a proper seal).

8.9.7   Return the culture tube to the field collection can and seal the can.

         NOTE: Previous experiments have shown that the organic vapours collected on Tenax GC are stable and can be quantitatively recovered up to at least 4 weeks after sampling, when the cartridges are tightly closed in culture tubes and placed in a second sealed container, protected from light and stored at $-20\,°C$.

8.9.8   Remove the exhale bag from the spirometer, place it in the wooden bag press and allow any remaining breath sample to flow out under the weight of the press. Hang the empty exhale bag on the hooks in the van. If additional breath samples are to be collected, leave the inhale bag in place.

14. ORIGIN OF THE METHOD

Analytical and Chemical Sciences
Research Triangle Institute
Research Triangle Park, NC 27709
USA

Contact point: Dr E.D. Pellizzari

METHOD 5 — DETERMINATION OF BENZENE, TOLUENE AND XYLENE IN BREATH SAMPLES BY GAS CHROMATOGRAPHY/MASS SPECTROMETRY

E.D. Pellizzari, R.A. Zweidinger & L.S. Sheldon

1. SCOPE AND FIELD OF APPLICATION

This method is suitable for the analysis of benzene, toluene and xylenes in breath (a description of breath sampling is given in Method 4).

The linear range for the analysis of a volatile organic compound depends mainly on the breakthrough volume of the compound on the Tenax GC sampling cartridge and on the sensitivity of the mass spectrometer. The linear range for quantification using fused silica capillaries on a gas chromatograph (GC)/mass spectrometer (MS)/computer is generally three orders of magnitude (5–5 000 ng). Table 1 lists measured detection limits for the title compounds. No interference has been observed. The analysis of a single breath sample requires 1.5 h.

2. REFERENCES

American Society for Testing and Materials, *Annual Book of ASTM Standards,* Part 11.03 *Atmospheric Analysis,* Philadelphia, PA

Atomic Energy Research Establishment, *Eight Peak Index of Mass Spectra* (1970) Vol. 1 (Tables 1 & 2) and II (Table 3) Mass Spectrometry Data Centre, Aldermaston, RG7 4PR, UK

Krost, K.J., Pellizzari, E.D., Walburn, S.G. & Hubard, S.A. (1982) Collection and analysis of hazardous organic emissions. *Anal. Chem., 54,* 810–817

Pellizzari, E.D. (1977) *Analysis of Organic Air Pollutants by Gas Chromatography and Mass Spectroscopy (EPA-600/2-77-100),* Cincinnati, OH, US Environmental Protection Agency

Pellizzari, E.D. (1980) *Evaluation of the Basic GC/MS Computer Analysis Technique for Pollutant Analysis (EPA Contract No. 68-02-2998),* Cincinnati, OH, US Environmental Protection Agency

Pellizzari, E.D., Bunch, J.E., Berkley, R.E. & McRae, J. (1976) Determination of trace hazardous organic vapor pollutants in ambient atmosphere by gas chromatography/mass spectrometry/computer. *Anal. Chem., 48,* 803–806

Pellizzari, E.D., Bunch, J.E., Berkley, R.E. & McRae, J. (1976) Collection and analysis of trace organic vapor pollutants in ambient atmospheres. *Anal. Lett., 9,* 45

Table 1. Approximate measured limits of detection and quantification limits for benzene, toluene and xylene in breath

Compound	m/z	LOD[a] (µg/m³)	QL[a] (µg/m³)
Benzene	78/50	0.01	0.05
Toluene	91	0.70	3.5
Xylene (m + p, o)	106/91	0.50	2.5

[a] The limit of detection (LOD) is defined as S/N = 4 for the ion selected for quantification. The quantification limit (QL) is defined as 5 × LOD. Limits are based on a collection volume of 15 L for 6.0 cm × 1.5 cm i.d. Tenax GC bed.

3. DEFINITIONS

Not applicable

4. PRINCIPLE

The breath sample is collected on a Tenax GC cartridge (see Method 4), dried over calcium sulfate and analysed by thermal desorption of volatile components into a GC/MS (Fig. 1).

5. HAZARDS

Benzene is a known carcinogen. Because of its volatility, care must be exercised to avoid its inhalation as well as dermal exposure. It should be handled cautiously in a well-ventilated fume hood and operators should wear protective face masks, clothing and gloves which do not readily absorb benzene and other aromatic compounds.

6. REAGENTS[1]

Compressed helium, 99.9% grade

Compressed nitrogen

Calibration standards:
    perfluorotoluene
    perfluorotributylamine (low mass)

---

[1] Reference to a company or product is for the purpose of information and identification only and does not imply approval or recommendation of the company or product by the International Agency for Research on Cancer, to the exclusion of others which may also be suitable.

Fig. 1. GC/MS analytical system for analysis of organic vapours trapped from air onto cartridges.

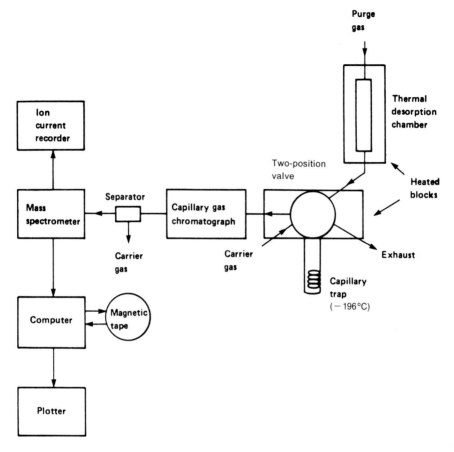

trisperfluoro-(heptyl)S-triazine (TRIS) (high mass for Finnigan 3300 MS) perfluorotributylamine (FC 43) for Finnigan 4021 MS

Pure analytes (see Table 1) in reagent bottles or permeation tubes (section 7)

Deuterated analytes for detecting breakthrough

7. APPARATUS[1]

Inlet manifold	Desorption chamber, valve and capillary trap interfaced to GC/MS system for thermal recovery of vapours trapped on Tenax sampling cartridges (see Fig. 1)
Gas chromatograph/mass spectrometer/computer	A Finnigan 9500 or Finnigan 9610 GC with a fused-silica capillary column, which is directly coupled to the ion source of the Finnigan 3300 or Finnigan 4021 MS system, respectively. A mass-flow controller (Tylan) is used to regulate the flow of carrier gas. Such an analytical system is shown in Figure 1. The characteristics of the GC/MS/computer system are specified in Tables 2 and 3.
Permeation system	See Figure 2.
Permeation tubes	Sealed plastic tubes with permeable walls, containing perfluorotoluene and analytes of interest (Metronics Corp., Santa Clara, CA, USA)
Tenax GC cartridges	See Method 4.

9.3 *Test portion*

Not applicable

9.4 *Preparation of standards*

9.4.1   System performance standards:

Load all of the compounds in Table 4 onto a single Tenax GC sampling cartridge (8.3), using the flash evaporation system (Fig. 3) and the following procedure[2]. Prepare standard solutions of the compounds in methanol (75 or 150 mg/L, see Table 4) and inject a 2-μL aliquot of each through the septum of the heated (250 °C) loading tube. Carry the vapour onto the Tenax cartridge with a stream of purified helium (60 mL/min) for 15 min. Store at −20 °C until required. System performance

---

[1] Reference to a company or product is for the purpose of information and identification only and does not imply approval or recommendation of the company or product by the International Agency for Research on Cancer, to the exclusion of others which may also be suitable.

[2] The 'void' (exit) end of all loaded cartridges should be marked and desorption (9.5) should take place with the carrier gas flowing in the opposite direction to that obtained during loading (see also Method 4, 8.7.2).

Table 2.   GC/MS specifications

Parameter	Finnigan 3300[a]	Finnigan 4021
Type	Low-resolution quadrupole	Low-resolution quadrupole
Resolution	Mass range to 1000 with unit resolution	Mass range to 1000 with unit resolution
Scan speed	1 s-10 min over entire range	0.1 s-10 min over entire range
Routine mass calibration standards	Perfluorotributylamine (low mass); trisper-fluoro-(heptyl)-*S*-triazine (high mass)	FC 43 (perfluorotributylamine)
Mode	Electron impact; chemical ionization (CH_4, NH_3, isobutane)	electron impact; chemical ionization, positive and negative
GC	Finnigan 9500	Finnigan 9610
GC columns	Glass capillaries (SCOT); packed; fused silica capillaries	Glass capillaries (WCOT, SCOT); fused silica capillaries; packed
GC injection	Glass capillaries; thermal desorption	Thermal desorption; splitter; Grob type; liquid
GC-MS	Single-stage glass jet; capillary direct coupling	Direct coupling or glass jet
Sample introduction	GC; direct probe interchangeable with molecular leak heated inlet	GC, interchangeable with direct probe
Computer	Data General NOVA 3	Data General NOVA 3
Computer hardware	32K central processor with Tektronix 4010-1 graphic terminal and keyboard	32K central processor with Tektronix 4010-1 graphic terminal and keyboard
	Versatec electrostatic printer/plotter	Versatec electrostatic printer/plotter
	4 Perkin-Elmer disk drives (5 megaword double density disks)	4 Perkin-Elmer disk drives (5 megaword double density disks)
	Wangco Model 1045 9-track 800 BPI, 45 IPS, industry-compatible magnetic tape	Wangco Model 1045 9-track 800 BPI, 45 IPS, industry-compatible magnetic tape
	External interface	External interface
Computer interface	Simultaneous dual mass spectrometer interface	Simultaneous dual mass spectrometer interface
Software capabilities	Control full scan mass spectral acquisition	Control full scan mass spectral acquisition
	Acquire multiple ion detection data for up to 25 ions	Acquire multiple ion detection data for up to 25 ions
	Reconstruct gas chromatograms	Reconstruct gas chromatograms
	Subtract background	Subtract background
	Reconstruct mass chromatograms	Reconstruct mass chromatograms

(Table 2. – cont'd)

Parameter	Finnigan 3300[a]	Finnigan 4021
	Calculate peak area from mass chromatograms	Calculate peak area from mass chromatograms
	Plot normalized or maximum intensity mass spectra	Plot normalized or maximum intensity mass spectra
	Library search (EPA/NIH)	Library search (EPA/NIH)
	Reverse library search	Reverse library search

[a] This equipment is employed by the authors.

Fig. 2. Permeation system for generating and loading air vapour mixtures[a]

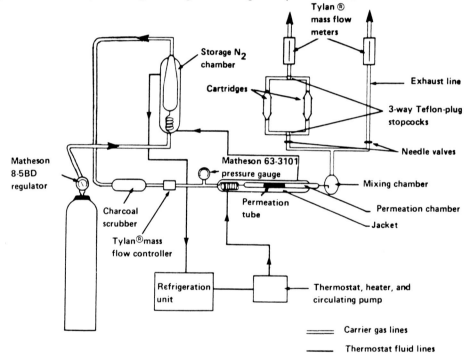

[a] The detailed operation of the permeation system is described by Krost et al. (1982).

standards are employed to determine the sensitivity and performance of the GC/MS/computer system on a daily basis (see also section 12.1).

9.4.2   Calibration (relative response factor) standards:

Using the permeation system (Fig. 2) or the flash-evaporator (see 9.4.1), load 250–450 ng of each of the analytes of interest, plus ~150 ng of perfluorotoluene (quantification standard), onto a single Tenax cartridge (8.3). If the permeation system is used, prepare a nitrogen/vapour mix-

Table 3. Mass (*m/z*) and relative ion abundances from perfluorotoluene acceptable for quantification with quadrupole instruments[a]

Perfluorotoluene (Finnigan 3300)

m/z	Relative abundance	
	Mean	Range
69	18	17–39
79	8	4–12
93	16	9–23
117	46	34–58
167	16	11–19
186	66	55–77
217	100	100
236	56	47–65

[a] To be achieved in the chromatography mode

Table 4. GC/MS/computer system performance and quantification standards

Compound	Quantity (ng)
Perfluorotoluene	150
Ethylbenzene	300
o-Xylene	300
n-Octane	300
n-Decane	300
1-Octanol	300
5-Nonanone	300
Acetophenone	300
2,6-Dimethylaniline	300
2,6-Dimethylphenol	300

Fig. 3. Scheme of vaporization unit for leading organic compounds dissolved in methanol onto Tenax GC cartridges.

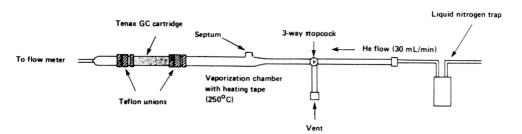

ture containing 1–4 ng analyte/mL and pass a known volume (∼ 200 mL) of the mixture through the Tenax cartridge. The amounts of the compounds loaded must be accurately known. Store at −20 °C until required.

Table 5. Operating parameters for GC/MS system

Parameter	Setting
Inlet manifold	
Desorption chamber and valve	270 °C
Capillary trap – minimum	– 195 °C (cooled with nitrogen)
– maximum	240 °C
Thermal desorption time	8 min
He purge flow	15 mL/min
GC	
60 m DB-1 wide-bore fused silica	40 °C (hold 5 min) → 240 °C, 4 °C/min
Carrier (He) flow	1.0 mL/min
Separator oven	240 °C
MS	
Finnigan 3300	
scan range	m/z 35 → 350
scan cycle, automatic	1.9 s/cycle
filament current	0.5 mA
electron multiplier	1 600 volts
analyser vacuum	18 mtorr
ion source vacuum	18 mtorr
inlet vacuum	25 mtorr
hold time	0.1 s

9.4.3   Using the permeation system, as in 9.4.2, add a known amount (~150 ng) of perfluorotoluene to the blank and to the five breath samples (8.2).

9.5 *Analyte determination*

NOTE: The operations described in 9.5 must be carried out in the order given.

9.5.1   Using the GC/MS operating conditions specified in Table 5, place the system performance standard (9.4.1) in the pre-heated desorption chamber and pass helium through the cartridge to carry the vapours into the capillary cold trap (Fig. 1).

9.5.2   When desorption is complete (8 min), rotate the inlet valve and raise the temperature of the capillary trap rapidly (> 100 °C/min), whereupon the carrier gas introduces the sample onto the GC column. When all analytes have eluted into MS, cool the column to ambient temperature.

9.5.3   Repeat 9.5.1 and 9.5.2 with the calibration standard (9.4.2).

9.5.4   Repeat 9.5.1 and 9.5.2 with the blank cartridge (8.2).

9.5.5   Repeat 9.5.1 and 9.5.2 with the five breath samples (8.2).

9.5.6   Repeat the cycle 9.5.1–9.5.5 until all breath samples have been analysed. If a cycle cannot be completed in a working day, each day must nevertheless begin with the analysis of a system performance standard (9.5.1–9.5.2) before completing the cycle.

9.6 *Data interpretation*

9.6.1 Qualitative analysis:
An ion chromatogram is constructed from the mass spectra. This will generally indicate whether the run is suitable for further processing, since it provides some idea of the number of unknown compounds in the sample and the resolution obtained using the particular GC column and conditions. See section 12.2 for compound identification procedures.

9.6.2 Quantitative analysis:
The time-dependent characteristic-ion spectra are employed to obtain chromatograms of breath samples and calibration standards (9.4.2). Both samples and standards contain known amounts of the quantification standard, perfluorotoluene. The ratios, peak area/mass loaded, for analyte and for perfluorotoluene, obtained with the calibration standard, are employed to calculate the relative response factor, F, which permits quantification of that analyte on the sample cartridge (see section 10).

10. METHOD OF CALCULATION

10.1 *Determination of relative response factor (F)*

The relative response factor, F_a, for a given analyte is obtained from,

$$F_a = A_a m_s / A_s m_a$$

where,

A_a = area of analyte peak on calibration standard chromatogram

A_s = area of quantification standard peak on calibration standard chromatogram

m_a = mass of analyte on calibration standard cartridge (μg)

m_s = mass of quantification standard on calibration standard cartridge (μg)

10.2 *Determination of analyte mass in sample*

Using the symbols employed in 10.1, the mass, m_a(μg), of the given analyte on the sample cartridge is obtained from,

$$m_a = A_a m_s / F_a A_s$$

where the values of A_a, A_s and m_s are those obtained from the sample cartridge.

NOTE: F_a is an average value, determined from at least three independent analyses carried out during analysis of a set of breath samples.

10.3 *Determination of mass concentration of analyte in sample*

The mass concentration of the given analyte in the breath sample, $\rho_a(\mu g/m^3)$, is obtained from,

$$\rho_a = 10^3(m_a - m_b)/V$$

where,

m_b = mass of analyte on blank cartridge (μg)

V = volume of breath sample (L)

and m_a is defined in 10.2.

11. REPEATABILITY AND REPRODUCIBILITY

The reproducibility of this method has been determined to range from ± 10 to $\pm 30\%$ (relative standard deviation) for different substances when replicate sampling cartridges are examined.

The accuracy of analysis is generally ± 10 to $\pm 30\%$, but depends on the chemical and physical nature of the compound.

12. NOTES ON PROCEDURE

12.1 *Assessment of chromatographic performance*

The quality of the chromatography is of the utmost importance for the accuracy and precision of qualitative and quantitative analysis. Glass or fused silica capillary columns are evaluated according to the following criteria:

(1) percent peak asymmetry factor (PAF)

$$\% \text{ PAF} = 100 \text{ B}/\text{F}$$

where
B = the area of the back half of the chromatographic peak

F = the area of the front half of the chromatographic peak (both measured 10% above baseline)

(2) height equivalent to an effective theoretical plate (HETP_{eff})

$$\text{HETP}_{eff} = L/[5.54 \ (X/Y)^2]$$

Table 6. Minimum performance specifications for glass capillary columns

Parameter	Test compounds	Value
Resolution	Ethylbenzene:*p*-xylene	>1.0
Separation number	Octane:decane	<40
% Peak asymmetry factor	1-Octanol	<250
	Nonanone	<160
	Acetophenone	<300
Acidity	2,6-Dimethylaniline: acetophenone	0.7–1.3
Basicity	2,6-Dimethylphenol: acetophenone	0.7–1.3

where

X = the retention distance (corrected for sweep time) of the compound,

Y = chromatographic peak width at one-half peak height,

L = column length (mm)

(3) separation number (SN)

$$SN = [D/(Y_1 + Y_2)] - 1$$

where

D = the distance between two peaks,

Y_1, Y_2 = widths at one-half height

(4) resolution (R)

$$R = 2 \, \Delta t/(W_1 + W_2)$$

where

Δt = distance between peak tops

W = peak width at base

(5) $\text{Acidity} = \dfrac{\text{weak base peak area (or height)}}{\text{acetophenone peak area (or height)}}$

$\text{Basicity} = \dfrac{\text{weak acid peak area (or height)}}{\text{acetophenone peak area (or height)}}$

The use of the compounds listed in Table 6 provides information regarding the degree of adsorption and the type of adsorption mechanism. The peak assymetry of 1-octanol and 5-nonanone serves to determine the extent of deactivation of the glass surface (PAF). The acidity and basicity of the glass or fused silica capillary column are assessed, respectively, by the adsorption of weak bases (e.g., 2,6-dimethylaniline) and acids (e.g., 2,6-dimethylphenol).

The resolution and separation number are determined for the compound pairs ethylbenzene:p-xylene and octane:decane, respectively. Table 6 lists the minimum performance specifications acceptable for breath analysis.

12.2 The computer automatically assigns masses during data acquisition by the use of the mass calibration table obtained for perfluorotributylamine. After the spectra are obtained in mass-converted form, processing proceeds either manually or by computer comparison with a library. Compound identification can involve several levels of certainty.

Level 1. The raw data generated from the analysis of samples are subjected only to computerized deconvolution/library search. Compound identification using this approach provides the lowest level of confidence. In general, it is reserved for those cases in which compound verification is the primary intent of the qualitative analysis.

Level 2. The plotted mass spectra are manually interpreted by a skilled interpreter and compared to spectra compiled in a data compendium. In general, a minimum of five masses and intensities ($\pm 5\%$) should match between the unknown and library spectrum.

NOTE: This level does not utilize any further information, such as retention time.

Level 3. The mass spectra are manually interpreted (as in level 2) and spectra and retention times are compared with those of the authentic compounds, using identical operating conditions.

13. SCHEMATIC REPRESENTATION OF PROCEDURE

Breath samples and blank cartridges
(one breath-sample cartridge in ten
is spiked with deuterated analytes
for breakthrough control)
↓
Add ~150 mg quantification
standard to each cartridge

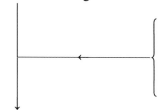

Prepare the following spiked
cartridges:
1. system performance standards
2. calibration (relative response
   factor) standards

Analyse system performance
standard, calibration standard,
blank and breath samples, in
that order, by GC/MS/computer
↓
Calculate relative response factor
from calibration standard
chromatogram.
Calculate analyte concentration
in sample using sample chromatogram
and relative response factor.

14. ORIGIN OF THE METHOD

Analytical and Chemical Sciences
Research Triangle Institute
Research Triangle Park, NC 27709, USA

Contact point: Dr E.D. Pellizzari

METHOD 6 — DETERMINATION OF PHENOL AND ITS GLUCURONO- AND SULFOCONJUGATES IN URINE BY GAS CHROMATOGRAPHY

J.P. Buchet

1. SCOPE AND FIELD OF APPLICATION

This method is suitable for the determination of the concentration of free plus bound phenol (in sulfo- and glucuronoconjugates) in urine, for the purpose of monitoring exposure to benzene (Lauwerys, 1983). Note, however, that some gastro-intestinal disorders (Duran *et al.*, 1973) and the absorption of certain drugs (Fishbeck *et al.*, 1975) can also give rise to positive responses.

Phenol concentrations ranging from 1 to 50 mg/L are easily detected in a 5-mL urine sample. Higher concentrations may be measured after sample dilution, while concentrations below 1 mg/L are almost never found, due to the background urinary excretion of phenol, even in the absence of exposure to benzene.

Excluding an overnight period required for the enzymatic digestion of phenol conjugates in the urine sample, the time required for analysis is 1 h. A well-trained technician can perform 50 phenol determinations per day using a dual-column gas chromatograph (GC).

Interference due to cresols, which is generally observed in colorimetric techniques for phenol measurement, is avoided by the use of gas chromatography (Buchet *et al.*, 1972; Dirmikis & Darbre, 1974).

2. REFERENCES

Buchet, J.P., Lauwerys, R.R. & Cambier, M. (1972) An improved gas chromatographic method for the determination of phenol in urine. *J. Eur. Toxicol., 1,* 27–30

Dirmikis, S.M. & Darbre, A. (1974) Gas-liquid chromatography of simple phenols for urinalysis. *J. Chromatogr., 68,* 169–187

Duran, M., Ketting, D., De Bree, P.K., Van Der Heiden, C. & Wadman, S.K. (1973) Gas chromatographic analysis of urinary volatile phenols in patients with gastro-intestinal disorders and normals. *Clin. Chim. Acta, 45,* 341–347

Fishbeck, W.A., Langner, R.R. & Kociba, R.J. (1975) Elevated urinary phenol levels not related to benzene exposure. *Am. Ind. Hyg. Assoc. J., 36,* 820–824

Lauwerys, R.R. (1983) *Industrial Chemical Exposure Guidelines for Biological Monitoring,* Davis, CA, Biomedical Publications, pp. 54–57

3. DEFINITIONS

Not applicable.

4. PRINCIPLE

Sulfo- and glucuronoconjugates of phenol are hydrolysed enzymatically for 18 h. An internal standard (nitrobenzene) and concentrated hydrochloric acid are then added and the mixture placed in boiling water for 30 min to complete the hydrolysis of the conjugates. After cooling, the total phenol is extracted in diethyl ether, an aliquot of which is analysed by gas chromatography. Freshly prepared aqueous phenol solutions of known concentration are similarly treated for calibration purposes.

5. HAZARDS

Phenol and nitrobenzene are toxic by ingestion, inhalation and skin contact.

Fuming hydrochloric acid is highly corrosive and can cause skin burns and irritation of the respiratory system.

Diethyl ether should be handled in a fume hood, since its vapours are easily inflammable and exert a narcotic action.

6. REAGENTS[1]

All reagents should be of analytical grade.

Hydrogen   99.99%, for flame-ionization detector (FID).

Nitrogen   99.999%, for GC mobile phase.

Air   99.999%, dry, for FID.

Phenol

Nitrobenzene

Diethyl ether

Fuming hydrochloric acid   ≥37%.

---

[1] Reference to a company and/or product is for the purpose of information and identification only and does not imply approval or recommendation of the company and/or product by the International Agency for Research on Cancer, to the exclusion of others which may also be suitable.

Disodium hydrogen phosphate	
Potassium dihydrogen phosphate	
β-Glucuronidase	Type H-2 crude solution (from *Helix pomatia*) containing ~ 100 000 U/mL at pH 5.0 and 37 °C as well as 1 000–5 000 U/mL sulfatase activity. Store at 4 °C (Sigma Chemical Co., St Louis, MO, USA).
Buffer solution	0.5 mol/L Na_2HPO_4/KH_2PO_4, pH 7.0.
Phenol standard solution	200 mg/L in deionized water. Prepare daily just before use.
Nitrobenzene internal standard solution	500 mg/L in deionized water. Prepare one day before first use, to allow for slow dissolution. Solution can be stored indefinitely in a refrigerator, since concentration changes do not affect quantification using calibration curves.
β-Glucuronidase working solution	Prepare a suitable volume daily by 10-fold dilution of the crude solution with deionized water.

7. APPARATUS[1]

Gas chromatograph	For isothermal analysis, equipped with FID
GC column	Stainless-steel, 1.5 m × 2 mm i.d., packed with 20% ethylene glycol succinate on Chromosorb W-AW-DMCS, 80–100 mesh
Water bath	37 °C, 100 °C
Test tubes	20-mL, glass-stoppered
Mechanical tube shaker	Vortex type
Syringe	Hamilton, 10 µL

8. SAMPLING

Urine samples collected in plastic containers can be stored at 4 °C up to one week before analysis. Control samples showed no change after several months at −20 °C.

---

[1] Reference to a company and/or product is for the purpose of information and identification only and does not imply approval or recommendation of the company and/or product by the International Agency for Research on Cancer, to the exclusion of others which may also be suitable.

9. PROCEDURE

9.1 *Blank test*

Analyse 5 mL of deionized water in place of urine (see 9.7.2).

9.2 *Check test*

Check the calibration of the apparatus during each work day by repeating the injection of the 40 mg/L working standard solution (9.7.1) at regular intervals.

9.3 *Test portion*

5.0 $\pm$ 0.05 mL of well-mixed urine sample.

9.4 *Hydrolysis and extraction*

9.4.1   Shake the sample container to suspend solids possibly settled during storage, then pipette a 5-mL aliquot into a 20-mL tube with a glass stopper.

9.4.2   Add 0.02 mL β-glucuronidase working solution. Mix well and place in a water bath at 37 °C for 18 h.

9.4.3   Add 0.25 mL of nitrobenzene internal standard solution and 2 mL of concentrated hydrochloric acid. Mix well and place in a water bath at 100 °C for 30 min. Take care to keep the tube tightly closed.

9.4.4   Cool to room temperature, then add 2 mL of diethyl ether. Stopper tube and shake with a mechanical shaker (e.g., 10 s with a Vortex).

9.4.5   Allow the tube to stand for a few minutes (if the emulsion is too stable, roll the tube between both hands until sufficient clear organic phase separates). Retain for GC analysis.

9.5 *GC operating conditions*

Column oven temperature   155 °C
Injection port temperature   250 °C
FID temperature   250 °C
Carrier gas (nitrogen) flow rate   40 mL/min.

At the start of each working day, condition the column by a few solvent injections.

9.6 *Analyte determination*

Inject about 5 µL of the organic extract (9.4.5) into the GC and record the heights (or areas) of the phenol and nitrobenzene peaks. Calculate the ratio of the peak height (area) of phenol to that of nitrobenzene.

9.7 *Calibration curve*

9.7.1   Dilute the freshly-prepared phenol standard solution with deionized water to obtain working standard solutions with phenol concentrations of 10, 20, 30 and 40 mg/L.

9.7.2   Analyse 5-mL aliquots of each of the working standard solutions and 5 mL of deionized water (blank) as indicated in sections 9.4–9.6, inclusive.

9.7.3   Applying the least-squares method, obtain the intercept and slopes of the first-order equation describing the variation of the peak height or area ratios with phenol concentration.

10. METHOD OF CALCULATION

Using the peak height (area) ratio obtained in 9.6 and the equation from 9.7.3, calculate the total phenol concentration in the urine sample.

11. REPEATABILITY AND REPRODUCIBILITY

11.1 *Repeatability*

The coefficient of variation for 25 determinations carried out over a five-month period was 6% at the 20 mg/L level.

Triplicate determinations performed on the same day gave a coefficient of variation of 2%.

No reproducibility data are available.

11.2 *Recovery*

Unlike phenylsulfate, phenylglucuronide cannot be completely hydrolysed by acid treatment alone. With the present method, the recovery determined in samples with free phenol (10 mg/L) was better than 98%. That obtained with phenylglucuronide at a level corresponding to 250 mg phenol/L was about 92%.

12. NOTES ON PROCEDURE

Not applicable.

13. SCHEMATIC REPRESENTATION OF PROCEDURE

Transfer 5 mL urine to glass-stoppered tube
↓
Add 0.02 mL β-glucuronidase solution
and hold at 37 °C for 18 h
↓
Add 0.25 mL internal standard (nitrobenzene) solution
+ 2 mL conc. hydrochloric acid
and hold at 100 °C for 30 min
↓
Cool and extract with 2 mL diethyl ether
↓
Inject several microlitres of organic phase into GC
↓
Determine ratio of peak height (area) of phenol
to that of nitrobenzene and obtain phenol
concentration in urine from calibration curve.

14. ORIGIN OF THE METHOD

Unité de Toxicologie Industrielle et Médecine du Travail
Université Catholique de Louvain
Clos Chapelle-aux-Champs 30, bte 30.54
1200 Bruxelles
Belgium

Contact point: Dr J.P. Buchet

METHOD 7 — DETERMINATION OF TOLUENE IN BLOOD BY HEAD-SPACE GAS CHROMATOGRAPHY

J. Angerer

1. SCOPE AND FIELD OF APPLICATION

This fused-silica capillary column gas chromatograph (GC) method for the determination of toluene in blood is highly specific. Interference by other volatile substances (acetone, acetic aldehyde, etc) present in blood has not been observed. Thus the method can also be used for the simultaneous determination of other aromatic hydrocarbons (e.g., benzene, xylenes, ethyl benzene) in blood.

The limit of detection is 5 µg/L, and the response is linear between 5 and 4 000 µg toluene per litre of blood.

The time necessary for analysis depends only on that required for the gas chromatographic separation, since there is practically no preparation of the sample; thus 30 to 40 analyses can be done per day.

2. REFERENCES

Angerer, J. (1985) Biological monitoring of workers exposed to organic solvents – past and present. *Scand. J. Work Environ. Health, 11,* 45–52

Sato, A., Nakajima, T. & Fujiwara, Y. (1975) Determination of benzene and toluene in blood by means of a syringe-equilibration method using a small amount of blood. *Br. J. Ind. Med., 32,* 210–214

3. DEFINITIONS

Not applicable.

4. PRINCIPLE

The blood sample is heated to 60 °C, and the volatile toluene accumulates in the vapour phase above the blood sample. After equilibration, an aliquot of the vapour phase is analysed on a fused-silica capillary column. A flame-ionization detector (FID) serves for the determination of toluene.

Blood solutions containing known amounts of toluene are used for calibration.

5. HAZARDS

Because of the risk of infection, gloves should be worn during the collection and handling of blood samples.

6. REAGENTS[1]

Ammonium oxalate	Purest available
Toluene	Reference substance for gas chromatography, purity 99.7% (Merck)
Bovine blood	GLD Gesellschaft für Labor und Diagnostik, D–4300 Essen 1, FRG
Nitrogen	99.999%, for mobile phase
Hydrogen	99.9%, for flame-ionization detector
Air	For flame-ionization detector
Stock standard solution	Bring the toluene used for the stock solution to 20 °C, at which temperature toluene has a specific gravity of 0.8669 g/cm^3. With a GC syringe, pipette 2.5 µL toluene into a 100-mL volumetric flask containing 20 mL bovine blood. While gently mixing the contents of the flask, make up to 100 mL with blood. The concentration of toluene in this stock solution is 21.6725 mg/L. Prepare just before use.
Working standard solutions	Dilute the stock standard solution by factors of 10, 25, 100 and 250 with bovine blood, to obtain toluene concentrations of 2 167, 867, 217 and 86.7 µg/L, respectively. Prepare 100 mL of each solution and store at −18 °C.

7. APPARATUS[1]

Gas chromatograph	Equipped with split injector and flame-ionization detector.
Capillary column	Fused-silica, 30 m × 0.25 mm i.d., bonded layer of cyanopropyl phenyl silicone (Durabond 1701) 0.25 µm thick

---

[1] Reference to a company and/or product is for the purpose of information and identification only and does not imply approval or recommendation of the company and/or product by the International Agency for Research on Cancer, to the exclusion of others which may also be suitable.

Thermostat, 60 °C   With bore holes for 20-mL injection vials (Grant Instruments, Cambridge, UK)

Thermostat, 20 °C

Injection (head-space) vials   20-mL, with polytetrafluoroethylene-coated butyl rubber stoppers

Hand-crimper   For butyl rubber stoppers

Gas-tight syringe   500-μL

8. SAMPLING

8.1 Take a 3-mL blood sample at the end of the work shift. Use disposable needles and syringes to take the blood from the cubital vein. Omit the usual disinfection of the puncture site because of possible interference from volatile organic solvents. Wash the forearm with soap, instead.

8.2 Immediately inject a 2-mL aliquot of the blood sample into an injection vial containing 50 mg ammonium oxalate to prevent coagulation. (Within wide limits, the toluene concentration in the vapour phase is independent of the volume of the sample.)

8.3 Close the 20-mL injection vial hermetically with a butyl rubber stopper, using a special hand-crimper. Mix the blood sample gently to dissolve the anticoagulant.

8.4 The samples can be shipped to the laboratory without further precautions and can be kept for at least three days without refrigeration. If the sample cannot be analysed immediately after arrival in the laboratory, it can be stored at -18 °C for at least six months without loss of the aromatic solvent.

9. PROCEDURE

9.1 *Blank test*

Analyse 2 mL of deionized water as described in 9.5. At least one blank should be analysed with each series. The blank test detects memory effects associated with any part of the analytical system.

9.2 *Check test*

9.2.1   Check the accuracy of the temperature setting of the thermostat by heating 2 mL of water in an injection vial. Measure the temperature of the water with a mercury thermometer. Repeat this check at intervals (e.g., every three months), especially when variable results are measured for the standard solutions.

9.2.2   Test the GC conditions at the beginning of each series of analyses by measuring the retention time of toluene and the sensitivity of the detector, using the working standard solutions.

9.3 *Test portion*

The injection vials containing 2 mL of blood (8.2) are used for analysis without further treatment.

9.4 *GC operating conditions*

Column temperature	60 °C
Injector temperature	250 °C
FID temperature	300 °C
Nitrogen carrier flow-rate	~2 mL/min
Hydrogen (FID) flow-rate	30 mL/min
Air (FID) flow-rate	300 mL/min
Make-up gas (N_2) flow-rate (Varian GC)	30 mL/min
Injection (split) ratio	1:25.

9.5 *Analyte determination*

9.5.1   Heat the injection vials in the thermostat at 60 °C for 30 min.

9.5.2   Warm the gas-tight syringe to 60 °C and rinse it with the vapour phase in the vial, lifting and pressing down the plunger several times. Take 500 µL of the vapour phase from the vial.

9.5.3   Inject 500 µL of the vapour phase into the GC and determine the peak area.

9.6 *Calibration curve*

9.6.1   Place 2 mL of each of the working standard solutions in a separate head-space vial and determine the GC peak areas as described in 9.5.1–9.5.3.

9.6.2   Draw a graph of the peak areas *versus* the toluene concentrations (µg/L), using the method of least-squares. Repeat 9.6 for each new series of blood analyses.

10. METHOD OF CALCULATION

Obtain the concentration of toluene in the blood sample using the calibration curve (9.6) and the peak area measured in 9.5.3.

11. REPEATABILITY AND REPRODUCIBILITY

11.1 *Repeatability*

Blood with toluene levels of 812 and 1 134 µg/L was repeatedly analysed to obtain coefficients of variation of 2.1 and 3.1%, respectively. Ten determinations were made at each concentration. When these 20 measurements were made on 20 different days, the respective coefficients of variation increased to 6.4 and 7.1%.

11.2 *Reproducibility*

The detection limit (section 1) and the results cited in 11.1 have been corroborated in another laboratory.

A blood sample containing toluene at a concentration of 1 084 µg/L was analysed 12 times and the average recovery was determined to be 110%.

12. NOTES ON PROCEDURE

Not applicable.

13. SCHEMATIC REPRESENTATION OF PROCEDURE

Not applicable.

14. ORIGIN OF THE METHOD

Zentralinstitut für Arbeitsmedizin
Adolph-Schönfelder-Strasse 5
D–2000 Hamburg 76
FRG

Contact point: Dr J. Angerer

METHOD 8 — DETERMINATION OF 2-METHYLPHENOL IN URINE BY GAS CHROMATOGRAPHY

J. Angerer

1. SCOPE AND FIELD OF APPLICATION

This method is suitable for the determination of 2-methylphenol in urine over the range 0.3–5.0 mg/L. These limits permit the detection of 2-methylphenol in the concentration range which is relevant for occupational health (a limit of 2.7 mg/L has been suggested for 2-methylphenol excretion in urine). To determine higher concentrations, the urine samples must be diluted.

The total amount of 2-methylphenol in urine is measured with this method; using simultaneous acid hydrolysis and steam distillation, conjugates are cleaved to yield free 2-methylphenol.

One operator can analyse ten urine samples per day.

2-Methylphenol is not normally present in urine and its detection constitutes a specific test for exposure to toluene. This method has been tested in several laboratories and is recommended by the German Commission for the Investigation of Health Hazards of Chemical Compounds in the Work Area.

2. REFERENCES

Angerer, J. (1985) Biological monitoring of workers exposed to organic solvents – past and present. *Scand. J. Work Environ. Health, 11 (Suppl.* 1), 45–52

Heinrich, R. & Angerer, J. (1985) Capillar-gas-chromatographische Bestimmung von Alkylphenolen in Harn. *Fresenius' Z. Anal. Chem., 322,* 766–771.

3. DEFINITIONS

Not applicable.

4. PRINCIPLE

The urine sample is spiked with 3-ethylphenol as internal standard and the mixture is steam-distilled under acidic conditions. The conjugates of 2-methylphenol and other phenols with glucuronic and sulfuric acids are cleaved and the phenols set free are separated from the urine. The steam distillate is acidified and extracted with methylene chloride. The reduced extract is analysed for 2-methylphenol using a capillary gas chromatograph (GC) with a flame-ionization detector (FID). The method is calibrated using solutions of 2-methylphenol in water.

5. HAZARDS

Avoid skin contact with 2-methylphenol and 3-ethylphenol because of their caustic properties. Protective spectacles should be worn during sublimation and distillation of 2-methylphenol and 3-ethylphenol, respectively, under reduced pressure.

All operations with methylene chloride should be carried out under a hood. Urine should be handled with gloves to avoid possible infection.

6. REAGENTS[1]

Methylene chloride	
Sodium sulfate	Anhydrous, purest available
Acetic acid	Purest available
Sulfuric acid	96%, purest available
Sulfuric acid	1 mol/L
2-Methylphenol	Purity >99% (sublimate commercial 2-methylphenol under reduced pressure). Store in brown bottle in refrigerator. Purify again if colour changes.
3-Ethylphenol	Purity >98% (distilled under reduced pressure). Store in brown bottle in refrigerator. Purify again if colour changes.
Nitrogen	99.999%, for GC and evaporation of solvent
Hydrogen	99.9%, for FID
Air	For FID
2-Methylphenol stock standard solution	100 mg/L. Place 100 mg 2-methylphenol in a 1-L volumetric flask and make up with distilled water. Prepare a fresh solution for each set of urine samples.

---

[1] Reference to a company and/or product is for the purpose of information and identification only and does not imply approval or recommendation of the company and/or product by the International Agency for Research on Cancer, to the exclusion of others which may also be suitable.

2-Methylphenol working standard solutions	0.5, 1.0, 2.0, 4.0 and 6.0 mg/L, prepared by dilution of stock standard solution with distilled water. Fresh solutions are required for each set of urine samples to be analysed.
3-Ethylphenol (internal standard) solution	100 mg/L. Place 100 mg 3-ethylphenol in a 1-L volumetric flask and make up with distilled water. Prepare a fresh solution for each set of urine samples.
Urine quality-control standard	1 mg 2-methylphenol/L. Pool at least 1 L of urine from unexposed subjects and cool for 16 h, then filter. Pipette 10 mL of 2-methylphenol stock standard solution into a 1-L volumetric flask and make up with pooled urine. Divide into 10-mL aliquots in disposable 20-mL plastic containers and store at $-18\,°C$.

7. APPARATUS[1]

Gas chromatograph	Equipped with split injector, temperature programme capability and FID
Capillary column	Fused-silica, 30 m × 0.32 mm i.d., bonded silicon phase SE-54, 0.25 μm thick
Steam generator and distilling apparatus	
Mechanical shaker	
Sublimation apparatus	
Roller mixer	For samples in 250-mL bottles
Vacuum distillation apparatus	
Test tubes	10-mL, graduated
Sample bottles	250-mL, polyethylene, with screw caps

---

[1] Reference to a company and/or product is for the purpose of information and identification only and does not imply approval or recommendation of the company and/or product by the International Agency for Research on Cancer, to the exclusion of others which may also be suitable.

Volumetric pipettes	1–10 mL
Separation funnel	100-mL
Volumetric flask	50-mL

8.   SAMPLING

Take the urine sample at the end of the work shift. Collect the urine in 250-mL polyethylene bottles which have been rinsed with distilled water. Add 1 mL of acetic acid/100 mL urine to adjust the pH of the sample to between 3 and 4 (a scrupulous volumetric dosage is not necessary because of the buffer capacity of urine and acetic acid). The sample can be shipped to the laboratory without further precautions and can be kept for at least three days without refrigeration. If it cannot be analysed immediately after arrival in the laboratory, it can be stored at $-18\,°C$ for at least six months without systematic bias of the result.

9.   PROCEDURE

9.1 *Blank test*

Analyse 10 mL of deionized water in place of urine, as described in sections 9.4–9.6.

It is not necessary to analyse the blank within each series of analyses if the glassware is known to be free from 2-methylphenol and 3-ethylphenol. This must be proved by several blank tests. (It has been shown that there is no memory effect due to the distilling apparatus.) Test the cleanness of the GC syringe by injection of the pure solvent.

9.2 *Check test*

Analyse the urine quality-control standard with each series of samples and check the retention times of 2-methylphenol and 3-ethylphenol and the sensitivity of the detector.

9.3 *Test portion*

10 mL of well-mixed urine sample. Frozen urine samples should be taken out of the refrigerator on the day before analysis and should be kept at room temperature.

9.4 *Analyte separation from urine*

9.4.1   Mix the urine sample in the 250-mL polyethylene bottle for 30 min, using a roller mixer.

9.4.2 Transfer a 10-mL aliquot of the urine sample to the distillation flask with a volumetric pipette. Add 1 mL of the internal standard solution (3-ethylphenol) and 3 mL 96% sulfuric acid.

9.4.3 Conduct steam through the distillation flask and collect 50 mL of the distillate in a 50-mL volumetric flask containing 2 mL of 1 mol/L sulfuric acid.

9.4.4 Transfer the distillate to a 100-mL separation funnel, add 15 mL methylene chloride and shake for 15 min on the mechanical shaker.

9.4.5 Transfer the organic layer to an Erlenmeyer flask, add 2 g anhydrous sodium sulfate and allow to stand for 1 h, with occasional shaking.

9.4.6 Filter the solution through a folded filter into a 25-mL flask. Wash the filter with 2.5 mL methylene chloride.

9.4.7 Evaporate the filtrate to about 5 mL under a stream of nitrogen.

9.4.8 Transfer filtrate (9.4.7) to a 10-mL graduated test tube and rinse the 25-mL flask with 1 mL methylene chloride.

9.4.9 Evaporate the combined organic phases (9.4.8) to 1 mL under a stream of nitrogen and retain for GC analysis.

9.5 *GC operating conditions*

Column temperature	5 min 60 °C, 5 °C/min to 110 °C, 20 °C/min to 200 °C, 10 min at 200 °C
Injector temperature	250 °C
Detector temperature	300 °C
Carrier gas (nitrogen) flow rate	2 mL/min
Hydrogen (FID) flow rate	30 mL/min
Air (FID) flow rate	300 mL/min
Make-up gas (N_2) flow rate (Varian GC)	30 mL/min
Injection (split) ratio	1:25.

9.6 *Analyte determination*

Inject 0.5 µL of concentrate 9.4.6 into the GC and record peak areas of 2-methyl- and 3-ethylphenol.

9.7 *Calibration curve*

9.7.1 Analyse 10 mL of each of the working standard solutions as described in sections 9.4–9.6.

9.7.2   Plot the ratios of the peak areas, 2-methylphenol/3-ethylphenol, *versus* the concentrations of the working standard solutions and draw a graph using the least-squares method.

10. METHOD OF CALCULATION

Obtain the concentration of 2-methylphenol in the urine sample using the calibration curve (9.7) and the ratio of the peak areas measured in 9.6.

11. REPEATABILITY AND REPRODUCIBILITY

11.1 *Repeatability*

A urine sample containing 2-methylphenol at a concentration of 2.4 mg/L was analysed 10 times, giving a coefficient of variation of 4.9%.

11.2 *Reproducibility*

The linear range (section 1) and the results cited in 11.1 were confirmed in another laboratory.

11.3 *Recovery*

The average 2-methylphenol recovery obtained with the 10 samples described in 11.1 was 104%. Hydrolysis of the glucurono-conjugate to liberate 2-methylphenol has been shown to be complete under the conditions described in section 9.4.

12. NOTES ON PROCEDURE

It has been shown that phenol, 3-methylphenol, 4-methylphenol, dimethylphenols and ethylphenol, 2-chlorophenol, 2-chloro-5-methylphenol, 2- and 3-nitrophenol, 3- and 4-chlorophenol and 3.4-dichlorophenol do not interfere with the GC separation of 2-methylphenol.

13. SCHEMATIC REPRESENTATION OF PROCEDURE

Mix sample 30 min and transfer 10-mL aliquot
to distillation flask
↓
Add 1 mL internal standard solution
+ 3 mL 96% sulfuric acid
↓
Steam distill and collect 50 mL in volumetric flask
containing 2 mL of 1 mol/L sulfuric acid
↓
Transfer distillate to 100-mL separation funnel,
add 15 mL methylene chloride and shake 15 min
↓
Transfer organic layer to Erlenmeyer flask
and dry for 1 h over 2 g anhydrous sodium sulfate
↓
Filter into graduated test tube,
wash filter with 2.5 mL methylene chloride
and evaporate filtrate to 1 mL under a stream of nitrogen
↓
Inject 0.5 μL of concentrate into GC
and determine peak areas of analyte and internal standard
↓
Determine analyte concentration in sample
using calibration curve obtained with standard solutions

14. ORIGIN OF THE METHOD

Zentralinstitut für Arbeitsmedizin
Adolph-Schönfelder-Strasse 5
D–2000 Hamburg 76
FRG

Contact point: Dr J. Angerer

METHOD 9 — DETERMINATION OF HIPPURIC ACID IN URINE BY HIGH-PRESSURE LIQUID CHROMATOGRAPHY

J. Angerer

1. SCOPE AND FIELD OF APPLICATION

The high-pressure liquid chromatographic method described here allows methyl hippuric acids, phenyl glyoxylic acid and mandelic acid to be determined together with hippuric acid in one run. (These aromatic carboxylic acids are metabolites of xylenes, ethyl benzene and styrene which are frequently used in mixtures with toluene.)

The limit of detection is 50 mg hippuric acid per litre of urine and the response is linear up to 2 000 mg/L. Higher concentrations may be determined by diluting the sample. The aromatic carboxylic acids which are excreted in urine do not interfere with the hippuric acid determination. Thirty samples can be analysed per day.

The Commission for the Investigation of Health Hazards of Chemical Compounds in the Work Area of the Deutsche Forschungsgemeinschaft has recommended this method for the determination of hippuric acid, methyl hippuric acids, mandelic acid and phenyl glyoxylic acid in urine.

2. REFERENCES

Lewalter, J., Schaller, K.H. & Angerer, J. (1985) Aromatische Carbonsäuren. In: Henschler, D., ed., *Analytische Methoden zur Prüfung gesundheitsschädlicher Arbeitsstoffe,* Band 2, *Analysen in biologischem Material,* Deutsche Forschungsgemeinschaft, Weinheim, Verlag Chemie, 8, Lieferung

Poggi, G., Giusiani, M., Palagi, U., Paggiaro, P.L., Loi, A.M., Dazzi, F., Siclari, C. & Baschieri, L. (1982) High performance liquid chromatography for the quantitative determination of the urinary metabolites of toluene, xylene and styrene. *Int. Arch. Occup. Environ. Health, 50,* 25–31

3. DEFINITIONS

Not applicable.

4. PRINCIPLE

The urine sample is spiked with 3-hydroxybenzoic acid (internal standard), and the acidified urine is then extracted with diethyl ether. An aliquot of the reduced organic extract is analysed with reversed-phase high-pressure liquid chromatography (HPLC) using a mixture of methanol:water (1:5) as the mobile phase. Ultraviolet detection is performed at a wavelength of 215 nm. Quantification is carried out by means of a calibration curve, using standard solutions of hippuric acid in water.

5. HAZARDS

5.1 To minimize exposure to diethyl ether and avoid ignition, operations with this solvent (extraction, evaporation) should be carried out in a hood.

5.2 Because of possible infection, gloves should be worn while handling urine samples.

6. REAGENTS[1]

Diethyl ether	Purest available
Hippuric acid	Recrystallize in water, then dry under reduced pressure to a constant weight over calcium chloride.
3-Hydroxybenzoic acid	
Hydrochloric acid	37%
Potassium orthophosphate trihydrate	Purest available
Phosphoric acid	95%, specific weight 1.71 g/cm^3
Methanol	For HPLC (Merck)
Deionized water	
Nitrogen	99.999%, for evaporation of the organic solvent
Buffer solution	Add 2.66 g of potassium orthophosphate to a 1-L volumetric flask and make up with deionized water. Adjust the pH to 3.5 with concentrated phosphoric acid.

---

[1] Reference to a company and/or product is for the purpose of information and identification only and does not imply approval or recommendation of the company and/or product by the International Agency for Research on Cancer, to the exclusion of others which may also be suitable.

Internal standard solution	5 g/L. Add 500 mg 2-hydroxybenzoic acid to a 100-mL volumetric flask and make up with a 1:1 solution of methanol:deionized water. This solution has a shelf-life of seven days.
Hippuric acid stock standard solution	5 g/L. Add 500 mg hippuric acid to a 100-mL volumetric flask and make up with 1:1 methanol:deionized water.
Hippuric acid working standard solutions	0.25, 0.5, 1.0 and 2.0 g/L, prepared by dilution of the stock standard solution with distilled water. Use freshly made up solutions for each calibration curve determination.
Urine quality control standard	2 g hippuric acid/L. Pool about 1.5 L urine from unexposed persons in a glass beaker, cool in a refrigerator for 16 h, then filter. Add 2 g hippuric acid to a 1-L volumetric flask and make up with the filtered urine. Divide into 10-mL aliquots and store at $-18\,°C$ in 20-mL disposable plastic containers.
HPLC mobile phase	0.01 mol/L phosphate buffer:methanol (3:1, v/v). Mix 750 mL phosphate buffer and 250 mL methanol in a glass beaker and filter through a membrane filter (Fluoropore, Millipore). Degas filtrate under reduced pressure (water jet).

7.   APPARATUS[1]

High-pressure liquid chromatograph (HPLC)	With 10-μL injection loop and ultraviolet detector
HPLC column	25 cm × 4.0 mm, steel, packed with Lichrosorb RP 18, 5 μm particle-size
Mechanical shaker	
Test tubes	10-mL, with caps
Disposable tubes	5-mL, polyethylene
Volumetric pipette	

---

[1] Reference to a company and/or product is for the purpose of information and identification only and does not imply approval or recommendation of the company and/or product by the International Agency for Research on Cancer, to the exclusion of others which may also be suitable.

8.   SAMPLING

Collect urine samples (≥ 100 mL) in 250-mL polyethylene bottles (rinsed with deionized water) at the end of the work shift.

For conservation, acidify the samples with acetic acid (1 mL acetic acid/100 mL urine). The sample can be shipped to the laboratory without further precautions and can be kept for at least three days without refrigeration. If the sample cannot be analysed immediately after arrival at the laboratory, it can be stored at $-18\,°C$ for at least six months without systematic bias of the results.

9.   PROCEDURE

9.1 *Blank test*

Anlayse 0.5 mL deionized water in place of urine, as described in sections 9.4–9.6.

9.2 *Check test*

Analyse the urine quality control standard with each series of samples and check the retention time of hippuric acid and the internal standard and the sensitivity of the detector.

9.3 *Test portion*

0.5 mL aliquot of well-mixed urine sample. Frozen urine samples should be taken out of the deep freeze on the day before analysis and should be kept at room temperature.

9.4 *Extraction of analyte*

9.4.1   Mix the sample in the 250-mL polyethylene bottle for 30 min, using a roller mixer.

9.4.2   Transfer a 0.5-mL aliquot of the urine sample to a 10-mL test tube. Add 50 µL of the internal standard solution and 25 µL concentrated hydrochloric acid. Mix well.

9.4.3   Add 3 mL diethyl ether and shake for 15 min on the mechanical shaker.

9.4.4   Transfer 2 mL of the organic layer to a 5-mL disposable polyethylene tube using a volumetric pipette.

9.4.5   Evaporate the organic extract to dryness under nitrogen stream.

9.4.6   Dissolve the residue in 0.5 mL of 1:5 (v/v) methanol:water and retain for HPLC.

9.5 *HPLC operating conditions*

Mobile phase flow rate	0.8 mL/min
Ultraviolet detector wavelength	215 nm

9.6 *Analyte determination*

Fill the 10-µL injector loop with concentrated extract (9.4.6) and record the peak areas of analyte and internal standard.

9.7 *Calibration curve*

9.7.1   Analyse 0.5 mL of each of the working standard solutions as described in sections 9.4–9.6.

9.7.2   Plot the ratios of the peak areas of hippuric acid/internal standard *versus* the concentrations of the working standard solutions and draw a graph using the least-squares method.

10. METHOD OF CALCULATION

Obtain the concentration of hippuric acid in the urine sample using the calibration curve and the ratio of the peak areas obtained in 9.6. Correct for the blank if necessary.

11. REPEATABILITY AND REPRODUCIBILITY

11.1 *Repeatability*

Pooled urine samples were spiked with hippuric acid to give additional concentrations of 0.25, 0.50 and 1.0 g/L and were analysed on ten different days. The coefficients of variation were 5.5, 12.8 and 3.4%, respectively.

11.2 *Reproducibility*

The linear range and repeatability data given in sections 1 and 11.1 have been confirmed in another laboratory.

11.3 *Recovery*

Hippuric acid was added to pooled urine to give an additional concentration of 6 g/L. The recovery was 99%.

12. NOTES ON PROCEDURE

Not applicable.

13. SCHEMATIC REPRESENTATION OF PROCEDURE

Mix sample 30 min and transfer 0.5 mL
to a 10-mL test tube
↓
Add 50 µL internal standard solution
+ 25 µL concentrated hydrochloric acid and mix well
↓
Add 3 mL diethyl ether and shake 15 min
↓
Transfer 2 mL of organic layer
to 5-mL polyethylene tube
↓
Evaporate to dryness under nitrogen stream
↓
Dissolve residue in 0.5 mL of 1:5 methanol:water
↓
Inject 10 µL into HPLC and measure peak areas
of analyte and internal standard
↓
Determine analyte concentration in sample
using calibration curve obtained with standard solutions

14. ORIGIN OF THE METHOD

Zentralinstitut für Arbeitsmedizin
Adolph-Schönfelder-Strasse 5
D–2000 Hamburg 76
FRG

Contact point: Dr J. Angerer

METHOD 10 — DETERMINATION OF XYLENES IN BLOOD BY HEAD-SPACE GAS CHROMATOGRAPHY

K. Engström & V. Riihimäki

1. SCOPE AND FIELD OF APPLICATION

This method is suitable for the determination of xylene isomers in blood specimens. The limit of detection is 0.5 µmol/L. Ethylbenzene, which normally accompanies xylene isomers in technical xylene (about 15%), does not interfere with the described determination of xylene.

2. REFERENCES

Riihimäki, V. & Pfäffli, P. (1978) Percutaneous absorption of solvent vapors in man. *Scand. J. Work Environ. Health, 4,* 73–85

3. DEFINITIONS

Not applicable.

4. PRINCIPLE

A head-space gas-chromatographic technique is employed. After equilibrium has been reached, a sample is drawn from the head-space and xylene is determined by gas chromatography (GC), with flame-ionization detection.

5. HAZARDS

Not applicable.

6. REAGENTS[1]

o-Xylene	purum, Merck
m-Xylene	purum, Merck
p-Xylene	purum, Merck
Xylene stock standard solution (1 635 µmol/L)	Prepare a mixture consisting of two parts *o*-xylene, six parts *m*-xylene and two parts of *p*-xylene. Inject 2 µL of the above mixture into 10 mL of mixed (pooled) human blood in a 10-mL vial and shake mechanically for 2 h.
Xylene working standard solutions	Prepare in appropriate Kimax® tubes (with minimum head-space volume) and shake mechanically for at least 1 h before use.
	Add 100 µL of stock standard solution to 50 mL of whole blood (3.3 µmol/L). Add 100 µL of stock standard solution to 20 mL of whole blood (8.1 µmol/L). Add 100 µL of stock standard solution to 10 mL of whole blood (16.2 µmol/L). Add 150 µL of stock standard solution to 10 mL of whole blood (24.2 µmol/L). Add 300 µL of stock standard solution to 10 mL of whole blood (47.6 µmol/L).

7. APPARATUS[1]

Vials	10-mL, 20-mL, 50-mL Kimax® tubes with Teflon-coated caps
Syringes	1-10 µL, Hamilton. 40–200 µL Digital Finn-pipette
Head-space bottles	25-mL, with airtight caps (Teflon-coated butyl rubber, secured by aluminium cap)
Pipettes	1.0 ± 0.01 mL
Gas chromatograph	With flame-ionization detector and vitreous silica column, 12.5 m × 0.2 mm i.d., coated with OV-101.

---

[1] Reference to a company and/or product is for the purpose of information and identification only and does not imply approval or recommendation of the company and/or product by the International Agency for Research on Cancer, to the exclusion of others which may also be suitable.

8. SAMPLING

See section 12.

8.1 For workers regularly exposed to xylene, assess their long-term xylene load by sampling at the beginning of a work day (*before* new exposure), towards the end of the work week.

8.2 Take a 10-mL sample of venous blood into a vial containing an anticoagulant. To avoid loss to air space in the tubes, fill the vials to the stopper. Refrigerate samples and do not open the vials until analysis. Ship the specimens to the analytical laboratory as soon as possible after collection.

9. PROCEDURE

9.1 *Blank test*

Perform a blank test with every analytical series by subjecting empty head-space bottles to the same procedure as the samples. No peak should be seen at the same retention times as the xylene isomers.

9.2 *Check test*

Not applicable.

9.3 *Test portion*

1.0 $\pm$ 0.01 mL, using a pipette.

9.4 *Xylene determination*

9.4.1   Pipette 1-mL portions of whole blood into 25-mL head-space bottles and seal with Teflon-coated butyl-rubber caps, secured by a pressed-on aluminium cap.

9.4.2   Maintain samples at 60 °C in an oven for 60 min, then transfer to thermostatted block of head-space injector system, maintained at 60 °C.

9.4.3   Inject a standard sample of head-space gas into GC.

9.5 *Gas chromatographic conditions*

Column temperature programme   Hold 5 min at 40 °C, then raise to 150 °C at 30 °C/min. Hold at 150 °C for 1 min.

Injector temperature	200 °C.
Detector temperature	300 °C.

Under the foregoing GC conditions, *m*-, and *p*-xylene have identical retention times and are eluted together.

9.6 *Calibration curve*

Follow procedure 9.4 with each of the xylene working standard solutions. For each concentration, sum the areas of the xylene peaks and plot the sum as a function of the total xylene concentration (μmol/L). The curve should be linear up to 200 μmol/L.

10. METHOD OF CALCULATION

For each sample, sum the areas of the peaks corresponding to the xylene isomers and obtain the total xylene concentration from the calibration curve.

11. REPEATABILITY AND REPRODUCIBILITY

The coefficient of variation was 7.3% for a standard solution with a total concentration of 24.2 μmol/L and 6.8% for a total concentration of 2.2 μmol/L. The results were calculated from 10 replicate determinations. No reproducibility data are available.

12. NOTES ON PROCEDURE

Xylene is absorbed into the body mainly through the lungs. Skin contact with liquid xylene may result in a notable absorption through the contaminated area and greatly elevate the concentration of xylene in the venous blood draining the contaminated part of the body. Thus, for workers handling liquid xylene with bare hands, the normal method of blood sampling (from the cubital vein) may yield spuriously high values.

Alterations of pulmonary uptake rates of xylene are mirrored by corresponding fluctuations of blood xylene. Cessation of exposure will result in a rapid initial decline of blood xylene. Thus during the first hours after exposure the half-time of blood xylene is about 0.5 h.

Since xylene is quite fat-soluble, some of the compound will be retained in the body, mainly in the adipose tissue, and slowly eliminated. This elimination follows a half-time of 1–2.5 days. Consequently, xylene reaches a steady-state in the body only after a week or two of repeated daily exposures.

13. SCHEMATIC REPRESENTATION OF PROCEDURE

Not applicable.

14. ORIGIN OF THE METHOD

Institute of Occupational Health
Department of Industrial Hygiene and Toxicology
Haartmaninkatu 1
SF–00290 Helsinki 29
Finland

Contact points: Dr K. Engström
Turku Regional Institute of Occupational Health
Hämeenkatu 10
SF–20500 Turku
Finland

Dr V. Riihimäki
Institute of Occupational Health
Department of Industrial Hygiene and Toxicology
Haartmaninkatu 1
SF–00290 Helsinki 29
Finland

METHOD 11 — DETERMINATION OF METHYLHIPPURIC ACIDS IN URINE BY GAS CHROMATOGRAPHY

K. Engström & V. Riihimäki

1. SCOPE AND FIELD OF APPLICATION

This method is suitable for the determination of methylhippuric acids in urine, for an assessment of human exposure to xylenes. The range of application is 0.1–20.0 mmol/L. No interference from the normal constituents of urine is seen in the specified range. Provided that the chromatographic step is automatized, one technician can prepare about 35 specimens (in duplicate) during a normal working day.

2. REFERENCES

Blatt, A.H. (1950) *Organische Synthesen,* Coll. Vol. 2, New York, John Wiley & Sons, p. 328

Engström, K., Husman, K. & Rantanen, J. (1976) Measurement of toluene and xylene metabolites by gas chromatography. *Int. Arch. Occup. Environ. Health, 36,* 153–160

3. DEFINITIONS

Methylhippuric acids: *o-*, *m-* or *p*-methylbenzoylglycine

BSTFA: *N,O*-bis-(trimethylsilyl)trifluoroacetamide

4. PRINCIPLE

Free and bound methylbenzoic acids in the urine are subjected to alkaline hydrolysis. The liberated acids are then extracted with diethyl ether, silylated and quantified using gas chromatography with flame-ionization detection.

5. HAZARDS

Concentrated sulfuric acid should be diluted by gently adding the acid to the water, not *vice versa.*

Diethylether and methylisobutylketone are volatile, easily inflammable solvents and should preferably be handled in a laboratory hood. Methylisobutylketone can react vigorously with reducing agents.

Fumes of BSTFA may be irritating to skin, eyes and mucous membranes.

6. REAGENTS[1]

2,3-Dimethylbenzoic acid	Fluka AG, purum.
Methanol	Merck, purest available
Diethyl ether	Merck, purest available
Methylisobutylketone	Merck, purest available
Sodium hydroxide	Merck, purest available, 11 mol/L
Sulfuric acid	Merck, purest available, 3 mol/L
Sodium chloride	Merck, purest available
BSTFA	Pierce Chemicals Co.
Glycine	Merck, purest available
Toluene	Merck, purest available
BSTFA in methyliso-butylketone	(1:1, v/v)
Internal standard solution	Dissolve 300.4 mg of 2,3-dimethylbenzoic acid in 100 mL of methanol.
Methylhippuric acid stock standard solution (20 mmol/L)	Weigh 77.2 mg of o-methylhippuric acid, 77.2 mg of p-methylhippuric acid and 231.6 mg of m-methylhippuric acid into 100 mL of urine (from an unexposed subject) containing a few drops of 11 mol/L sodium hydroxide solution. The o-, m- and p-methylhippuric acids (purity >98%) are prepared from the respective methylbenzoic acids, which are transformed to corresponding acid chlorides, then reacted with glycine under alkaline conditions (Blatt, 1950). The methylhippuric acids obtained are purified by recrystallization from toluene. (The structures and purities of the acids were confirmed with proton nuclear magnetic resonance spectrometry.)

---

[1] Reference to a company and/or product is for the purpose of information and identification only and does not imply approval or recommendation of the company and/or product by the International Agency for Research on Cancer, to the exclusion of others which may also be suitable.

| Methylhippuric acid working standard solutions | Urine from unexposed subject.
0.5 mL stock solution made up to 20 mL with urine (0.5 mmol/L).
2.0 mL stock solution made up to 20 mL with urine (2.0 mmol/L).
5.0 mL stock solution made up to 20 mL with urine (5.0 mmol/L).
10.0 mL stock solution made up to 20 mL with urine (10 mmol/L).
Stock standard solution (20 mmol/L). |
| | Divide the working standard solutions into suitable portions (e.g., 3 mL) and store at $-20\,°C$ until required. The solutions can be stored without deterioration for at least 4 months. |

7. APPARATUS[1]

Gas chromatograph (GC)	With flame-ionization detector and an autosampler. Glass capillary column, 50 m × 0.7 mm i.d., coated with SE-30.
Micropipettor	1.0 ± 0.01 mL
Test tubes	15-mL, with Teflon-coated screw caps
Thermo-block	To hold test tubes, 80 °C
Centrifuge	To handle 15-mL tubes

8. SAMPLING

See section 12.

In cases of continuous, steady exposure, the peak of the methylhippuric acid excretion is usually reached after several hours. It is thus possible to use spot samples voided at the end of the work day to assess the xylene uptake during the preceding hours. A minimum sample of 5 mL from a single voiding is required, but 100 mL of urine is recommended in order to obtain a representative sample. Store the specimens at $+5\,°C$ until required for analysis.

---

[1] Reference to a company and/or product is for the purpose of information and identification only and does not imply approval or recommendation of the company and/or product by the International Agency for Research on Cancer, to the exclusion of others which may also be suitable.

9.   PROCEDURE

9.1 *Blank test*

To check the purity of the reagents, carry out a blank test using the procedure described in 9.4, except that water is used in place of the urine sample.

9.2 *Check test*

Not applicable.

9.3 *Test portion*

1.0 ± 0.01 mL, using the SMI micropipetter.

9.4 *Methylhippuric acids determination*

9.4.1   Prepare an adequate number of 15-mL test tubes by adding 0.5 mL of internal standard solution and evaporating to dryness in a thermo-block (80 °C). Cap the tubes and store at +5 °C until required. (The tubes can be stored without deterioration for at least one month.)

9.4.2   In duplicate, pipette 1.0-mL portions of the sample urine and 1 mL of 11 mol/L sodium hydroxide into the tubes containing the internal standard and place for 1.5 h in an oven at 140 °C.

9.4.3   Cool the hydrolysate, then acidify with 2.5 mL of 3 mol/L sulfuric acid and saturate with sodium chloride.

9.4.4   Extract the hydrolysed methylbenzoic acids from the urine with 5 mL of diethylether by mechanically shaking for 20 min, followed by centrifuging for 5 min at 1 000 × *g*.

9.4.5   Pipette 1.0 mL of the diethylether phase into the autosampler bottle (1.8 mL) and evaporate to dryness, preferably by keeping it at room temperature in a laboratory hood overnight.

9.4.6   Prior to the GC analysis, silylate the residue by adding 100 μL of BSTFA in methylisobutylketone (1:1, v/v).

9.4.7   Add 500 μL of methylisobutylketone and inject 1 μL into the GC by means of the autosampler.

9.5 *Gas chromatography conditions*

Column temperature	150 °C
Injector temperature	200 °C
Detector temperature	200 °C

9.6 *Calibration curve*

9.6.1 Follow procedure 9.4, using the working standard solutions (section 6) in place of the urine test portions in step 9.4.2.

9.6.2 Divide the area of each methylhippuric acid peak by the area of the internal standard peak. Plot the resulting quotients as a function of the methylhippuric acid concentrations. The plots are normally linear over the concentration range employed here.

9.7 *Recovery*

Recovery was estimated by analysing the three isomers of methylbenzoic acid according to steps 9.4.5–9.4.7 and comparing the GC peak areas with those obtained after hydrolysis of the corresponding methylhippuric acids. The comparison showed that the glycine conjugate can be hydrolysed almost completely with the alkaline treatment. The total recovery of the three isomers varied from 95% to 105%, when standard solutions with concentrations from 5 to 10 mmol/L were tested.

10. METHOD OF CALCULATION

Divide the area of the peak corresponding to each isomer by the area of the internal standard peak. The methylhippuric acid concentrations (mmol/L) which correspond to each quotient may then be read from the appropriate calibration curve.

11. REPEATABILITY AND REPRODUCIBILITY

The coefficients of variation were 1.2% for a specimen with a total concentration of 9.2 mmol/L, and 3.4% for a specimen with 0.8 mmol/L. The results were calculated from ten replicate determinations. No reproducibility data are available.

12. NOTES ON PROCEDURE

Xylene is absorbed into the body mainly through the lungs. Absorption through the skin is also possible, but is rarely significant in magnitude. About 95% of the absorbed xylenes are rapidly metabolized to methylbenzoic acids, then to the respective glycine conjugates, methylhippuric acids. Methylhippuric acids are efficiently and rapidly excreted by the kidneys, probably *via* an active secretion mechanism; tubular reabsorption is unlikely. In the post-exposure phase, the initial elimination half-time of methylhippuric acid is about 1 h.

13. SCHEMATIC REPRESENTATION OF PROCEDURE

Add internal standard to 15-mL tube
and evaporate to dryness
↓
Pipette 1.0-mL sample + 1.0 mL of 11 mol/L sodium hydroxide
into tube and hold for 1.5 h at 140 °C
↓
Cool, acidify with 2.5 mL of 3 mol/L sulfuric acid
and saturate with sodium chloride
↓
Extract with 5 mL diethyl ether
and centrifuge for 5 min
↓
Pipette 1.0 mL of diethyl ether phase into autosampler bottle
and evaporate to dryness at room temperature overnight
↓
Silylate residue with 100 μL of BSTFA
in methylisobutylketone,
then add 500 μL of methylisobutylketone
↓
Inject 1 μL into gas chromatograph

14. ORIGIN OF THE METHOD

Turku Regional Institute of Occupational Health
Hämeenkatu 10
SF–20500 Turku
Finland

Contact points: Dr K. Engström
Turku Regional Institute of Occupational Health

Dr V. Riihimäki
Institute of Occupational Health
Department of Industrial Hygiene and Toxicology
Haartmaninkatu 1
SF–00290 Helsinki 29
Finland

PUBLICATIONS OF THE INTERNATIONAL AGENCY FOR RESEARCH ON CANCER

SCIENTIFIC PUBLICATIONS SERIES

(Available from Oxford University Press)
through local bookshops

No. 1 LIVER CANCER
1971; 176 pages; out of print

No. 2 ONCOGENESIS AND HERPESVIRUSES
Edited by P.M. Biggs, G. de-Thé & L.N. Payne
1972; 515 pages; out of print

No. 3 N-NITROSO COMPOUNDS: ANALYSIS
AND FORMATION
Edited by P. Bogovski, R. Preussmann & E. A. Walker
1972; 140 pages; out of print

No. 4 TRANSPLACENTAL CARCINOGENESIS
Edited by L. Tomatis & U. Mohr
1973; 181 pages; out of print

*No. 5 PATHOLOGY OF TUMOURS IN
LABORATORY ANIMALS. VOLUME 1.
TUMOURS OF THE RAT. PART 1
Editor-in-Chief V.S. Turusov
1973; 214 pages

*No. 6 PATHOLOGY OF TUMOURS IN
LABORATORY ANIMALS. VOLUME 1.
TUMOURS OF THE RAT. PART 2
Editor-in-Chief V.S. Turusov
1976; 319 pages
*reprinted in one volume, Price £50.00

No. 7 HOST ENVIRONMENT INTERACTIONS IN
THE ETIOLOGY OF CANCER IN MAN
Edited by R. Doll & I. Vodopija
1973; 464 pages; £32.50

No. 8 BIOLOGICAL EFFECTS OF ASBESTOS
Edited by P. Bogovski, J.C. Gilson, V. Timbrell
& J.C. Wagner
1973; 346 pages; out of print

No. 9 N-NITROSO COMPOUNDS IN THE
ENVIRONMENT
Edited by P. Bogovski & E. A. Walker
1974; 243 pages; £16.50

No. 10 CHEMICAL CARCINOGENESIS ESSAYS
Edited by R. Montesano & L. Tomatis
1974; 230 pages; out of print

No. 11 ONCOGENESIS AND HERPESVIRUSES II
Edited by G. de-Thé, M.A. Epstein & H. zur Hausen
1975; Part 1, 511 pages; Part 2, 403 pages; £65.-

No. 12 SCREENING TESTS IN CHEMICAL
CARCINOGENESIS
Edited by R. Montesano, H. Bartsch & L. Tomatis
1976; 666 pages; £12.-

No. 13 ENVIRONMENTAL POLLUTION AND
CARCINOGENIC RISKS
Edited by C. Rosenfeld & W. Davis
1976; 454 pages; out of print

No. 14 ENVIRONMENTAL N-NITROSO
COMPOUNDS: ANALYSIS AND FORMATION
Edited by E.A. Walker, P. Bogovski & L. Griciute
1976; 512 pages; £37.50

No. 15 CANCER INCIDENCE IN FIVE
CONTINENTS. VOLUME III
Edited by J. Waterhouse, C. Muir, P. Correa
& J. Powell
1976; 584 pages; out of print

No. 16 AIR POLLUTION AND CANCER IN MAN
Edited by U. Mohr, D. Schmähl & L. Tomatis
1977; 311 pages; out of print

No. 17 DIRECTORY OF ON-GOING RESEARCH
IN CANCER EPIDEMIOLOGY 1977
Edited by C.S. Muir & G. Wagner
1977; 599 pages; out of print

No. 18 ENVIRONMENTAL CARCINOGENS:
SELECTED METHODS OF ANALYSIS
Edited-in-Chief H. Egan
VOLUME 1. ANALYSIS OF VOLATILE
NITROSAMINES IN FOOD
Edited by R. Preussmann, M. Castegnaro, E.A. Walker
& A.E. Wassermann
1978; 212 pages; out of print

No. 19 ENVIRONMENTAL ASPECTS OF
N-NITROSO COMPOUNDS
Edited by E.A. Walker, M. Castegnaro, L. Griciute
& R.E. Lyle
1978; 566 pages; out of print

No. 20 NASOPHARYNGEAL CARCINOMA:
ETIOLOGY AND CONTROL
Edited by G. de-Thé & Y. Ito
1978; 610 pages; out of print

No. 21 CANCER REGISTRATION AND ITS
TECHNIQUES
Edited by R. MacLennan, C. Muir, R. Steinitz
& A. Winkler
1978; 235 pages; £35.-

Prices, valid for October 1987, are subject to change without notice

SCIENTIFIC PUBLICATIONS SERIES

No. 22 ENVIRONMENTAL CARCINOGENS:
SELECTED METHODS OF ANALYSIS
Editor-in-Chief H. Egan
VOLUME 2. METHODS FOR THE MEASUREMENT
OF VINYL CHLORIDE IN POLY(VINYL
CHLORIDE), AIR, WATER AND FOODSTUFFS
Edited by D.C.M. Squirrell & W. Thain
1978; 142 pages; out of print

No. 23 PATHOLOGY OF TUMOURS IN
LABORATORY ANIMALS. VOLUME II.
TUMOURS OF THE MOUSE
Editor-in-Chief V.S. Turusov
1979; 669 pages; out of print

No. 24 ONCOGENESIS AND HERPESVIRUSES III
Edited by G. de-Thé, W. Henle & F. Rapp
1978; Part 1, 580 pages; Part 2, 522 pages; out of print

No. 25 CARCINOGENIC RISKS: STRATEGIES
FOR INTERVENTION
Edited by W. Davis & C. Rosenfeld
1979; 283 pages; out of print

No. 26 DIRECTORY OF ON-GOING RESEARCH
IN CANCER EPIDEMIOLOGY 1978
Edited by C.S. Muir & G. Wagner,
1978; 550 pages; out of print

No. 27 MOLECULAR AND CELLULAR ASPECTS
OF CARCINOGEN SCREENING TESTS
Edited by R. Montesano, H. Bartsch & L. Tomatis
1980; 371 pages; £22.50

No. 28 DIRECTORY OF ON-GOING RESEARCH
IN CANCER EPIDEMIOLOGY 1979
Edited by C.S. Muir & G. Wagner
1979; 672 pages; out of print

No. 29 ENVIRONMENTAL CARCINOGENS:
SELECTED METHODS OF ANALYSIS
Editor-in-Chief H. Egan
VOLUME 3. ANALYSIS OF POLYCYCLIC
AROMATIC HYDROCARBONS IN
ENVIRONMENTAL SAMPLES
Edited by M. Castegnaro, P. Bogovski, H. Kunte
& E.A. Walker
1979; 240 pages; out of print

No. 30 BIOLOGICAL EFFECTS OF MINERAL
FIBRES
Editor-in-Chief J.C. Wagner
1980; Volume 1, 494 pages; Volume 2, 513 pages;
£55.-

No. 31 N-NITROSO COMPOUNDS: ANALYSIS,
FORMATION AND OCCURRENCE
Edited by E.A. Walker, L. Griciute, M. Castegnaro
& M. Börzsönyi
1980; 841 pages; out of print

No. 32 STATISTICAL METHODS IN CANCER
RESEARCH. VOLUME 1. THE ANALYSIS OF
CASE-CONTROL STUDIES
By N.E. Breslow & N.E. Day
1980; 338 pages; £20.-

No. 33 HANDLING CHEMICAL CARCINOGENS IN
THE LABORATORY: PROBLEMS OF SAFETY
Edited by R. Montesano, H. Bartsch, E. Boyland,
G. Della Porta, L. Fishbein, R.A. Griesemer,
A.B. Swan & L. Tomatis
1979; 32 pages; out of print

No. 34 PATHOLOGY OF TUMOURS IN
LABORATORY ANIMALS. VOLUME III.
TUMOURS OF THE HAMSTER
Editor-in-Chief V.S. Turusov
1982; 461 pages; £32.50

No. 35 DIRECTORY OF ON-GOING RESEARCH
IN CANCER EPIDEMIOLOGY 1980
Edited by C.S. Muir & G. Wagner
1980; 660 pages; out of print

No. 36 CANCER MORTALITY BY OCCUPATION
AND SOCIAL CLASS 1851-1971
By W.P.D. Logan
1982; 253 pages; £22.50

No. 37 LABORATORY DECONTAMINATION
AND DESTRUCTION OF AFLATOXINS
B_1, B_2, G_1, G_2 IN LABORATORY WASTES
Edited by M. Castegnaro, D.C. Hunt, E.B. Sansone,
P.L. Schuller, M.G. Siriwardana, G.M. Telling,
H.P. Van Egmond & E.A. Walker
1980; 59 pages; £6.50

No. 38 DIRECTORY OF ON-GOING RESEARCH
IN CANCER EPIDEMIOLOGY 1981
Edited by C.S. Muir & G. Wagner
1981; 696 pages; out of print

No. 39 HOST FACTORS IN HUMAN
CARCINOGENESIS
Edited by H. Bartsch & B. Armstrong
1982; 583 pages; £37.50

No. 40 ENVIRONMENTAL CARCINOGENS:
SELECTED METHODS OF ANALYSIS
Edited-in-Chief H. Egan
VOLUME 4. SOME AROMATIC AMINES AND
AZO DYES IN THE GENERAL AND INDUSTRIAL
ENVIRONMENT
Edited by L. Fishbein, M. Castegnaro, I.K. O'Neill
& H. Bartsch
1981; 347 pages; £22.50

No. 41 N-NITROSO COMPOUNDS:
OCCURRENCE AND BIOLOGICAL EFFECTS
Edited by H. Bartsch, I.K. O'Neill, M. Castegnaro
& M. Okada
1982; 755 pages; £37.50

No. 42 CANCER INCIDENCE IN FIVE
CONTINENTS. VOLUME IV
Edited by J. Waterhouse, C. Muir,
K. Shanmugaratnam & J. Powell
1982; 811 pages; £37.50

SCIENTIFIC PUBLICATIONS SERIES

SCIENTIFIC PUBLICATIONS SERIES

SCIENTIFIC PUBLICATIONS SERIES

No. 85 ENVIRONMENTAL CARCINOGENS:
METHODS OF ANALYSIS AND EXPOSURE
MEASUREMENT. VOLUME 10. BENZENE
AND ALKYLATED BENZENES
Edited by L. Fishbein & I.K. O'Neill
1988; 318 pages; £35.-

No. 86 DIRECTORY OF ON-GOING RESEARCH
IN CANCER EPIDEMIOLOGY 1987
Edited by D.M. Parkin & J. Wahrendorf
1987; 685 pages; £22.-

No. 87 INTERNATIONAL INCIDENCE OF
CHILDHOOD CANCER
Edited by D.M. Parkin, C.A. Stiller, G.J. Draper,
C.A. Bieber, B. Terracini & J.L. Young
(in press) 1988; approx. 400 pages; £35.-

No. 88 CANCER INCIDENCE IN FIVE
CONTINENTS. VOLUME V
Edited by C. Muir, J. Waterhouse, T. Mack,
J. Powell & S. Whelan
1988; 1004 pages; £50.-

No. 89 METHODS FOR DETECTING DNA
DAMAGING AGENTS IN HUMANS:
APPLICATIONS IN CANCER EPIDEMIOLOGY
AND PREVENTION
Edited by H. Bartsch, K. Hemminki & I.K. O'Neill
1988; approx. 520 pages; £45.-

No. 90 NON-OCCUPATIONAL EXPOSURE TO
MINERAL FIBRES
Edited by J. Bignon, J. Peto & R. Saracci
(in press) 1988; approx. 500 pages; £45.-

No. 91 TRENDS IN CANCER INCIDENCE IN
SINGAPORE 1968-1982
Edited by H.P. Lee, N.E. Day &
K. Shanmugaratnam
1988; approx. 160 pages; £25.-

No. 92 CELL DIFFERENTIATION, GENES
AND CANCER
Edited by T. Kakunaga, T. Sugimura,
L. Tomatis and H. Yamasaki
1988; approx. 220 pages; £25.-

No. 93 DIRECTORY OF ON-GOING RESEARCH
IN CANCER EPIDEMIOLOGY 1988
Edited by M. Coleman & J. Wahrendorf
1988; approx. 650 pages; £26.-

IARC MONOGRAPHS ON THE EVALUATION OF THE CARCINOGENIC RISK OF CHEMICALS TO HUMANS

(English editions only)

(Available from booksellers through the network of WHO Sales Agents*)

Volume 1
Some inorganic substances, chlorinated hydrocarbons, aromatic amines, N-nitroso compounds, and natural products
1972; 184 pages; out of print

Volume 2
Some inorganic and organometallic compounds
1973; 181 pages; out of print

Volume 3
Certain polycyclic aromatic hydrocarbons and heterocyclic compounds
1973; 271 pages; out of print

Volume 4
Some aromatic amines, hydrazine and related substances, N-nitroso compounds and miscellaneous alkylating agents
1974; 286 pages;
Sw. fr. 18.-

Volume 5
Some organochlorine pesticides
1974; 241 pages; out of print

Volume 6
Sex hormones
1974; 243 pages;
out of print

Volume 7
Some anti-thyroid and related substances, nitrofurans and industrial chemicals
1974; 326 pages; out of print

Volume 8
Some aromatic azo compounds
1975; 357 pages; Sw.fr. 36.-

Volume 9
Some aziridines, N-, S- and O-mustards and selenium
1975; 268 pages; Sw. fr. 27.-

Volume 10
Some naturally occurring substances
1976; 353 pages; out of print

Volume 11
Cadmium, nickel, some epoxides, miscellaneous industrial chemicals and general considerations on volatile anaesthetics
1976; 306 pages; out of print

Volume 12
Some carbamates, thiocarbamates and carbazides
1976; 282 pages; Sw. fr. 34.-

Volume 13
Some miscellaneous pharmaceutical substances
1977; 255 pages; Sw. fr. 30.-

Volume 14
Asbestos
1977; 106 pages; out of print

Volume 15
Some fumigants, the herbicides 2,4-D and 2,4,5-T, chlorinated dibenzodioxins and miscellaneous industrial chemicals
1977; 354 pages; Sw. fr. 50.-

Volume 16
Some aromatic amines and related nitro compounds — hair dyes, colouring agents and miscellaneous industrial chemicals
1978; 400 pages; Sw. fr. 50.-

Volume 17
Some N-nitroso compounds
1978; 365 pages; Sw. fr. 50.

Volume 18
Polychlorinated biphenyls and polybrominated biphenyls
1978; 140 pages; Sw. fr. 20.-

Volume 19
Some monomers, plastics and synthetic elastomers, and acrolein
1979; 513 pages; Sw. fr. 60.-

Volume 20
Some halogenated hydrocarbons
1979; 609 pages; Sw. fr. 60.-

Volume 21
Sex hormones (II)
1979; 583 pages; Sw. fr. 60.-

Volume 22
Some non-nutritive sweetening agents
1980; 208 pages; Sw. fr. 25.-

Volume 23
Some metals and metallic compounds
1980; 438 pages; Sw. fr. 50.-

Volume 24
Some pharmaceutical drugs
1980; 337 pages; Sw. fr. 40.-

Volume 25
Wood, leather and some associated industries
1981; 412 pages; Sw. fr. 60.-

Volume 26
Some antineoplastic and immunosuppressive agents
1981; 411 pages; Sw. fr. 62.-

*A list of these Agents may be obtained by writing to the World Health Organization, Distribution and Sales Service, 1211 Geneva 27, Switzerland

IARC MONOGRAPHS SERIES

*From Volume 43 onwards, the series title has been changed to IARC MONOGRAPHS ON THE EVALUATION OF CARCINOGENIC RISKS TO HUMANS

INFORMATION BULLETINS ON THE
SURVEY OF CHEMICALS BEING
TESTED FOR CARCINOGENICITY

(Available from IARC and WHO Sales Agents)

No. 8 (1979)
Edited by M.-J. Ghess, H. Bartsch
& L. Tomatis
604 pages; Sw. fr. 40.-

No. 9 (1981)
Edited by M.-J. Ghess, J.D. Wilbourn,
H. Bartsch & L. Tomatis
294 pages; Sw. fr. 41.-

No. 10 (1982)
Edited by M.-J. Ghess, J.D. Wilbourn
& H. Bartsch
362 pages; Sw. fr. 42.-

No. 11 (1984)
Edited by M.-J. Ghess, J.D. Wilbourn,
H. Vainio & H. Bartsch
362 pages; Sw. fr. 50.-

No. 12 (1986)
Edited by M.-J. Ghess, J.D. Wilbourn,
A. Tossavainen & H. Vainio
385 pages; Sw. fr. 50.-

NON-SERIAL PUBLICATIONS

(Available from IARC)

ALCOOL ET CANCER
By A. Tuyns (in French only)
1978; 42 pages; Fr. fr. 35.-

CANCER MORBIDITY AND CAUSES OF
DEATH AMONG DANISH BREWERY
WORKERS
By O.M. Jensen
1980; 143 pages; Fr. fr. 75.-

DIRECTORY OF COMPUTER SYSTEMS
USED IN CANCER REGISTRIES
By H.R. Menck & D.M. Parkin
1986; 236 pages; Fr. fr. 50.-